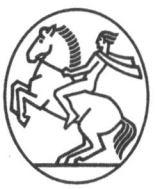

N. Loimer, R. Schmid, A. Springer (eds.)

Drug Addiction and AIDS

Springer-Verlag Wien New York

DDr. Norbert Loimer
Univ.-Doz. Dr. Rainer Schmid
Univ.-Prof. Dr. Alfred Springer
Department of Psychiatry, University Hospital of Vienna
Austria

The printing of this publication has been supported by a grant of the
Austrian Ministary of Science and Research.

Printed on acid-free paper

With 52 Figures

ISBN-13:978-3-211-82298-2   e-ISBN-13:978-3-7091-9173-6
DOI: 10.1007/978-3-7091-9173-6

Foreword

Drug abuse and AIDS present a new and unparalleled challenge to our society. The fatal combination of the two calls for an urgent incentive for new ideas and strategies to be developed in the fight against this until recently seemingly indomitable enemy.

HIV-prevalence among drug abusers has increased markedly during the late eighties. Whereas the proportion of AIDS cases among that population had been 1% in 1984, it had jumped up to 29% in 1989. This percentage, as we know from epidemiological studies, varies greatly for different countries. The highest percentage of cumulative AIDS cases among drug abusers in Europe has been found in the southern region, while in Scandinavian countries, with the exception of Denmark, this percentage is very low. Austria belongs to those countries with a relatively high prevalence.

This development has had a strong impact on the social response towards drug abuse and has caused a marked change among health authorities: WHO experts, for instance have proposed that, controlling drug abuse and promoting a healthy life style should remain the long term objectives with highest priority but that otherwise, in the short term, the priority should be prevention of AIDS transmission. Most European countries have adopted new goals in the direction of harm reduction in line with this new approach. Strategies most prominently used in harm reduction include:
- low treshhold counseling and treatment facilities to attract as many drug users as possible at an early stage in their career;
- the availability of clean needles and syringes;
- AIDS counseling, counseling in safe sex and safe use practices;
- the availability of condoms;
and
- substitution treatment to limit risk-taking behavior.

Not all European countries have adopted all of these objectives but most of them have implemented at least one or the other, according to their needs and possibilities. In contrary in the United States the goal of drug policy is to keep people away from drugs and to fight a war on drugs rather than to shift towards harm reduction strategies.

Clearly enough these new objectives are accelerating a change of paradigms. To implement them one has to shift from the sociological/criminological paradigm of deviancy to a medical paradigm, identifying the former „drug fiend" as a medical case and accepting him as a patient. A certain „re-medicalization" in the treatment of drug abusers proves that these major changes have taken place.

In most countries health professionals are not well equipped for these new tasks which they are confronted with. There is a desperate need for further information and postgraduate training. Meetings such as the Vienna Symposium on Drug Abuse and AIDS therefore may act as important mediators to bring together outstanding experts to present their results and to discuss their experience in front of a large audience of scientists and practitionars in a very open way.

Information about even radical treatment schemes and discussion of different strategies in the fight against drug abuse and AIDS is of vital importance at a time when much more research is needed to understand the epidemiology of drug use and of HIV-infection among drug users and the relationship between HIV-prevalence and certain behavioral patterns of drug users. Moreover, discussion is, particularly important in a situation where no common philosophy about priorities exists and, last but not least, no effective cure for AIDS is in sight. Discussions such as we have attended in Vienna are stimulating our intellectual capacities, support unconventional thinking and, on the whole, are highly motivating. They will definitely help us to develop ideas, which in the long run may prove helpful to the individuals we are caring for and to the society we are part of.

Prof. Alfred Springer, M. D.
Director, Ludwig Boltzmann Institute for Addiction Research, Vienna

Contents

Epidemiology

Methadone Treatment

Management and Treatment

Prevention

Observations on the Stabilization of HIV Seroprevalence Among Injecting Drug Users

D. C. Des Jarlais

Beth Israel Medical Center, 11, Beach Street, New York 10013, NY USA

Introduction

HIV seroprevalence among injecting drug users (IDUs) has stabilized in a large number of cities, including New York,[1] Stockholm,[2] Vienna,[3] Amsterdam,[4] San Francisco,[5] and Innsbruck.[6] This stabilization has occurred at very different levels of HIV seroprevalence, from the 50% in New York to the 12% in San Francisco. The precise reasons why the stabilization has occurred at such differing levels have yet to be determined, but probably include: the extent to which HIV had already spread among the local group of IDUs (prior to large-scale AIDS risk reduction); and the extent to which the local legal, geographic, and social organization of the "community" of IDUs facilitates the multi-person use of injection equipment. Stabilization of HIV seroprevalence among IDUs in various cities has now occurred often enough that it can be considered a "normal" outcome of an HIV epidemic among IDUs.

The question then arises as to how long such stabilization is likely to endure. Should it be considered a cresting of the epidemic—to be followed by substantial declines in seroprevalence—as was the case with traditional epidemics of infectious diseases? Or should it be considered a temporary plateau, with seroprevalence eventually rising to a full "saturation" of the local population of IDUs? In this paper, I will examine the question of "enduring" stabilization of HIV among IDUs, using preliminary data from a number of our studies of IDUs in New York City. The overall conceptualization of stable HIV seroprevalence that I will use in this paper sees stabilization as a balance of dynamic factors, rather than as a static situation. I also want to note the exploratory nature of this conceptualization. It is presented here more as a framework for generating testable hypotheses, rather than as a scientifically documented set of conclusions.

Large-Scale AIDS Risk Reduction

The first important factor in stablization of HIV seroprevalence among IDUs is large-scale AIDS risk reduction/behavior change. In all cities where stable HIV seroprevalence has been observed, it has followed large-scale AIDS risk reduction by IDUs. Typically, half or more of the IDUs in a city have to change their injection practices before stabilization will occur. "Safer" drug injection practices are usually found to have been incorporated as new social norms within the local subculture of IDUs, so that safer injection does not depend only upon the individual drug injector's motivation to avoid exposure to HIV. The semi-independence of these new social norms from individual motivation to avoid HIV is particularly important, since reduction in HIV transmission may require behavior change by IDUs who already know (or suspect) that they have been exposed to the virus. These norms will also have a self-perpetuating quality, rather than being limited to a specific time period.

This large-scale risk reduction must, however, be thought of as risk reduction, rather than total risk elimination. Everyone in the group who continues to inject illicit drugs must still be considered to be at risk for exposure to HIV. Whether or not an IDU shares injection equipment will always have situational determinants (primarily, the availability of clean equipment at the time of injection), and even among the most highly motivated safer injectors there will always be the possibility of at least temporarily "relapsing" back to high-risk injection. Thus, even with large-scale risk reduction, a low to moderate rate of new HIV infections among the local group of IDUs will be a statistical certainty.

Loss to the Population of Injecting Drug Users

There are other factors that will serve to offset the increase in HIV seroprevalence that would be expected with a low to moderate rate of new HIV infections. A major offsetting factor will be loss of HIV seropositves to the population of active IDUs. The loss of seropositives would have both an immediate, direct effect of lowering HIV seroprevalence—because they would no longer be in the population—and an indirect, extended effect, because they would not be present to transmit HIV to seronegative IDUs.

One way in which HIV seropositives would be lost to the population of IDUs would be for them to permanently abstain from any further injection of illicit drugs. This might occur through their own efforts, probably with strong informal support systems (*** Waldorf and Biernacki book),[7] or through participation in formal drug abuse treatment programs. The frequency at which formal drug abuse treatment leads to permanent abstention from further drug injection is not known. Commonly used estimates are that, in an area with a (relatively) large-scale treatment system, about 15% to 20% of a population of IDUs in an area will recieve drug abuse treatment in any given year—and that 15% to 20% of those who receive such treatment will permanently cease to inject illicit drugs. Formal drug abuse treatment would thus result in a modest annual reduction in the number of persons actively injecting drugs. The number of persons who permanently stopped injecting illicit drugs through means other than formal treatment systems is exceedingly difficult to estimate. It may depend, in large part, on how one defines an active IDU; i.e., whether any injection would qualify, or whether high-frequency injection (addiction) is needed for inclusion in the population of IDUs.

While estimating the numbers of persons who permanently stop injecting illicit drugs is quite difficult, determining the likely HIV serostatus of these persons is even more problematic. HIV-seronegative drug injectors may also stop injecting illicit drugs. Thus, it is not possible to know the net effect on HIV seroprevalence of persons permanently stopping their injection of illicit drugs . The net effect might be zero, an increase, or a decrease in HIV seroprevalence.

It is much easier to estimate the effect of deaths among IDUs on HIV seroprevalence. Our current studies of deaths among drug injectors in New York indicate an annual death rate of about 3% per year, with the death rate among HIV seropositives approximately twice that of seronegatives. While a higher death rate among seropositives would always serve to lower HIV seroprevalence, the actual net effect of the deaths on seroprevalence will depend upon the initial seroprevalence rate. In New York City, with a seroprevalence of approximately 50%, the net effect of deaths would be to lower seroprevalence by approximately one percent per year.

Entry of New Injectors

A second factor which would tend to lower HIV seroprevalence among a population of IDUs is the entry of new persons into the group. With only a few exceptions—such as a gay man starting to inject drugs, or a long-term sexual partner of a drug injector starting to inject drugs—all of the new injectors would be HIV-seronegative at the time they begin injecting. Thus, the entry of new injectors into the population would reduce the seroprevalence rate. In our New York City studies, about 15% to 20% of the subjects are "new drug injectors", persons who have begun injecting within the last five years.

Paradoxically, while the net effect of entry of new injectors will usually be to reduce the overall seroprevalence rate, the actual seroconversion rate among the new injectors themselves is likely to be relatively high. For the new injectors, any "effective" exposure to HIV would result in a seroconversion, while among more experienced injectors, many "effective" exposures will be re-infections, and thus not be seen as seroconversions. Reaching new injectors with AIDS prevention programming is often quite difficult. They frequently do not identify as "addicts" and are less likely than more experienced injectors to seek assistance at syringe-exchange programs. Moreover, it will often be several years before their drug injection reaches a level where they would seek assistance at drug treatment programs.

Summary

Stable HIV seroprevalence can be conceptualized as a balance between opposing trends: low to moderate rate of new HIV infections, against differential death rates and entry of new injectors into the local group of IDUs. It is possible that such a stable seroprevalence situation might continue indefinitely. In a situation of stable seroprevalence, major public-health priorities are: to reduce the number of new injectors, and to develop ways of preventing HIV exposure among persons who do begin injecting illicit drugs. It would also be very helpful to develop new methods for assisting drug injectors to stop injecting. Even with a low to moderate seroconversion rate, the cumulative probability that an IDU would become infected with HIV over a decades-long career may still approach unity.

References

1. Des Jarlais DC, Friedman SR, Novick D, et al: HIV-1 Infection among intravenous drug users in Manhattan, New York City. JAMA 1989;261(7):1008-1012.

2. Kall K, Olin R: HIV status and changes in risk behavior among intravenous drug users in Stockholm 1987-88. AIDS 1990;4(2)153-157.

3. Loimer N, Presslich O, Hollerer E, Pakesch G, Pfersman V, Werner E: Monitoring HIV-1 infection prevalence among intravenous drug users in Vienna 1986-1990. AIDS Care 1990;2(3):281-286.

4. Van Haastrecht HJA, van den Hoek JAR, Bardoux C, Leentvaar-Kuypers A, Coutinho RA: The course of the HIV epidemic among intravenous drug users in Amsterdam, the Netherlands. Am J Public Health 1991;81(1):59-62.

5. Watters JK, Cheng Y, Segal M, Lorvick J, Case P, Carlson J: Epidemiology and prevention of HIV in intravenous drug users in San Francisco, 1986-1989. Read before the Sixth International Conference on AIDS, San Francisco, June 22, 1990.

6. Fuchs D, Unterweger B, Hausen A, et al. Anti-HIV-1 antibodies, anti-HTLV-1 antibodies and neopterin levels in parenteral drug addicts in the Austrian Tyrol. JAIDS 1988;1(1):65-66.

7. Waldorf D, Biernacki P: Natural recovery from heroin addiction: A review of the incidence literature. J of Drug Issues 1979;9:2, 281-289.

HIV-Antibody Testing and Risk-Prone Behaviour Amongst IVDU's in Oslo, Norway

G. WELLE-STRAND

Uteseksjonen, Akuttinstitutsjonen, Postboks 9017 Vaterland, N-0134 Oslo 1, Norway

The objective of the study was to find the HIV-sero-conversion rate amongst two different populations of mainly IVDUs in Oslo and relate it to the self-reported risk-prone behaviour.

Oslo, the capital of Norway, has approximately 500 000 inhabitants and there are 3-5000 IVDUs in this city. All treatment programs in Norway are drugfree; that is there have been no methadone maintenance programs in Norway. The only IVDU's who get methadone are approximately 10 HIV-infected persons who have developed severe immunodeficiency.

Up to December 31st 1990 approximately 200 IVDUs in the Oslo region were found to be HIV-positive. Most of the HIV-positive drug abusers were infected between 1983 and 1987; in the last 3 years few newly discovered HIV-positive IVDUs have been found (20 to 30 each year). Several investigations have shown that about 90 % of the IVDUs have been HIV-tested; so we do have a pretty good view of the overall situation. Up to December 31st 1990 only 15 IVDUs in Norway have been diagnosed as having AIDS, but reports from the hospitals in Oslo show that an increasing proportion of the HIV-positive IVDUs are getting sicker. More than 30 HIV-positive IVDUs have died for reasons other than HIV-associated sickness; the majority of these 30 persons have died from an intoxication(overdose).

Uteseksjonen is a municipal outreach program in the center of Oslo. At the daycenter there is a doctor 2 1/2 days a week, and there is a possibility to take a HIV-antibody test on a voluntary basis. Uteseksjon's aim is to reach "drifting youth in the center of Oslo" and a large proportion of these young persons are drug abusers.

Akuttinstitusjonen is a detoxification and evaluation clinic for drug abusers over the age of 18 in the center of Oslo. When the patients get there, they have a compulsory doctor's examination and they are offered a HIV-antibody test if they have engaged in risk-prone behaviour.

About 15 % of the patients in both places are HIV-antibody positive. In 1987 and 1988 only one new HIV-positive individual was found through the HIV-testing at the two places, although the patients reported considerable risk-prone behaviour.

We therefore designed a questionnaire in order to describe the risk-prone behaviour more thoroughly and relate it to the test results. The questionnaire is filled in together with the doctor performing the test who is the same person in both institutions.

Table 1 shows how many tests have been performed on different patients each year and for the two years put together. The results of the two different institutions have here been combined.

Table 1

1989	205 tests on 157 persons
1990	156 tests on 130 persons
TOTAL	361 tests on 250 persons 124/250 women(50%) and 126/250 men(50%)

Table 2. Average age when tested

	Akuttinstitusjonen	Uteseksjonen
1989	27.7 years	22.5 years
1990	28.7 years	24.4 years

Table 2 shows that an older age group has been tested at Akuttinstitusjonen (the detoxification clinic) than at Uteseksjonen (the municipal outreach program). The results from the two institutions will be put together in the rest of the presentation.

Table 3. Rate of response to the questionnaire (the patients are asked to fill in the questionnaire every time they have the HIV-test, so some patients have answered more than once)

1989	202/205 (99%)
1990	154/156 (99%)

Table 4. How many of the responders who take the HIV-antibody test for the first time

1989	15/157 (10%)
1990	13/130 (10%)

Table 4 shows that the vast majority of the patients have been HIV-antibody tested before; and a lot of the patients

Table 5. Certain characteristics of the persons being tested

	1989 N=157	1990 N=130
IVDU after 1979	90 %	91 %
IVDU last 3 months	80 %	81 %
Prostitution after 1979	40 %	33 %
-female	64 %	60 %
-male	13 %	6 %
Gonorrhea	33 %	36 %

Table 6. Results of the HIV-antibody test, hepatitis B antigen and antibody test and hepatitis C antibody test

	1989 N=205	1990 N=156
HIV-antibody positive	0*	0
Hepatitis B antigen positive	3	1
Hepatitis B antibody positive	96(47%)**	97(62%)**
Hepatitis C antibody positive	– ***	81(52%)

*   1 test positive screening; but negative Western Blot; later completely negative.

**   12 persons have received hepatitis B vaccine.

*** Hepatitis C antibody test was only available from the end of 1989.

     The period covered by the questionnaire is from 3 months prior to the last HIV-antibody test taken up to the moment of the actual test. The average time from the last HIV-antibody test was in 1989 9.1 months and in 1990 8.9 months; the period in question is on average one year prior to the actual test.

Table 7. Sexual practice and use of condoms in the period asked for (N is here the number of tests)

	1989 N=205	1990 N=156
Sexual contact with stable partner -Use of condoms	153 (75%)	116 (74%)
-never/almost never	95 %	91 %
-half of the time	1 %	2 %
-always/almost always	4 %	6 %
Prostitution -Use of condoms	70 (34%)	33 (21%)
-never/almost never	13 %	3 %
-half of the time	3 %	3 %
-always/almost always	80 %	94 %

12

Use of condoms during sexual contact with a person other
than a stable partner who is not buying sex is almost identical to the use of condom with a stable partner. More than 90 %
of the total population have had sexual contact with one or
several partners during the last year.

Table 8. Sex with a known HIV-antibody positive person in the
actual period

		1989	1990
Sexual contact with known HIV-positive person		19/157 (12%)	10/130 (8%)
Female		12/19	7/10
Male		7/19	3/10
Number of sexual contacts with known HIV-positive person	1-3	10/19	6/10
	4-6	4/19	0
	7-14	0	0
	>15	5/19	4/10
Use of condoms -never/almost never		13/19	4/10
-half of the time		0	2/10
-always/almost always		6/19	4/10

It seems to be more common for female IVDUs to engage in
risk-prone sexual behaviour with a HIV-positive person. There
is also a tendency towards less risk-prone behaviour in 1990
than in 1989, especially when it concerned having sexual
contact with a person known to be HIV-positive.

Table 9. Borrowing of syringe/needle amongst the respondants who have been IVDU's in the given period (N is here the number of tests where the person being tested has been an IVDU in the period we are asking for)

	1989 N=176	1990 N=139
Borrowed needle/syringe from stable partner -average number of times	72 (41 %) 17	50 (36 %) 17
Borrowed needle/syringe from person other than stable partner -average number of times	72 (41 %) 4	62 (45 %) 2
Borrowed needle/syringe from known HIV-positive	13 (7 %)	7 (5 %)

Table 9 gives an overview of how many persons have borrowed needle/syringe from other persons in the actual period, and how many times this has occured. In addition the respondants were asked how the needle and/or syringe was cleaned. The results
have not been systematized, but the main impression is that the vast majority have cleaned their needle/syringe once or several times in water.

I will go into further details about the persons reporting to have borrowed needle and/or syringe from a person known to be IIIV-positive. In 1989 11 different persons borrowed needle/syringe from a person known to be HIV-positive. 9 of the respondants had borrowed needle/syringe from a HIV-positive person 1-3 times in that period; the two others 10 and 90 times respectively. Only one of the 11 persons had cleaned the equipment in chlorine, the 10 others had cleaned the equipment in cold water or claimed that the needle/syringe "looked clean".

In 1990 6 different persons borrowed needle/syringe from a person known to be HIV-positive. 5 of the respondants had borrowed needle/syringe from a HIV-positive person 1-2 times in that period; the last person 5 times. 3 of the 6 persons had cleaned the equipment in chlorine; the 3 others had cleaned the equipment in cold water or not at all.

There seems to be some reduction in risk-prone behaviour related to intravenous drug abuse from 1989 to 1990, notably more persons report better disinfection procedures for their equipment.

The results show that amongst IVDUs in Oslo there is a low incidence of HIV-antibodies even though there is a considerable amount of risk-prone behaviour.

Possible reasons why the situation in Norway is so favourable in comparison with a lot of other countries in Europe are:

1. The prevalence of HIV is still low (approximately 5 %) amongst Norwegian IVDUs.
   -amongst the "heavy" heroin addicts the prevalence of HIV-antibody is 15-20 %.
2. The majority of the HIV-infected IVDUs know their serostatus.
   - our impression is that IVDUs knowing that they are HIV-antibody positive try to prevent the virus spreading to other persons.
3. Relatively few of the HIV-positive IVDUs are newly infected or have developed immmunodeficiency.
   -they are not in the stage of their HIV-infection where they are most infectious.
4. The standard among Norwegian IVDU's even before the HIV epidemic was to use clean syringes/needles.
   -this was learned during the years with a high prevalence of acute hepatitis B (1975-1986).
5. The Norwegian health authorities very quickly produced good quality practical information for people involved with risk-prone behaviour on how to avoid getting infected.
6. The availability of clean needles and syringes has most of the time been good.
   -needles and syringes have most of the time been on free sale from the pharmacies.
   -in the center of Oslo there is a bus delivering free needles and syringes during the evenings and nights.
7. Could the HIV-strain in Norway be less contagious than virus strains in other countries ?

Our investigation shows, however, that the situation is not stable; and we can therefore expect increasing incidence as the population of HIV-positive IVDUs gets sicker. In particular the IVDUs are not protecting themselves against sexual transmission; the use of condoms is extremely low apart from when the IVDUs are engaged in prostitution. A large proportions of the IVDUs still borrow injection equipment from other persons, even though this is probably less frequent than during previous years.

HIV-Prevalence and Mortality in Relation to Type of Drug Abuse Among Drug Addicts in Stockholm 1981–1988

A. Annell[1], A. Fugelstad[2], and G. Ågren[3]

[1] Department of Toxicomania Sabbatsberg Hospital, Behandlingsgruppen i City,
S. t Eriksgatan 40, S-11234 Stockholm
[2] Department of Psychiatry, S. t Görans Hospital
[3] Social Welfare Administration, Stockholm, Sweden

Background

HIV infection was introduced among the intravenous drug abusers in Stockholm in the summer in 1983 and subsequently began to spread. The infection was clinically detected by testings beginning in October 1984. (Pehrson 1988) Most of the intravenous drug abusers in Stockholm have been tested for HIV antibodies and thereby they have been informed about the test result. The vast majority of the HIV positive cases were detected before 1986, or 319 addicts. After that there was a decline of the rate of spread of HIV and at the end of 1988 they were 410. At the end of 1990 there were 456 cases in Stockholm county. The first case of aids occurred in the end of 1987.

Thus, as reported from several other cities, in Stockholm there has been a phase of rapid spread of HIV followed by a levelling off at a lower level of incidence as shown by "Fig. 1". It is notable that, in contrast to other big cities, in Stockholm exchange or delivering of syringes and needled is forbidden by a resolution of the parliament. Furthermore, the decline in incidence began before an expansion of the Methadone maintenance treatment program was decided by the authorities and performed in practice. The decline can be attributed to behavioural changes following intensive information from the end of 1984 to drug abusers and drug abuse workers about HIV transmission and ways to protect oneself and others. There has been an extensive HIV testing. The Stockholm laboratories have

performed tests in more than 7000 individuals with a previous or present
drug abuse (Blaxhult, Böttiger, Janzon 1989). There is a persistent high
frequency of testing. Combined with counselling it enhances the awareness
an knowledge of risks, which is our main weapon against the spread of
HIV.

Testing is voluntary. Some abusers have been tested more than twenty
times. Among IVDU:s there is a certain amount of social pressure to be
tested. They want to know the serostatus of persons, with whom they have
to share injecting equipements. Most of them are honest about it. Among
IVDU:s it seems to be accepted to ask a casual sex partner about HIV
test results (Käll 1990).

Fig. 1 (from the National Bacteriological Laboratory)

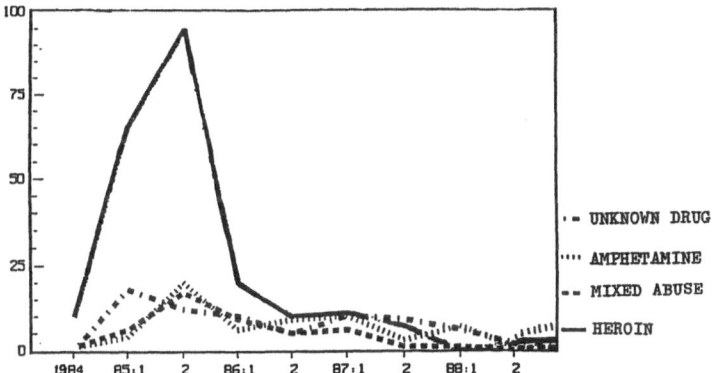

**NUMBER OF NEW HIV-POSITIVE INDIVIDUALS
AMONG IVDU:S IN STOCKHOLM COUNTY**

About 2/3 of the HIV positive IVDU:s in Stockholm use heroin as their
main drug, 1/4 use amphetamine and the rest have a mixed abuse. The decline in incidence is most striking for heroin abusers, whereas there is
a fairly constant incidence among amphetamine abusers. The most plausible
explanations are two. The HIV infection reached the heroin abusing population one or two years before the amphetamine using population and at a
time, before we had got a knowledge about the spread. Secondly, these two
populations have different patterns of injecting habits, the amphetamine
users being less inclined and stressed to share equipements (Annell 1989,
Käll, Olin 1990).

The total IVDU population in the Stockholm region is estimated through repeated investigations to be around 3000. Out of these about 40% use heroin. In Sweden heroin abuse is concentrated to the the Stockholm region and the province of Skane in southern part of the country. Most IVDU:s combine their main drug with cannabis, bensodiazepines or alcohol.

Compared to sex proportions in the total IVDU population there are more HIV seropositive males (Annell 1989).

In Sweden there were 2007 seropositive persons known in total at the end of 1988. At the end of 1990 there were 2655 cases. 504 of them had contracted aids. The aids cases among IVDU:s were 18 (13 in the Stockholm area).

Prevalence studies in Stockholm

The National Bacteriological Laboratory has estimated that the 300 - 350 seropositive IVDU:s reported to be heroin addicts is about one third of the total population of heroin users (Annell 1989).

During the period October 1984 - December 1985 half of the heroin addicts and one third of patients with a mixed abuse at the detoxification clinic at Sabbatsberg Hospital were seropositive (Helgesson 1986).

A study conducted at the Remand Prison in Stockholm from January to October 1987 showed a seroprevalence of 63.4% among heroin addicts and 6.3% among amphetamine abusers. In both these studies there is a methodological problem, constituted by the relatively short observation period. This gives a prevalence figure, which is too high. Abusers frequently admitted are more often seropositive. Women tend to be under-represented in prison. When the study in the Remand Prison was extended to December 1989, prevalence figures decreased to 36.8% among heroin abusers, 5.3% among amphetamine abusers and 11.1% for all abusers. 96% of the in-mates had been tested for HIV antibodies (Käll, Olin, Laurén 1990).

Repeated reports during 1988 and 1989 on drug abusers in contact with the social wellfare in the city of Stockholm show that 282 out of 3173 known abusers were seropositive. 168 out of the 666 heroin users were seropositive and 66 out of 1412 amphetamine users (Ågren, Anderzon, Berglund,

Fugelstad 1990). In a cohort of 152 drug addicts under coercive care in 1986 - 1988 58 were seropositive (Fugelstad 1989).

Objective

The aim of this study is to follow up a representative cohort of drug abusers attending a hospital during a period, when HIV infection was being introduced among the drug abusers in Stockholm, and to study the HIV prevalence and mortality in the group in relation to dominating type of drug and sex.

Material

The study includes all patients attending the drug abuse clinic at Sabbatsberg Hospital during the period 1 January 1981 to 31 December 1988. Totally 1677 patients, 1163 men and 514 women, were under care during this time. 1001 of them were referred more than one time to the wards.

Representativeness

In Stockholm county there are three clinics for medical detoxification of narcotic drug abusers. The clinic at Sabbatsberg Hospital is the biggest one and responsible for the central part of the region, primarily the city of Stockholm, including the down town area. In 1986 an inventory showed, that 90% of all drug abusers treated in hospital in the city of Stockholm attended the department at Sabbatsberg Hospital (Johansson 1987).

The material comprises more than half of the HIV positive drug abusers at this time in the Stockholm region, that is 220 cases. Moreover, of them 194 were seropositive already in 1984 - 85, that is the vst majority of those first infected in the region. Most of them were well known by the staff of the clinic.

Method

From information in journals the main drug used, summing up all admissions, was categorized in heroin, amphetamine, mixed and others.

From the Swedish Population Register the patients, who were deceased, were identified. The annual mortality is calculated out from the number of deaths and the observed person-years for each category.

Results

The average age at their first referral is for the opiate abusers 28.2 years old and for the central stimulants abusers 29.7 years old.

The distribution of main drug and tests and HIV status is demonstrated in "Fig. 2" illustrating "Table 1". 405 patients are not tested, the majority of them belonging to the group admitted to the clinic before 1985 and no later returned. Including only patients admitted after 1984 tests are performed in 90.8% of them.

The HIV seroprevalence for the total material is 17.3%. For heroin users it is 31.9%, for amphetamine users 5.1% and for mixed intravenous drug users 7.3%. Separating those in care before and after 1984 respectively makes no difference.

Fig. 2 and Table 1.

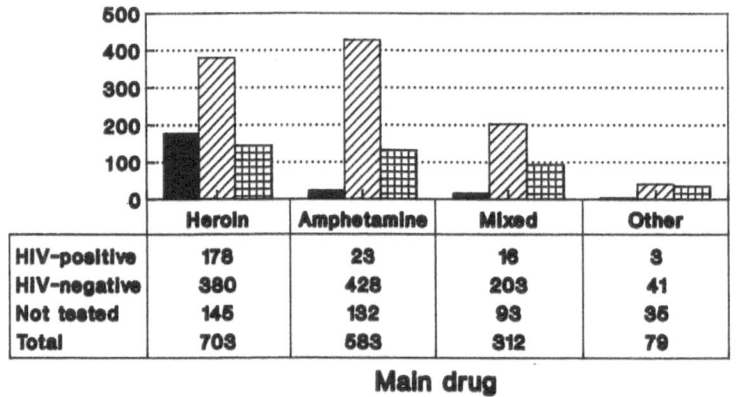

HIV-status and main drug
N=1677

	Heroin	Amphetamine	Mixed	Other
HIV-positive	178	23	16	3
HIV-negative	380	428	203	41
Not tested	145	132	93	35
Total	703	583	312	79

Main drug

■ HIV-positive ▨ HIV-negative ▦ Not tested

Sabbatsberg 1981-1988

There is no significant disproportions in distribution between sexes.
There is a tendency for women to be tested more often.

Totally 147 patients have died at the end of the study period in December
1988. 39 of them were HIV positive. All those four, who had got an aids
diagnosis were alive. The mortality related to HIV status was uneven in
different years as seen in "Fig. 3".

Fig. 3.

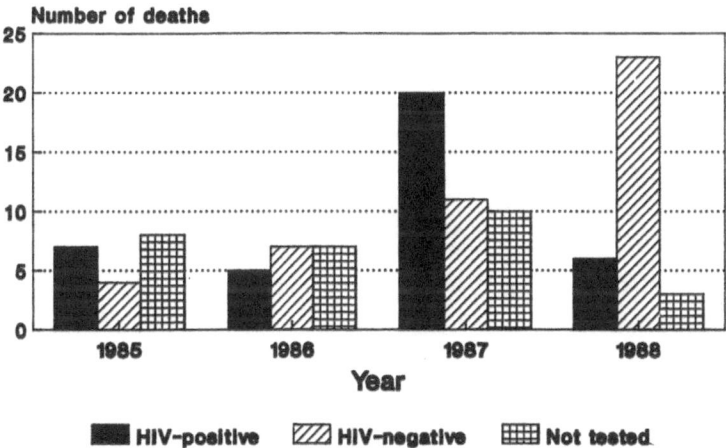

Annual mortality
related to HIV-status

Annual mortality for all heroin addicts both for the whole observation
period and separately for the parts of it before and after November 1984,
when HIV tests were started, is 3.3%. However, for the HIV positive heroin addicts it is 5.3%, that is considerably increased. For the amphetamine abusers it is 1.2%. Causes of death are dominated by death by injection of narcotic illegal drugs. Only one suicide occurred among the HIV
positive patients.

Conclusions

This cohort is representative for drug abusers in central Stockholm requiring hospital care. Most of them are injecting abusers.

The HIV seroprevalence found corresponds to other studies in Stockholm with similar extremely high test frequency and consolidates the figures previously given.

The mortality is very high, especially among heroin addicts. There is no general increase in mortality rates in the months following HIV testing. However, during an extended observation period the following few years there is a significantly increased mortality among HIV positive abusers. The causes of death are not directly related to the HIV infection.

Reference List

Annell A (1989) Behandling av aidssjuka narkomaner. Rapport från nordiskt seminarium 1989. Nordiska kontaktmannaorganet för narkotikafrågor, Soc. Depart.(Ministry of Health an Social Affairs), Stockholm

Blaxhult A, Böttiger M, Janzon R (1989) HIV-infektion bland injektions-missbrukare i Sverige. Swed Med J (Läkartidningen) 86:28-29, 2518-2519

Fugelstad A (1989) LVM-vård av narkomaner. Kartläggning av narkomaner in-skrivna på Serafens LVM-hem 1986-1988. FoU-byrån, Social Wellfare Admini-stration, Stockholm

Helgesson B (1986) Hälften av en grupp heroinister i Stockholm LAV/HTLV-III-positiva. Swed Med J (Läkartidningen) 83:23, 2147

Käll K (1990) Providing care for HIV-infected drug users in Swedish pri-sons. Unpubl. oral pres. at WHO-meeting in Vienna

Käll K, Olin RG (1990) HIV status and changes in risk behaviour among intravenous drug users in Stockholm 1987-1988. AIDS 4:153-157

Käll K, OlinRG, Laurén K (1990) HIV status and changes in risk behaviour among intravenous drug users in Stockholm 1987-1989. Unpubl.

Pehrson PO (1988) HIV-infection among IV drug abusers in Stockholm. IV International Conference on AIDS, Stockholm 1988, abstract 4510

Ågren G, Anderzon K, Berglund E, Fugelstad A (1990) Narkotikasituationen i Stockholm. FOU-byrån, Stockholm Social Wellfare Administration

HIV-Related Drug Addict Deaths Outside Medical Institutions in Stockholm

A. Fugelstad[1] and J. Rajs[2]

[1] Department of Psychiatry, S. t Görans Hospital,
S. t Göransgatan 141, S-112 81 Stockholm
[2] Department of Forensic Medicine, Karolinska Institutet, Stockholm, Sweden

INTRODUCTION

The main objective of this report is to study mortality and cause of death among HIV infected drug addicts in the Stockholm area over a five year period (July 1, 1985 - June 30, 1990).

There are approximately 3000 active intravenous drug users (IVDUs) in the area. About 40% of these use heroin as their main drug, while the remaining 60% use amphetamine. The number of IVDUs has been rather constant for the last ten years.

At the end of 1984, HIV was discovered among drug users in the Stockholm area for the first time. Böttiger M (1991), personal communication. Approximately 7000 persons were screened, and 220 HIV seropositive cases had been detected among drug addicts by the end of 1985.

By analyzing frozen blood samples, it could be demonstrated that some drug addicts were infected already in 1983. Käll et al. (1990).

In the last years, 20-30 new HIV-positive drug addicts have appeared annually. In the beginning of 1991, there were 425

known seropositive IVDUs in the Stockholm area. 17 addicts
had developed AIDS.

The majority of the seropositive addicts are heroin users,
but the number using amphetamine as their main drug is
rising.

The mortality rate among Swedish drug addicts varies
depending on the dominating drug. Ågren et al.(1990). The
mortality among amphetamine users is about 1% annually. The
corresponding rate among heroinists is 3% per year. Heroin
users often die in connection with the injection of the drug.
Addicts mainly using amphetamine show more varied causes of
death.

During the last part of the 1980s, the organization for
treatment capacity and care of drug addicts has expanded.
Both medical and social services have been granted greater
funds. A number of social field workers have been appointed.
Their main task is to detect new drug addicts and convince
them to seek treatment.

The city of Stockholm recently started a new program for
methadone maintenance treatment, presently helping 220
patients, 50% of which are seropositive.

In Sweden there are two laws on compulsory care which can be
applied in order to force drug addicts to undergo treatment.
One is the law on care of alcohol and drug abusers, ruling
that addicts maybe sent to involuntary care for a period of
up to 6 months, if they are actually risking their health and
refuse voluntary treatment. The other is the law on
infectious diseases according to which it is possible to
isolate persons who do not comply with the public health
security measures specified by the chief medical officer.

Several questions can be asked in this context. Do the
changes in the treatment system influence the mortality among
drug addicts? Does the HIV infection interfere with mortality

rates and causes of death? Do HIV infected drug addicts acquire a more destructive pattern of drug abuse with an increased mortality? Are they dying at a later stage from their infection? What is the proportion of suicide among the deaths?

The aim of the present report is to answer or shed light on, the above questions.

PATIENTS AND METHODS

The study was carried out at the Government Institute for Forensic Medicine in Stockholm during a 5-year period (July 1, 1985 to June 30, 1990). Persons dying outside hospitals as a result of violent action, poisoning, or otherwise suddenly and unexpectedly, under unclear or suspicious circumstances, including most users of opiates and central stimulants, were examined in this institute. A total of 16,948 bodies of all ages and both sexes were examined during the study period.

There were, in all, 1,912,499 residents in the service area (the counties of Stockholm and Södermanland, and the community of Gotland) in 1987 i.e. at an intermediate time point of the study period. The population in Stockholm County amounted 1,606,157 this year. The same year 1,156 HIV-positive persons were registered in Stockholm County, i.e. 2/3 of all known cases in Sweden; 386 or 1/3 of these were drug addicts.

Prior to autopsy, blood samples were analyzed for HIV antibodies at the National Bacteriological Laboratory (SBL). Cases with samples positive in ELISA-screening and Western blotting were counted as HIV-positive. Forensic chemical analyses were made at the Government Laboratory for Forensic Chemistry in Linköping. In known or suspected drug addicts, forensic chemical analyses were designed to disclose presence of alcohol, barbiturates, tranquilizers, opiates, central stimulants and cannabis.

In HIV-positive cases, a thorough external inspection of the
body was done and forensic chemical analyses were made on
blood obtained by puncture of deep veins, as well as on urine
- when available. With the consent of the police authorities
requesting our services, and considering the findings at the
external inspection and the results from the forensic
chemical analyses, we refrained from autopsy in cases of
obvious suicide or in those dying suddenly in connection with
drug injection. When information and observations were
unequivocal, autopsy was performed, including histopatho-
logical investigation. Following to these criteria, about one
third of all the HIV-positive casualties were subjected to
complete and one third to incomplete (excluding examination
of the brain) autopsy. In one third of the cases no autopsy
was made.

Information about deceased persons was obtained from police
and hospital records and was, when possible, supplemented
with information available from their families and friends as
well as from social workers.

Particular effort was made in cases of drug addicts having
died in connection with intravenous drugadministration, in
order to find out whether the casualty was of accidental,
suicidal or homicidal origin.
The study was approved by the ethical committee of the
Karolinska Institute.

RESULTS

During the five-year period July 1, 1985 - June 30, 1990 331
drug addicts died outside a hospital. Figure 1 shows a nearly
even distribution of deaths of drug addicted victim during
the study period, with a peak during the first half of 1990.
Positive results of HIV-testing were obtained in 57 of 331
deaths. All of these - except two - were already registered
by the National Laboratory before death. However, information
in records available before the time of autopsy was found in

less than half of the cases. The distribution of the drug addict deaths in relation to the results of HIV-testing is shown in Fig. 2, demonstrating a peak in the first half of the 1987.

Deaths among drug addicts in Stockholm
Deaths outside hospital 1985-1990.

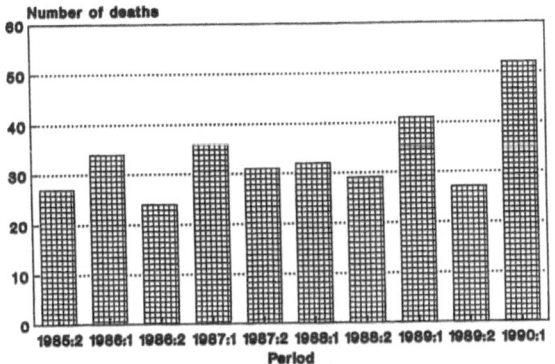

Govern. Institute for Forensic Medicine.

Fig. 1. Distribution of drug addict deaths outside medical institutions in Stockholm during five years, July 1, 1985 - June 30, 1990, divided into six month periods.

Mortality and HIV-status
Deaths outside hospital 1985-1990.

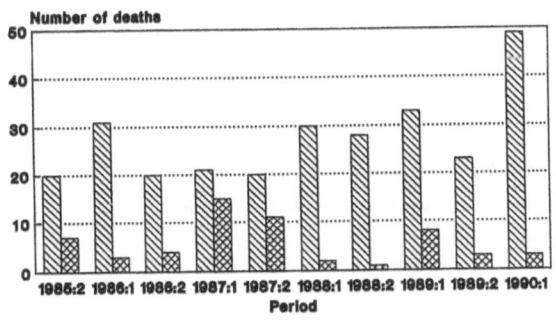

Govern. Institute for Forensic Medicine.

Fig. 2. Mortality and HIV-status of drug addicts in Stockholm during five years, July 1, 1985 - June 30, 1990, divided into six month periods.

Of the 57 HIV-positive drug addicts, 44 were males and 13
females (Fig. 3), the sex ratio being approximately 3:1. The
HIV-positive female drug addicts were 23-29 years old, with
an average age of 26.4. The infected male drug addicts were
21-44 years old, with an average age of 32.2. They showed
greater age span and higher age than their female
counterparts.

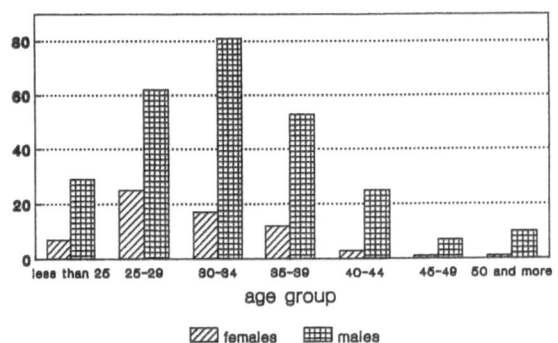

Fig. 3.   Age and sex distribution of HIV positive drug addict
          deaths.

Of the 331 drug addicts, 245 (74%) used opiates as the main
drug, 59 (17.2%) mainly central stimulants, and 6 (1,8%)
cocaine; in 21 cases (6.3%), it was not possible to find out
whether the dominating drugs were opiates or central
stimulants. The main drug status in relation to occurrence of
HIV-infection is shown in Table I.

Toxicological examinations were made in 55 of the total of 57
HIV-positive drug addict deaths. The results are shown in
Table II. There was no death case with negative toxicological
findings. The most common findings were opiates in
combination with medicinal drugs and/or alcohol or
amphetamine (demonstrated in 36 of 55 analyzed postmortem

TABLE I.

MAIN DRUG AND HIV-STATUS OF 331 DRUG ADDICTS DYING OUTSIDE
HOSPITALS IN STOCKHOLM 1985 - 1990.

Main drug	HIV-negative n (%)	HIV-positive n (%)
Opiates, n = 245	193 (79)	52 (21)
Amphetamine, n = 59	57 (96)	2 (4)
Cocaine, n = 6	6 (100)	0
Not known, n = 21	18 (86)	3 (14)
TOTAL: 331	274 (83)	57 (17)

samples). Findings of only opiates, or central stimulantia,
were less common, occurring in 3 and 1 of 55 examined
instances, respectively. Alcohol was found in the blood of
more than half of the 55 analyzed cases (29/55). However,
there was no addict in which alcohol was the only drug found
in the blood. The most common medicinal drugs were
benzodiazepines (demonstrated in 34 of 55 analyses).

48 HIV-positive drug addicts died in connection with
intravenous heroin administration or its sequelae; only two
of these deaths were classified as suicides. One of these had
a blood morphine level of 1.3 ug/g, another one 0.5 ug/g,
both in combination with medicinal drugs. The remaining 46
deaths were classified as accidental or of otherwise
undetermined cause. Among these 46 heroin addicts, 42 deaths
were instantanenous, the addicts collapsed in immediate
connection with the heroin administration, and died
immediately, or where found right where they had made the
injection with the syringe still in the vein. Their
postmortem blood morphine concentrations showing that 28 of
42 (66%) had less than 0.30 ug morphine per gram blood. There
were also two methadone suicides, with blood methadone
concentrations of 1.1 ug/g and 3.5 ug/g, respectively.

TABLE II.

TOXICOLOGICAL FINDINGS IN POSTMORTEM SAMPLES TAKEN FROM 57
HIV-POSITIVE DRUG ADDICTS DYING OUTSIDE HOSPITALS IN
STOCKHOLM 1985 - 1990

Findings	n	(%)
Opiates	3	(5.3)
Opiates + alcohol	6	(10.5)
Opiates - medicinal drugs	11	(19.3)
Opiates, alcohol + medicinal drugs	14	(24.6)
Opiates, alcohol + amphetamine	2	(3.5)
Opiates, alcohol, medicinal drugs + amphetamine	5	(8.7)
Opiates, medicinal drugs + amphetamine	6	(10.5)
Amphetamine	1	(1.7)
Amphetamine + medicinal drugs	1	(1.7)
Amphetamine, alcohol + medicinal drugs	2	(3.5)
Medicinal drugs	4	(7.0)
No examination done	2	(3.5)
TOTAL:	57	(100)

TABLE III.

CAUSES OF DEATH OF HIV-POSITIVE DRUG ADDICTS

Cause of death		n (%)
Non-violent death, total		1 (1.7)
Liver cirrhosis (303)	1 (1.7)	
External violence and poisoning, total		56 (98.3)
Collapse and death following heroin injection (E 980)	48 (84.2)	
Suicide (E 950 - E 958)	7 (12.3)	
Homicide (E 960)	1 (1.7)	
TOTAL:		57 (100)

However, it could not be ascerteined, whether the methadone
in these instances was taken intravenously or orally.

Table III shows the causes and manner of death in HIV-
positive drug addicts. This table demonstrates that the only
instance classified as "natural death" was an addict dying as
a result of alcohol abuse. Death from intravenous
administration of heroin was the dominating manner of death
of HIV-positive addicts, suicide being the second (but much
less common) manner.

The exterior examination of the bodies showed unspecific
changes of the skin, like injection marks and scars, and,
occasionally, acne or furunculosis, while stigmata indicative
of a specific disease process were lacking. The HIV-positive
persons looked no more emaciated than the HIV-negative.

DISCUSSION

This study can be said to give an almost complete picture of
the extent of HIV infection among drug addicts having died
outside medical institutions in the Stockholm area - the area
in Sweden with the highest incidence of HIV. The possibility
that some the drug addict deaths could have escaped detection
was considered minimal. Karlsson t et al (1988)). The number
of newly discovered cases - 2/57 was low, attesting to the
efficiency of the anti-HIV-measures in Sweden. As illustrated
by our survey, the spread of the HIV infection has, after an
advance during the first two years (1985 - 1987) reached a
peak during the first half of 1987, and then continuously
abated.

The crucial moment in the life of a heroinist comes with the
abrupt collapse brought about by the heroin injection,
especially if the abuser is HIV infected. The reason for the
collapse is usually, according to the principle of least
resistance, ascribed to an "overdose". The literature states
that 0.3 microgram morphine/gram blood can be considered as a

lethal concentration. Monforte JR (1977). A suddenly arising
depressive effect of the drug on the CNS following the
inravenous injection, pulmonary edema resulting from
anaphylactic shock, and a variety of heart arrythmias
probably are important causative factors of the life
threatening collapse. Steinberg AD (1968), Duberstein et al
(1971), Frand et al (1972), Karliner JS et al (1969), Lipski
et al (1974), Urthaler et al (1975) and Glauser et al (1977).
In our study 28 of the 42 HIV-positive drug addicts (60%)
dying in connection with the injection had concentrations
lower than 0.3 microgram morphine/gram blood. However, as
illustrated in Table II, that the heavy drugs - like heroin
and amphetamine - seldom occur as the only drugs associated
with a fatal outcome, suggesting that the combined action of
the drugs may be of significance for the death of the addict.
Another plausible explanation relates to the assumption that
the HIV positive heroinists to a greater extent than the noninfected ones were "weaned", i.e. detoxified, and
consequently - at a relapse - no longer were adapted to their
previous, "normal" dose.

In the public debate, the theory of concealed suicides is
often brought up; this notion is not confirmed by the present
study. The peak of deaths in the first 6 months of 1987 (see
Fig. 2) received much attention; even the homicide theory was
consi-dered but was not corroborated in any instance.

When treating pneumocystis carinii in AIDS patients, drug
allergy is seen remarkably often following use of sulfa
preparations. Hopewell PC et al (1986), Hughes WR (1987) and
Leport et al (1988). An increased risk of developing
anaphylaxis caused by HIV virus could possibly explain the
excess mortality among the seropositive but otherwise symptom
free heroinists, when the drug is injected.

Infection with HIV has, so far, not resulted in any epidemic
of suicides among drug addicts, even though occasional
suicides have occurred, apparently triggered by a HIV
infection or fear thereof. The decrease in suicides among HIV

negative drug abusers could be interpreted as showing that
not even actual knowledge of a recent exposure to the
infectious agent is a common motive for suicide for a not yet
seroconverted person. Manifestations of AIDS symptoms seem to
be more suicide stimulating than the information that
infection has really occurred. Rajs et al (1991). The drug
addicts in Sweden became the objects of HIV infection several
years later than the homo- and bisexual males. Thus, an
increase of suicides among the HIV-infected drug addicts is
to be expected.

REFERENCES

Böttiger, M (1991). National Bacteriological Laboratory
(SBL). Personal communication.

Duberstein J L, Kaufman D M (1971) A clinical study of an
epidemic of heroin intoxication and heroin-induced pulmonary edema. Am J Med 51:704-714

Frand U I, Shim C S, William M H (1972) Heroin-induced
pulmonary edema. Ann Intern Med 77:29-356

Glauser F L, Downie R L, Smith W R (1977) Electrcardio-
graphic abnormalities in acute heroin overdosage. Bull Narc
1:85-89

Hopewell P C, Luce J M (1986) Pulmonary manifestations of the
acquired immunodeficience syndrome. Clinics in immunology
allergy. Aids and HIV Infection. Ed Pinching AJ 6:489-518

Hughes W T (1987) Pneumocystis carinii pneumonitis. N Engl J
Med 317:1021-1023

Karliner J S, Steinberg A D, Williams M H (1969) Lung
function after pulmonary edema associated with heroin
overdose. Arch Intern Med 124:350:353

Karlsson T, Eklund B, Rajs J (1988) HIV-relaterade dödsfall
utanför sjukvårdsinrättningar i Stockholm. Läkartidningen
85:22, 1990-1993

Käll K I, Olin R G (1990) HIV status and changes in risk
behaviour among intravenous drug users in Stockholm
1987-1988. AIDS 4:153-157.

Leport C, Raffi F, Matheron S, Katlama c, Regner B, Saimot
A G, Marche C, Vedrenne C, Vilde J L (1988) Treatment of
central nervous system toxoplasmosis with pyrimetha-
nine/sulfadiazine combination in 35 patients with the
acquired immunodeficience syndrome. Am J Med 84:94-100
Lipski J, Stimel B, Donoso E (1974) The effect of heroin
and multiple drug abuse on the electrocardiogram. Am Heart
J 86:663-668

Monforte J R (1977) Some observations concerning blood
morphine concentrations in narcotic addicts. J Forensic Sci
22:718-722

Pehrson P O, Gaines H, Gyllensten K, Moberg L G, Struve J,
von Sydow M, Sönnerborg A, Åkerlund B (1988) HIV-infection
among IV drug abusers in Stockholm. Abstract 4510. IV
International Conference on AIDS, Stockholm.

Steinberg A D, Karliner J S (1968) The clinical spectrum
of heroin pulmonary edema. Arch Intern Med 122:122-127

Urthaler F, Isobe J H, James T N (1975) Direct and vagally
mediated chronotropic effects of morphine studies by
selective perfusion of the sinus node of awake dogs. Chest
68:222-228

Rajs J, Fugelstad A (1991) HIV-related suicides in Stockholm.
Manuscript in preparation

Ågren G, Anderzon K, Berglund E, Fugelstad A (1990)
Narkotikasituationen i Stockholm. FoU-byrån Socialtjänsten
 i Stockholm

HIV infection in 403 Female Prostitutes in Italy

U. Tirelli[1], M. Spina[1], G. Rezza[2], E. Vaccher[1], F. Caprilli[3],
M. Giuliani[2], A. Saracco[4], A. Lazzarin[5], D. Serraino[1], G. Gentili[3],
V. Accurso[6], S. Mancuso[6], and R. De Marcato[7]

[1] Centro di Riferimento Oncologico di Aviano, Unità AIDS, V. Pedemontana Occ.,
I-33081 Aviano (PN), Italy
[2] Centro Operativo AIDS, Istituto Superiore di Sanità, Roma
[3] Istituto Dermosifilopatico, Ospedale San Gallicano, Roma
[4] CNR, Milano
[5] Clinica Malattie Infettive L. Sacco, Milano
[6] Istituto di Clinica Medica e Malattie Cardiovascolari Università degli Studi di Palermo
[7] II Facoltà di Medicina – Università degli Studi di Napoli

INTRODUCTION

Since the beginning of HIV epidemic, it became clear that the modality of transmission was different between Western Countries and Africa (1). Infact, in Africa heterosexual contact is the most important factor in the spread of HIV infection and female prostitutes are considered to be the major reservoir of HIVinfection (2).

The first studies on the prevalence of HIV infection among female prostitutes were published in 1984 and were carried out in Africa. They found that among the female prostitutes tested, 1% of them were HIV-seropositive in Ghana (3), 56% in Kenya (4) and 80% in Rwanda (5). On the other hand, in Western Countries it appeared soon very important the role played by intravenous drug addiction in the spread of HIV infection. Infact all published studies showed that seroprevalence was very low among non-intravenous drug users prostitutes (non-IVDU) and very high among IVDU-prostitutes.

In New York 31.3% of those who used intravenous drugs were found to be seropositive in comparison with 6.9% of the non-IVDU (6). Other studies carried out in USA showed a seroprevalence among non-IVDU of 1% in Atlanta (7). In Europe the prevalence of HIV infection among female prostitutes showed the same pattern as in the USA.

Studies carried out in Holland found 5% of the non-IVDU prostitutes were HIV-seropositive that and 34% of the IVDU (8); in Spain 2.4% among non-IVDU were seropositive and 54.6% among IVDU (9).

The aim of our cross-sectional multicentre study, supported by a grant of Ministry of Health, is to estimate the HIV seroprevalence among selected female prostitutes in Italy.

MATERIALS AND METHODS

Between Jannuary 1988 and November 1990 we have collected data on HIV serological testing of 403 female prostitutes including non-IVDUs and IVDUs living in five italian towns: Milan, Rome, Naples, Pordenone and Palermo. Sexually transmitted disease (STD) clinics and HIV-outpatient facilities were used as sources of data on women engaged in prostitution. HIV serological testing was offered on voluntary basis and demographic data were collected, ensuring confidentiality of information. Serology for HIV was performed using ELISA test with confirmation by Western blot.

RESULTS

Four hundred and there prostitutes were tested. Table 1 shows the country of origin of our female prostitutes.

COUNTRIES OF ORIGIN OF 403 FEMALE PROSTITUTES LIVING IN ITALY

TABLE 1

COUNTRY OF ORIGIN	NON-IVDUs	IVDUs
ITALY	215	118
SPAIN	2	–
COLOMBIA	50	–
BRASIL	3	–
MEXICO	3	–
URUGUAY	2	–
VENEZUELA	2	–
REPUBLIC DOMINICANA	2	–
ARGENTINA	2	–
TUNISIA	4	–
TOTAL	285	118

Overall, 50 (12.4%) were infected: 6 out of 285 non-IVDUs (2.1%) and 44 out of 118 IVDUs (37.2%). The median age was 33.4 years in the non-IVDU group (range 19-63) and 25.6 years in the IVDU group (range 17-40). Non-IVDU prostitutes were significantly older than the IVDU prostitutes (p 0.01).
Two of the six HIV-seropositive non-IVDU prostitutes were regular sexual partners of seropositive male IVDUs. For the other four women no Known risk factors were reported other than prostitution. One of these patients died of CDC-defined AIDS.
Table 2 shows the distribution of HIV by risk group and age class.

TABLE 2   HIV ANTIBODIES IN 403 FEMALE PROSTITUTES

AGE (YR)	NON-IVDUs HIV+/TOTAL (%)	IVDUs HIV+/TOTAL (%)	TOTAL HIV+/TESTED (%)
< 20	0/4	5/11 (45.4)	5/15 (33.3)
20 - 29	0/111	30/84 (35.7)	30/195 (15.4)
30 - 39	3/126 (2.3)	9/22 (40.9)	12/148 (8.1)
40 - 49	2/31 (6.5)	0/1	2/32 (6.2)
> 50	1/13 (7.7)	-	1/13 (7.7)
TOTAL	6/285 (2.1)	44/118 (37.2)	50/403 (12.4)

Condoms were reported to be used routinely and correctly by the vast majority of non-IVDU prostitutes while few IVDU prostitutes used them.
Moreover a number of non-IVDU prostitutes reported to have sex with their non payant partners without condoms and some of then had IVDU partners or seropositive partners.

CONCLUSIONS

This study shows that, athough at very low level, HIV infection is present among non IVDU female prostitutes and this seroprevalence is increasing with years (10,11) However, it is in known wetter seroprevalence among non-IVDU female prostitutes is significantly higher than that of the non prostitute women of the same age group. Our data show high prevalence of HIV infection among IVDU female prostitutes. These data were obtained on a voluntary basis: had anonymous testing been done, the results may well have been different and in all probability the level of infection would have been higher. Few clients (of prostitutes) realize that HIV seropositivity is widespread among female IVDU prostitutes and that it is not easy to distinguish between IVDU and non-IVDU prostitutes.

Moreover, it is well known that most cliants prefer to have sex without condoms. All these findings emphasize the possible role played by IVDU prostitutes in the spread of HIV in the heterosexual population.

REFERENCE

1. Goedert JJ, Sarngadharan MG, Biggar RJ, et al.
   Determinants of retrovirus (HTLV-III) antibody and immunodeficiency condition in homosexual men.
   Lancet 1984; 2: 711-6.

2. Quinn TC, Mann JM, Curran JW, et al.
   AIDS in Africa: an epidemiologic paradigm.
   Science 1986; 234: 955-63.

3. Neequaye AR, Neequaye J, Mingle JA, Ofori Adjeid D.
   Preponderance of females with AIDS in Ghana (Letter).
   Lancet 1986; 2: 978.

4. Kreiss JK, Koech D, Plummer FA, et al.
   AIDS virus infection in Nairobi prostitutes.
   N. Engl. J. Med. 1986; 314: 414-8.

5. Van De Perre P, Clumeck N, Carael M, et al.
   Female prostitutes: a risk group for infection with Human T-Cell Lymphotropic virus Type III.
   Lancet 1985; 2: 524-7.

6. Wallace J, Mann J, Beatrice S.
   Survey of streetwalkers in New York City for anti-HIV-I antibodies.
   IV International Conference on AIDS, Stockholm 1988, Abstract 4046.

7. CDC.
   Human Immunodeficiency in the United States: a review of current Knowledge.
   MMWR 1987; 36: 1-48.

8; Praats C, Laga M, Van Royen P, Peeters N, Hendrickx C, Piot P.
   Female Prostitutes in Antwerp: a risk group for HIV infection.
   V International Conference on AIDS, Montreal 1989, Abstract MAP
   49:86.

9. Estebanez P, Zunzunegui V, Najera R, Colombo C.
   Study of the prevalence of HIV infection Among Spanish Female
   Prostitutes
   In Press.

10. Tirelli U, Vaccher E, Carbone A, De Paoli P, Santini GF,
    Monfardini S.
    HTLV-III Antibody in prostitutes (Letter).
    Lancet 1985; 2: 1424.

11. Tirelli U, Rezza G, Giuliani M et al.

How to Explain the Low Figures of AIDS Cases Among Intravenous Drug Addicts in Belgium?

J.-P. Roussaux and J.-P. Jacques

Comité de Concertation pour l'Alcool et les Drogues, 55 rue du Président,
B-1050 Brussels, Belgium

INTRODUCTION

In Belgium, the figures of AIDS cases and HIV seropositive patients among intravenous drug addicts are still remarkably low compared to neighbouring countries.

However, three methodological issues have to be pointed out and impair the validity of our data. First, as for any kind of outlaw behaviour, precise measures are impossible, the target population being obliged to hide and sometimes to avoid contacts, even with therapeutic facilities. A second important limit comes from recruitment bias, since most of our prevalence studies took place within specific sub-populations, such as methadone clients, inmates, drug users who voluntarily submitted to HIV screening, and street contacts. Thirdly, as usual in Belgium where epidemiological studies are in general rather scarce, there are no large scale prevalence surveys among drug users or abusers. Nevertheless, the complementarity of the different sub-populations involved in the studies we shall soon review, and the convergence of the results make us assume that the actual figures must not be very far from the figures we shall infer from our partial data.

REVIEW OF EXISTING STUDIES

The first study conducted in Belgium took place in 1985, in a outpatient methadone clinic where 14 seropositive drug addicts were found within a screened population of 75 patients (DE WIT S., 1986), raising the prevalence percentage to 18.8 % .

A second publication (ROELANDT M., 1987) concerned 302 drug addicts treated in 2 psychiatric hospitals in Brussels, in the same methadone clinic, in 3 therapeutic communities and within the drug addict clients of 3 general practitioners who did frequently prescribe substitution opiates. This study concluded to an average percentage of 10.9 % HIV seropositives among this treatment seeking sub-group.

A third study involved all the 3126 inmates prosecuted or convicted for drug related crimes in Brussels in 42 months from may 1985 (DONOT A., 1988, 1989), and gave an incidence rate varying along the time, with a maximum of 7.7 % in 1986 and a minimum of 3.1 % in 1987, showing a significant trend to a lower incidence in the more recent months !

In a survey performed in 1988 by the C.C.A.D. (1989), a written questionnaire was sent to 156 prevention and treatment facilities of the Belgian French speaking Community. The return rate was fair (33 %), involving mainly the specialised treatment facilities . Among 51 centres or services answering, a total of 3610 addicts in treatment were identified, among them 883 injecting drug addicts (24.5 %). Within this sub-population of intravenous drug addicts, 59 were affected with AIDS (6.68 %) and 42 were detected asymptomatic HIV seropositives (4.75 %). The figures of all HIV affected intravenous drug addicts in treatment (asymptomatic, ill or dead) rose to 11.4 % .

In the ELISA study (1990), drug addicts appear only marginally, as 3.1 % of the applicants within a context of anonymous and free testing (59 /1920 tests). But it shows that the drug addicts living in Brussels are rarely found seropositive, since the prevalence hardly reach a 5 % (3 cases) of the 59 seropositives discovered, they represent 11.5 % of all the seropositives found (3/26).

The "BOULE-DE-NEIGE" (Snow-Ball) campaign conducted in 1989-90 in three major cities of the Belgian French speaking Community was designed to enhance level of interest and information about HIV transmission among I.V.D.U. and to gather information about their awareness, opinions, information and practice as far as aids is concerned. During the first campaign, the best analysed until now, 163 street drug addicts were enquired by means of a questionnaire administred by a team of 20 hired drug addicts, called "jobists" who were drilled and paid for the prevention and enquiry work ("job").
Within the questionned population, 80 % uses drugs parenterally, 55.8 % shares their equipment at least once in their carreer, 47.9 % shares at least once in the last 4 weeks; 51 % are in contact with a G.P. or a clinic, leaving 49 % of this population out of reach of any treatment, counselling social service. 54 % declares that they personnally know a friend or relative who is HIV seropositive, and 61 % submitted to a HIV screening test, more or less recently (last test : 8 1/2 months, mean). Within this 163 street drug addicts sample, only 3.1 % declares to be found HIV seropositive (with an important methodological bias : suspicion about confidentiality).

Since then, three other "BOULE-DE-NEIGE" campaigns have been launched and one is still on the run, involving more than 400 street drug addicts. An overview of the results to be published shows a quite similar pattern (JACQUES J.P., 1990, 1991).

In the Belgian Dutch speaking Community, a survey is performed every 6 months since 1988, to investigate HIV status of all patients treated in outpatient and residential programs for drug addiction treatment (PEETERS, 1990). For the 1988-89 period, 1619 drug addicts in treatment (853 intravenous, i.e. 52.7 %) were enrolled. Data about HIV status were recorded for 73 % of I.V.D.U. and for 41 % of non injecting drug addicts. For the last sub-group, none (0 %) were found HIV seropositive, while 4 % of the I.V.D.U. screened were found seropositives.

These results are confirmed by a very exhaustive and interesting study, performed also in the Dutch speaking Community by Dr. S.TODTS and his team (TODTS S., 1990). They questionned 200 street drug addicts, of whom 60 % use to inject daily. Out of these, 76.5 % use to share their equipment. TODTS found a 4.5 % prevalence of HIV infection, which was correlated first with homosexual contacts and second with long stay in high prevalence countries (Southern Europe).

In a study to be published, VALETTE M. (1991) found a 13.2 % prevalence of HIV infection in a screened population of 197 patients in an outpatient treatment centre, with methadone and buprenorphine experimental substitution programs. This study also evoques the concentration of seropositive patients within this type of treatment program ; AIDS and other symptomatic HIV infected patients tend to stay longer in substitution treatment or in psychosocial support treatment than HIV seronegative patients. Therefore,the proportion of HIV affected patients tend to increase in a restricted cohort of patients ("numerus clausus") because they are admitted less reluctantly.

Finally, the general overview of AIDS and HIV infected people in Belgium, is stated in the half-yearly report of the Institut d'Hygiène et d'Epidemiologie (1990). For all the 400 known cases of AIDS in Belgium, I.V.D.U. account for no more than 13 cases (<3.5 %).

The same report also focuses on the 6042 HIV seropositive reported cases, confirmed by Western Blot test, 59 % of which being of European origin (when nationality known, N = 2016). For 1698 people, the risk category is known, revealing that I.V.D.U. account for 8 % of transmission cause, which is a far more significant figure than for AIDS cases. Out of these, 59 cases involved Belgian and 130 involved other nationalities, including people who cumulate more than one risk (e.g. I.V.D.U. and homosexual contacts).

We can then assume that the prevalence of HIV infection among drug addicts in Belgium must be found between 3.1 % and 11.4 %. There may be a slight trend towards higher prevalence in the French speaking Community (with figures up to 11.4 %) than in the Dutch speaking Community (where figures raise up to 4.5 %).

It has been advocated that French speaking drug users had more contacts with higher prevalence countries of Southern Europe, and that Dutch speaking drug users had easier access to Methadone maintenance in the Netherlands.

Risk behaviour

Some studies were designed to describe risk behaviour among the I.V.D.U.'s . Four major items have been considered:

  - sexual behaviour (multiple and/or homosexual partners,   refuse of condoms)
  - injecting or not injecting habits
  - renewal and/or desinfection of material (syringes)
  - needle sharing (frequency, and type of partner)

In a study conducted with drug addicts both in jail and in a substitution program, PASCUAL-SALCEDO M. (1989) tried to identify by a questionnaire based on the STIMSON model (1989) risk behaviour and to indicate trends to a shift towards safer behaviour. All subjects were "hard" drug users and injected on a daily basis. The same equipment was re-used up to 4.9 times . Among I.V.D.U. up to 89 % shared at least occasionnaly their equipments.

Most of sharing occured with friends and with sexual partner, rarely with an occasionnal person. Sharing implicated up to 2.0 people .

Cleaning of material occured in about 80 %, but with plain water in a large majority; only a third of those who clean their material used antiseptics or bleach.

Within the 6 last months, subjects had up to 3 sexual partners, of whom a fifth are drug addicts themselves. Around half of the partners were occasionnal partners. Homosexual partners accounted for up to 14 % of respondents. A condom was used by a third of the subjects.

Street addicts were questionned about risk behaviour related to HIV transmission in the "BOULE-DE-NEIGE" campaigns (JACQUES, 1990, 1991). As expected from the recruitment instructions given to the "jobists", intravenous drug use was largely predominant (80 %) within the sample ; 118 among the 131 I.V.D.U. reached an impressive mean of 5 injections daily !

In an already mentioned study, TODTS (1990) explored the same features with convergent results. Three-quarters of the subjects declared having shared their equipment and recognize only one reason : lack of supply, mainly for financial reasons. Ritual reasons are not aknowledged.

Some new findings have to be stressed, such as the negative influence of **low schooling**, and **social exclusion**. For instance, 20 % of the subjects declared to be homeless and 25 % declared to live without any income; among these two subgroups, share of needles occurs significantly more often. Other factors correlated with prominent sharing behaviour are : young and unexperienced drug users, particularly among amphetamine users and opiate users who are just beginning to inject. The study also showed that young non-opiate users and chronic heroin abusers fortunately do not mix together, keeping the first group, however more careless, far away from the virus reservoir of the latter.

Sharing of needles was reported by 56 % of respondents, of whom 46 % within the last month. Sharing mostly involves a close friend (74 %) or a sexual partner (49 %), and only a short 6 % share with someone unknown.

The pattern of needle and seringe sharing in Belgium, as depicted by street based studies
(JACQUES, 1990, 1991; TODTS, 1990), is rather different than in other countries, especially in southern Europe and in the U.S.A. (FRIEDLAND G.H., 1985). Sharing individuals are very seldom unknown to each other : at the opposite, they use to be very close related individuals, such as regular sexual partner and close friends (buddies). Even with a dealer, sharing is rather uncommon. All Belgian street based studies recommand enhanced availability of new syringes at any time of day and night, at cheap price. If ritual sharing does play a role, it is either unconscious or not aknowledged by the subjects interviewed, with a remarkable exception of the first injections by the very beginner which is still at high risk, even in a large availability environment.

Shooting galleries do not exist in our country, and this lack of anonymous and large scale sharing pattern could largely explain the relatively low figures of HIV infection, even if other risky behaviours are well represented in our country.

Cleaning of material occurs in 68 % of subjects, but only up to 18 % use efficient desinfectants, while only 9 % declare throwing their equipment away after one use.

Fear of prosecution is another important reason of sharing and is often reported. This sounds legitime since the possession of needle is a sufficient reason to be jailed.

As in other studies, like the "BOULE-DE-NEIGE" study, sexual behaviour shows serious risks of transmission, since condom, if used, is never used with a "good-looking" partner. Homosexual prostitution account for 4 % of male subjects, and this sub-group shows high marginalisation and high risk behaviour.

Study also focsed on Hepatitis B and S.T.D., and discovered a very high incidence of both.

All these data stress on the lack of behavioural changes until now, that is the virtual conditions for further transmission of HIV among a large part of Belgian drug users.

TODTS concluded that Belgium is still in the virus introduction phase, that the virus dissemination is still limited to male homosexual contacts and to people having travelled from high prevalence areas. Fortunately, he could point out some encouraging signs of awareness and concern.

General impression of all clinicians (see for instance DEWIT, 1986) in the drug and aids field is that ethnic factors also play an important role, with drug abusers of Spanish, Italian and Morrocan origin, living in limited areas, being more often affected.

Some hypothesis to explain the Belgian situation :

In addition to the already mentiones low needle sharing, we would like to consider three main factors which could explain the low figures described above.

1. Easy access thoughout the 80ies to social security

During the post 1st world war period, the political orientation in Belgium was coined by the constant governemental participation of center-left (christian democrats and socialists) movements. It has been a priority for these administrations to build up an easily accessible system of social welfare and medical coverage, practically state-founded.

Even if it has been reported that up to 40 % of I.V.D.U's applicants for methadone program were not actually insured, the correction of this situation was carried out by social workers attached to the different programs, who were able to restore the full assurability of the applicant, and therefore, his full acceptability to any treatment program.

In cases of total lack of personal or family financial ressources, Social Welfare Public Center are habilited to grant regular modest but sufficient allowance during the treatment period.

2. Easy access to a large range of treatment facilities

We should distinguish here three periods partially overlapping :

2.1. period : **1970-1983** : first epidemic spread of heroin abuse.
The only two answers to the problem were classical inpatient detoxification (ROUSSAUX, 1983) followed by outpatient psychiatric treatment or "wild" methadone sustitution carried out by isolated G.P. or psychiatrist working in unspecific settings.

Lack of control on the large quantities of prescribed injectable opiates with the development of a black market, brought the intervention of justice (BAUDOUR, 1987) as well as the opening of a methadone program and an extreme reduction of isolated prescribers. So even before the implementation of a specific answer to the new phenomenon, a rather easily accessible treatment possibility was in fact available.

2.2. 2nd period : **1979-1987** : caracterized by a drastic appliance of the existing repressive law which increased dramatically the number of emprisonment (up to 17˙%). An alternative to jail was largely proposed by a rather authoritarian self-help organisation (known as "Le Patriarche") which exerced a real appeal at least t wards judges and some families.

2.3. 3rd period : **1980-1983** : implementation of a specific network. With variable support of political and administrative authorities, a specific network (ranging from Therapeutic Communities to Drug Free outpatient Treatment, Methadone maintenance Program, Day Clinics, specialized detoxification wards, orientation and documentation agencies) has been implemented in a few years, actually just when the HIV was probably introduced in our country.

3. Easy access to methadone maintenance through the G.P.'S

Since 1983, most of the G.P., altough discouraged to practice opiate substitution, went on with a massive non opiates and particularly BZD prescription.

It has been already argumented by M. REISINGER (1990) that easy access to methadone maintenance through the general practioners had played a major role in reducing AIDS cares. This author stresses the easy access to isolated practioner for "the more problematic, the more marginalized, the more suicidal drug addicts who generally don't adapt to the bureaucratic restraint".

Event if methadone treatment does play an important role, where and when it is prescribed, M. REISINGER's hypothesis deserve some restrictions. When "wild" prescription was so massive in Belgium (1979-1983), injectable methadone was far more common than oral form and therefore the needle sharing was likely. As a proof, serological markers of Hepatitis B was regularly found, up to 75 % by street heroïn as well as by methadone users, clearly indicating that sharing was persistent.

Anyhow, clinical evidence shows clusters of drug addicts in medical waiting rooms and by local pharmacies, where encounters may occur leading to risky behaviors, either with injectable drugs, relapse and needle sharing or with occasional sexual intercourse.

Actually, these critics could be matched by a limitation of the number of treated cases by each prescriber.

A last indication that Methadone Program alone cannot explain low prevalence of HIV in Belgium is to be found in the observation that although methadone was less available in the Dutch-speaking community, its prevalence rate is less elevated than in the French-speaking part of the country.

Conclusions

We may conclude that the prevalence of HIV infection among drug addicts in Belgium must be found between 3.1 % and 11.4 % .
The studies which explored risk behaviour among the I.V.D.U.'s confirmed that the four major risks of HIV transmission are still highly implicated :
- hetero- and homosexual transmission through unprotected sexual intercourses with occasional or multiple partners
- injection habits
- lack of renewal and/or desinfection of syringes
- needle sharing

Street based studies have indicated that the pattern of needle sharing involves quite never unknown individuals, but only very close related individuals, such as regular sexual partner and close friends and is attributed to lack of supply, for financial reasons.

The virtual conditions for further spread of HIV among a large part of Belgian drug users are met, in particular by the very beginners which are still at high risk, even when new needles are available.

Belgium is still in the virus introduction phase, but the virus spread is still limited to male homosexual and to travellers from high prevalence areas. Some encouraging signs of awareness and concern are observed.

Social welfare and the full range of treatment programs, with a probable specific role of methadone substitution, when available, contribute to the fortunate pre-epidemic situation described in Belgium.

Frequently consulted by every drug user, general practitioners play probably an important role, by prescription of methadone and non-opiate substitutes, and therefore contributing to an informal harm reduction policy.

References

BAUDOUR J. - L'amour condamné. Pierre Mardaga Ed., 1987

Comité de Concertation sur l'Alcool et les Autres Drogues (C.C.A.D.) - Actualisation du sondage toxicomanie et sida, 22 mai, 1989.

DE WIT S., JACQUES J.P., CLUMECK N. - Toxicomanie intraveineuse et infection à HIV en . Belgique, Psychotropes, Vol. III, N° 2, automne 1986, p. 7-10.

DONOT A., VERHOEVEN-LESPAGNARD L., Screening for HIV antibodies in high risk groups among the inmates of Brussels prisons, Abstract of the communication presented in the 3rd Intern. Conf. on AIDS, STOCKHOLM, 1988 (pre-study involving the first 1785 inmates prosecuted or convicted for drug related crimes in Brussels from may 23, 1985 to may 22 1987 ; half-year incidence (new cases) of 7.1, 7.1, 7.7, 3.2 %).

DONOT A., VERHOEVEN-LESPAGNARD L., Screening for HIV antibodies in high risk groups among the inmates of Brussels prisons, Abstract of the communication presented in the 5th Intern. Conf. on AIDS, MONTREAL, june 1989.

ELISA, Centre de dépistage anonyme et gratuit de Médecins Sans Frontières, Rapport oct. 1990.

FRIEDLAND G.H. & al. - Intravenous drug abusers and the AIDS. Demographic, drug use, and needle-sharing pattern, Arch. Intern. Med, Vol. 145, Aug. 1985, pp. 1413-1417.

Institut d'Hygiène et d'Epidémiologie - S.I.D.A. en Belgique, n° 22, Situation au 30 septembre 1990.

JACQUES J.P., GOESDEEL A. - "Snowball", communication at the International Expert Meeting : AIDS, Drug abuse and Mass migration", 19-21/11/1990, Berlin.

JACQUES J.P. - "BOULE-DE-NEIGE" 1989-1990, Rapport général d'activités et développements, C.C.A.D., fevr. 1991.

PASCUAL-SALCEDO M. - Analyse des comportements à haut risque vis-à-vis du sida chez des toxicomanes intraveineux. Mémoire de Licence Spéciale en Santé publique,

Université Libre de Bruxelles, 1989.

PEETERS R. - Resultaten HIV-enquête 1988/89, unpublished report, 1990.

RESINGER M. - Arrêter l'héroïne. Ed. Complexe, Bruxelles, 1990.

ROUSSAUX J.P. - Toxicomanie aux opiacés : techniques de sevrage et thérapeutiques de substitution. J. Pharm. Belg., 1983, 38, 1, 47-52.

ROELANDT M., ZOMBEK S. - Sida, séropositivité et toxicomanes à Bruxelles, Psychotropes, vol. III, n°3, hiver 1987, pp. 27-30.

STIMSON G.V. & al. - Injecting equipement exchange schemes; a preliminary report on research. Monitoring Research Group, University of London Goldsmith's College, London, 1989.

TODTS S. - Risicogedrag bij injecterende druggebruikers in Vlaanderen, V.Z.W. Free Clinic, Antwerpen, 1990.

VALETTE M., de LA MALLE J.P. & al. - Protocole d'évaluation du Projet LAMA, 1991, under press.

Drug Addiction and AIDS in Republic of Croatia and Yugoslavia

S. SAKOMAN[1] and A. HEĆIMOVIĆ[2]

[1] Center for Drug Addiction, Clinical Hospital „Dr. M. Stojanović, Vinogradska c. 29, YU-41000 Zagreb, Croatia
[2] Health Center „Novi Zagreb", Primary Health Care, Scientific Unit, Naselje februras-kih žrtava 29, YU-41000 Zagreb, Croatia

The Yugoslav socio-cultural area varies a great deal. The organization of the society in the last decades has not decreased them but has in many spheres turned the differencec into antagonisms that has caused a deep crisis that is leading to the desintegration of the postwar federation. Croatia, one of the six Yugoslav republics, is from the cultural point of view nearer to the west european countries and belongs with Slovenia to the most developed. It has approx. 4,500.000 inhabitants, the capital is Zagreb (approx. 1,000.000 inhabitants). The epidemiological situation in regard to drug addiction as well as the organization of the control of this socio-pathological appearance in the republics as well as in reagions within the republics greatly differ. This country has no uniform doctrine for coping with drug addiction and a lot of attitudes concerning prevention as well as treatment and rehabilitation of the drug addicts are not brought into accord and coordinated. So in Belgrade for example the programme for drug addiction control is primarely based on the use of Metadon (in the last fifteen years) while the programme in Zagreb has favoured prevention through primary care using an interdisciplinary coordinated approach and a drug-free programme has been used in treatment. The results of the Zagreb and Belgrade programmes can be evaluated and compared with the situation in some other urban centers with practically no programme. So now there are thousands of drug addicts in Belgrade (the number of the HIV positive patients among drug addicts is very high - up to 50 %), in comparison with hundreds in Zagreb (whereas the the number of HIV seropositive drug addicts among them is very low not more than 1 to 2%).

Characteristics of Epidemiological Situation in Yugoslavia

The forms of drug abuse among the young population are registered since mid sixties. The first groups appear in the public as a problem in early seventies in Belgrade, Zagreb and some places along the Adriatic coast (Pula). In spite of the fact that Republic of Macedonia is a traditional opium producer the first groups of drug addicts appear there much later. The use of opium (domestic growing) and canabis, heroin increasingly dominates the illegal market. In late eighties misuse of cocain is sporadic (in the western Republic of Slovenia) however the main problem is caused by heroin opiates respectively. Heroin is imported from Turkey or via Turkey. At the beginning of the drug addcition Yugoslavia has been only a transit region for illegal smuggling of heroin on the way to Western European countries, lately considerable quantities of that drug are smuggled for the domestec market. As a substitute for heroin in urban area and even more in smaller places the use of opium tea made by cooking of dry poppy capsules, the growing of which is widely spread in the agricultural regions of Croatia and Vojvodina, is spreading. Farmers earn a lot of money by illegigal sale of poppy capsules much more than by sale of poppy seeds. In many places, especially in the southern parts of Croatia and islands the illegal growing of bhang is spread and significant quantities of hashish arrive by sea (from Maroco or from Near East). Glue sniffing or taking of "pep pills" (sedatives, analgetics, antiparkinsonics) belong to other abuses. The interest in abuse of hallucinogens (LSD) is decreasing while the abuse of amphetamines and its derivatives has not been significant.

Epidemiologic research has not been systematic in this country, however on the basis of data of the Public Health Service, police and canvassing it can be concluded that the drug addiction is growing especially in places with poorer quality of living and lack of preventive programmes in schools and better standards of living the police has not been succsessfull in privention of organized illegal offer of drugs.

Epidemiological research is continously organized in Zagreb since 1978 and the data are entered in the register of the treated drug addicts of Croatia. So in mid eighties it was found that in the population of the secondary school students the number of them who have tried at least once a drug ranges between 10 and 20 % depending on the area. They have most frequently experimented with marijuana and then with pills and solvents. The number of adolescents who have consumed these drugs has been between 2 and 3 %. In the last ten years the interest of young people in Zagreb for taking drugs has not significantly increased although the number of them who continued to use drugs after the initial experiments has increased. According to estimation the number of periodical consumers (most frequently of canabis) has increased about 5 %. The number of young people who have experienced with narcotic drugs stayed on the same level i.e. 0.3 and 0.5%.

Developement of Drug Abuse Control Programme in Croatia

In contrast to other republics the first specialized program for treatment of drug addicts in Clinical Hospital "Dr. M. Stojanović" started in Croatia already in 1971. Beside the famous Center for Alcoholism the drug abuse control programme started developing on the Clinic. The Institute for Dependences was opened in Belgrade in 1986, aldough years ago the use of Methadone was widely used for treatment of drug addicts. Still today within the frame of their hospitalisation even HIV positive and some HIV negative heroin addicts spend several months in the hospital and most of them are treated with relatively high daily doses of Methadone. The Zagreb school of drug adiction treatment prefers the drug -free approach and Methadone has not been used even in the detoxification phase that is done in the Intensive Care Unit (Clonidine and Tramadole are used) in a programme of specifically guided therapeutic community with approx. 25 patients and a relatively short stay at the hospital (about 40 days). The team for the intensive therapetical procedure (individual and group, mostly reality therapy, family group therapy, education, recreative therapy and help in solving a series of personal and other problems of each drug addict and necessary pharmacotherapy) consists of three psychiatrists, behavioural therapist, social worker and 8 nurses or medical technologists.

An indiviadual long-term outpatient follow-up and treatment programme is made for each drug addict, who asked for help of this only specialized programme in Croatia in ambulatory care oferring every help in solving uncountable crisis and dificult situations in which either the addict or addict and his family find themself in. The work with an addict is characterized by highly differential psychotherapeutical approach from the therapist requiring a lot of skill, patient and philantropy towards the man "who has chosen a process of decay by taking drugs". So, although the programme is restrictive concerning use of methadone and pharmacotherapy it has been attractive to the addicts as a new experience of interpersonal relationship with the therapy team whose members have accepted them, strenghtened their dignity and self–respect, arouse in them responsibility and wish to try to change their behaviour and a lot of them have been stopped in the process of alienation from society and their families and although a permanent abstinence from drugs is not achieved, the pathology of their behaviour and their addiction severity index has been considerably mitigated.

For a small number of cases the addicts were suied, it was tried to discharge them on probation or to punish them with shorter imprisonment. In of of the prisons has been organized a treatment programme guided by psychiaters of the Clinic since 1980.

While about 160 addicts have been treated in hospital and in treatment community yearly, approx. 220 hospitalizations, a considerably greater number of younger addicts have been included in an exclusively outpatient, family treatment in cooperation with the school, local Public health service and Social Service. This outpatient programme covered mostly the Zagreb region. Lately because of HIV infections in Zagreb individual programmes for treatment with methadone under continuous supervision of the Center for Dependences of the Clinic has been intoduced for uncurable addicts, mostly older than 30 years or for addicts, completly unmotivated for absinence, long–term heroin addicts (5 or more years of addiction), whose behaviour is dangerous for their surrounding, and treated by general practitioners chosen as family doctor. 80% of all the treated addicts in 1991 are heroin dependent.

In order to get an insight into some characteristics of the group of addicts treated in 1990 in the therapeutic community of the Zagreb Center for Dependences a survey from the hospital register in the form of tables. The programme has covere d 156 persons from Croatia. All the cases have been tested on HIV twice and all have been found HIV seronegative.

Table 1

Addicts treated in Center for Dependences
of the Clinical Hospital "Dr. Mladen Stojanović" in 1990

Drug Addiction (IV-G)
(Source: Clinical Register)

age group	males	females	total
<=20	10 = 8.9%	7 = 15.9%	17 = 10.9%
21 - 30	68 = 60.7%	23 = 52.3%	91 = 58.3%
31 - 40	29 = 25.9%	9 = 20.5%	38 = 24.4%
41 - 50	3 = 2.7%	2 = 4.5%	5 = 3.2%
=>51	2 = 1.8%	3 = 6.8%	5 = 3.2%
T O T A L	112 = 100.0%	44 = 100.0%	156 = 100.0%

blank entries for the current question: 0

It is evident that the addicts in Croatia, except those cometing from Split and Dalmatia are getting older. They used marijuana, drugs and solvents, starting using narcotics at the age of 15, after three years they start experimenting with narcotics. After 4 - 5 years the heroin addiction is developed and the parents finally face the truth. The first organized professional treatment starts about the age of 25 forced by family or most frequently legal circumastances.

Table 2

Legal status of addicts treated in the Center for Dependences
in the clinical hospital "Dr. M. Stojanović " in 1991

Addiction (IV-G)
(Source: Clinical Register)

legal standing	male	female	total
clean record	29 = 25.9%	31 = 70.5%	60 = 38.5%
minor criminal offences	14 = 12.5%	4 = 9.1%	18 = 11.5%
conditional penalty	13 = 11.6%	1 = 2.3%	14 = 9.0%
inprisonment prior to treatment	15 = 13.4%	0 = .0%	15 = 9.6%
several imprisonments	27 = 24.1%	2 = 4.5%	29 = 18.6%
legal proceedings introduced	14 = 12.5%	6 = 13.6%	20 = 12.8%
T O T A L	112 =100.0%	44 =100.0%	156 =100.0%

blank entry for current question: 0

Although practically all heroin addicts commited a criminal act and after more than 5 years of taking this expensive drug (1 gram costs approx. 150 DM), about

40% of them have had no problems with the police. About 30% of them have been in prison and the rest have been conditionally punished or committed minor criminal offences or the first treatment took place during the time they have been on trial.

Table 3
The financial standing of the families of the addicts treated in the Center for Dependences of the Clinical Hospital "Dr. M. Stojanović " in 1990

Addiction (IV-G)
(Source: Clinical Register)

financial standing	male	female	total
imperilled standing	9 = 8.0%	4 = 9.1%	13 = 8.3%
poor	43 = 38.3%	12 = 27.3%	55 = 35.3%
good financial stand.	52 = 46.4%	24 = 54.5%	76 = 48.7%
rich	8 = 7.1%	4 = 9.1%	12 = 7.7%
T O T A L	112 =100.0%	44 =100.0%	156 =100.0%

blank entries for a question : 0

According to the data in the table 3 one can see that the addicts come from rich families (about 8%) as well as from very poor ones. About 50% of them come from families with average financial standing and 35% of the addicts from poor ones. The Financial status is seen from the housing standard, about 27% have inadequate, too small or without standard facilities, while 65% have good dwelling conditions (among them somewhat less than a half of them have individual apartments of family houses and the rest live in state apartments). The family relationship has influenced the personality in the pre-adolescent period. So among the addicts treated in 1990 30% of the addicts have a parent (mostly the father) who is an alcoholic,, 7% have parents suffering from mental illnesess or mental disturbances, 20% of them are children of devorsed parents, one or both of their parents died before the addict's age of 14 in 6 % of cases and in 20% of cases the family relationships have been heavily distroyed or inadequate, the parents have an impersonal relationship towards their children. In most of the families the father does not participate in the family life and took no part in the upbringing of children while the mother has been overpatronizing so that the children suffered a separation crisis as adolescents.

Table 4

Participation of the family in the treatment of the addict in the Center for Dependences in the Clinical Hospital "Dr. M. Stojanović" in 1990

Addiction (IV-6)
(Source: Clinical register)

participation of the family	man	woman	total
cooperative	53 = 47.7%	29 = 67.4%	82 = 53.2%
react only on calls	25 = 22.5%	5 = 11.6%	30 = 19.5%
reject cooperation	5 = 4.5%	1 = 2.3%	6 = 3.9%
absent	14 = 12.6%	2 = 4.7%	16 = 10.4%
without family	14 = 12.6%	6 = 14.0%	20 = 13.0%
T O T A L	111 = 100.0%	43 = 100.0%	154 = 100.0%

blank entries for a question: 2

The data from the table 4 show that the traditional family is still preserved in Croatia that will not easily separate from its member regadless of the fact that he is a very serious addict. About 53% of the addicts has a family that wants to help him in any way. About 23% cases lack any family help and their prospects are less favourable.

About 23% of the treated addicts are married and about 16% are divorced and about 40% have one or two children. About 44% of the addicts have only primary education, 56% have secondary and about 8% graduated from a college or university. This population is mostly older and they have been treated because of drug addiction (pills). 46% of the addicts are employed and only about 3% of them are farmers. For 47% of the treated addicts it was their first treatement. Significant improvment is found in 36% cases and 22% of the addicts have left the therapeutic community in the course of the treatment. Beside drug addiction 15% of them have been alcoholics and 7% of them drink more that moderate amounts of alcohol. 98% of them are smokers. Cigarettes have been their first drug. About 60% of the treated juvenile addicts have had no striking signs of behavioural or psychological disturbances. Considerable improvement and motivation has been found at 34% of addicts while at 38% no way of treatment managed to cause wanted changes in their behaviour including inevitable abstitency from drugs. The therapeutic team exptected complete results in 25% cases at discharge from the therapeutic community and at making appointments for further treatment at outpatient department.

The Treatement Plan of The Zagreb School of Drug Control

This plan should be accepted for the whole territory of Croatia and even in Zagreb it should be "decentralised" i.e. to organize the treatment at the level of manucipalities what was done in Zagreb in the last 12 years. A comission consisting of professionals in several fields (public health care , police, courts, schools, social work and journalists), elected at the Republic level has to coordinate and evaluate the results of the mutual agreed doctrine. The members of the commission coming from various parts of Croatia are in charge of the regional organization. It is the first time that the Ministry of Health and the Croatian Government are willing to support the programme. The programme included privention, treatment and control of drug addiction.

Role of Police

Beside the usual tasks of the police to stop illegal trade and smuggling of drugs the task of special trained policemen is to be a sort of social workers on the spot to keep an eye on the addicts and inform the general practitioner. The aim is early diagnose and early treatment. In the municipality Novi Zagreb out of 182 registered addicts the police detected 112 and informed the primary care about them. The police has nothing to do with the family and school. The police stops the formation of groups of addicts in the streats and public places. The police works on reducing the risk of contact of addicts with non-addicts. The police has to control the keeping and writing of prescriptions for narcotics. Such a cooperation with the police was not possible in all the cities of Croatia and especially not in other parts of Yugoslavia.

Role of Schools

The teachers are continuously trained to detect an addict and to reduse the interest for drugs educating and informing their students about adrugs and make them understand drug addiction in order to stop their fascitation by a "dope friend". They are tought healthy way of living and how to take an attitude towards addiction and how to say no when offered by friends. The teachers chose students to wach their friends especially those who belong to the population with high risk. The aim of the cooperation with schools is to prevent drop out. The class takes the role of a therapeutic community.

Judiciary

Jucidiary plays a significat role in various drug abuse supression programmes. Special attention is payed to each individual case regarding the motive of the especially juvenile deliquent for crime commitment. The punishment should be more repressive in cases when the deliquent is a drug dealer selling drugs to other addicts and an addict who buys drugs only for his own use should be punished less severe motivating him for appropriate treatment. In the prison Lepoglava the compulsory treatment of addicts is organized since 1980 including regular visits of the doctors of the Center for Dependences. An detoxication treatment is organized The treatment with methadone is possible in a hospital and drug free treatment is only used in prison.

Social Work

Social workers have very important role as cooperators of schools where they will be included in family therapy for pupils with biheivioral, psychical or drug problems. Social worker will colaborate with family doctor in solving problems in family pathology, especially when a member of the family need support in dealing with alcoholism. In supervising minor drug addicts, social worker will cooperate with the team and coordinate the work of specialist, general practitioner and judge for juvenal delinquents.For the cases treated in penal institutions, in cooperation with them, he will organize postpenal treatement and help in finding job for the addicts. Also he will help in maintaining the relations between addict and his family, especially if the addicts themselves have children.

Health Care

Primary health care in very important in programms for addiction control. In this papper we described a psrt of activities of the Center for Dependences of Zagreb of the Clinical Hospital "Dr M. Stojanović", which along with practical work on treating the addicts,developed and carried out a lot of preventive activities and coordinated work of other institutions in Zagreb and other parts of Croatia. As the headmaster of this Center became the chairman of the Croatian Comission for supressing drug abuse, we expect that society will show more interest for further development of the Center.

As it is practically impossible to centralize the treatement of addicts and other activities on prevention, last year a local programm for suppressing the drug abuse started in Novi Zagreb. Data were collected out of several sources (police, Center for Dependences, schools, general practitioners).By data processing we found out that police discovered 112 cases out of 182. Part of them was unknown to any other institution and even to their families. As the family doctor is the only one person who have posibility and duty to enter a family, a special methodology was made to enable the general practitioners and members of their teams in cooperation with other institutions to give a more active help to the addicts (especially adolescents who just started using drugs) and their families. That would shorten the period till the start of intervention. In lots of families group therapy would hava very impertant in prevention.

If a special Commision of the Center for Dependences finds out that the only solution left is to keep the patient on methadone, the general practitioner will carry out that procedure under the supervision of the specialists of the Center. Patient must report to his doctor every day because of the taking of daily dose of methadone. For realisation of that programm more doctors must be educated in this field and work on that is one of the most important tasks of this Center.

Alternative Programms

By democratisation of life in croatia there are more possibilities for organising all kinds of Societies dealing with drug abuse and other dependences. In Split a process of forming of therapy communes started in connection with religious communities.

Drug Addiction and HIV Infection

When first cases of HIV infection were reported in Europe, specialists of the Center organized a special program for protection of addicts. Since the testing of all addicts who come to the Center started, no new cases have been reported for last four years in Croatia. In past three years just seven cases were reported.

In 1989 the following results are found in Croatia:

- homo and bisexuals   tested   9   – HIV seropositive 3
- heterosexuals   tested   1681   – "   "   1
- drug addicts   tested   118   – "   "   1
- haemophylics   tested   40   – "   "   2
- dialysed   tested   321   – "   "   0
- newborns(mother HIV pos.) "   6   – "   "   0
- others   tested   2030   – "   "   0

In Zagreb, Croatia prevention of HIV infection has started very early, even before appearing HIV seropositive infection among the drug addict groups. In the last three years hospitalized drug addicts have no HIV seropositive test results. Also among drug addicts treated in outparient departments no HIV seropositive patients were found in the last three years.

Programme of Drug Addiction and AIDS Treatement in Community Novi Zagreb Health Center "Novi Zagreb" Primary Health Care

Novi Zagreb ist one of the communities of the City of Zagreb with approx. 160.000 inhabitants. This area is characterized by many varieties that cannot be easily explained concerning the addiction to drugs and the attitute towards this serious socio-pathologic phenomenon. There is no unique doctrine in strategy of prevetion of addiction, methods of treatment and rehabilitation.

Increase of number of drug addicts and their increasing criminal activity linked with addiction initiated this experimental program in the community of Novi Zagreb.

Because of lack of cumulative data we have gathered all the relevant data from all the possible sources and services visited by drug addicts irrespective of the reason: out-patient departments, Clinical hospital for treatment of drug addicts, Police and Social Service of the community. Data about all the known and indentified cases have been gathered in the course of the last five years.

We have decided that Primary Health Care should be the carrier of the Program of drug addiction. It is agreed that a data base should be organized there that correpondeds to the organization of the health protection in this country.

A Questionaire for drug addicts (herewith enclosed) has 20 basic questions and 64 possible answers. A great number of data for each interviewed addict is gathered in such a way. The data are entered in the data base. We can demostrate very interesting and significant characteristics of this high risk population valid for this area.

It is important to emphasized that the most cases of the addicts and drug dealer have been gived by the police after they have comitted a crime. This fact means that the health care is inadequate. It is interesting to stress that more than 60 per cent of the addicts have never contacted the social service of the community!

The listings of addicts is not made only according to alphbetic order but also according to addreses so that certain building and streets can be easily recognized as "epidemic points". Identification number of each citizen is the best way to find them because it is well known that they often change addresses.

This experimental program developed in Novi Zagreb needs a direct active approach in order to cover as big number of cases as possible. A speacially trained team together with the families of the addicts should help the addicts in solving their often very complicated situations. This is a way to prevent further separation and allienation of drug addicted persons towards social margins. Otherwise they would endanger society by spreading addiction, crime and AIDS.

According to variable list in "Questionnaire for narcotics and drug eddicts in the municipality of New Zagreb" a simple database structure and computer program in dBASE III PLUS compatible language were created. Differences were estimated with Chi-square test.

Data about 177 examinees was entered into computer database. SPSS PC+ standard software package on IBM PC XT/AT personal computer was applied for statistical analysis of data. There were 60.9% males and 39.1% females between examined persons. Mean age for males was 29.9 years

(S.DEV=5. 8; N=106) and for females 33.1 years (S.DEV=13.3; N=66). Frequency distribution according to age groups is as follows: <20 y: 2.3%,; 20-24 y: 16.9%; 25-29 y: 34.3%; 30-34 y: 24.4%; 35-39 y: 10.5% and 40 and more years 11.6% of examinees. There were significant differences in age between male and female drug abusers in our sample (Chi-sq.=16.1; p=0.0064; D.F.=5). (See Table 5.).

According to source of data about abusers, frequency distribution is as follows: 18.9% from primary health care, 56. 1% from police; 4.9% from hospital psychologist, 4.9% from general practitioner and police, 9.1% from primary health care doctor and hospital psychologist and 6.1% from all three sources of data.

There were significant differences in sex distribution of drug abusers according to source of data (Chi-sq.=18.8; p=0.002; D.F.=5). (See Table 6.) With incoplete primary school there were 2.6% examinees, with complete 24.4%, 25.6% with incomplete secondary school, 37.2% with complete secondary school, 7.7% with incomplete high school and only 2.6% with complete high education. There was no significant difference in education between males and females in our sample (p=0.71).

According to employment picture, there were 18.8% pupils and students, 17.2% unemployed persons who left school, 53.1% employed persons and 10.9% persons who threw up their job. There was no difference between males and females (p=0. 45). (See Table 7.).

Marital status of examinees is as follows: 63% were single, 24.7% married, 9.6% divorced, 1.4% with compassionate marriage and 1.4% separated. There was no difference between males and females (See Table 8)

According to housing conditions, there were 54.9% examinees with their parents, 33.8% in their own flat, 2.8% as subtenant, 1.4% in dormitory and 7.0% were homeless. There was significant difference between males and females (p=0.04). With their parents there were 68.4% of males and only 39.4% of females. In addition, there were 48.5% females in their own flat, and only 21.1% males (See Table 9).

According to military service, there were 12.5% of persons liable to military service, 59.4% served, 15.6% temporary disabled and 12.5% disabled(N=32).

Frequency distribution according to use of social wellfare facilities is as follows: 66.7% never, 12.5% have been under supervision, 1.4% are on feleaf and for 19.4% of drug abusers in our sample social worker took part in the treatment of the addict. There were 60.9% of drug abusers in our sample with legal problems, 23.4% commited a violation, 7.8% vere in prison, 3.1% were in prison and under accusation, and 4.7% were punished under conditional judgement. There were significant difference between males and females (p=0.019). There were 82. 8% females with no legal problems and only 42.9% males (See Table 2.).

Frequency distributions according to diagnoses of type of addition (ICD) are shown in Table 7.

According to use of alcohol, frequency distribution was as follows: 30.9% mainly abstinent, 19.1% with abuse of alcohol, 30.9% not treated alcoholics, 10.3% unsuccesfuly treated alcoholics and 7.4% recovered alcoholics. There was not significant difference between males and females.

According to interval of drug taking, there were 27.4% drug abusers with less than 5 years of drug taking, 37.1% with 5 to 9 years and 35.5% abusers with 10 or more years of drug taking. There were no significant differences between examinees in duration of drug taking interval according to alcohol abuse (p=0.20), sex (p=0.65), education (p=0.09), legal problems (p= 0.52) and treatment (p=0.49).

Finally, according to treatment of addiction, there were 22.1% never treated drug abusers in our sample, 19.5% treated by general practitioner and 58.4% treated in hospital (N=77). There was signifficant difference between males and females in "prospect of treatment" (p=0.03; N=66). About 18.9% males rejected the treatment and only 10.3% females. There were 8.1% males with succesful adjustment and only 3.4% females.

An adviser-psychiatrist started working two time a week in the Health Center "Novi Zagreb", Zagreb. He has received 286 individuals, couples, families and groups (160 man and 126 women). As because of psychological problems some persons hardly manage to come. During consultations it has been decided that it would be the best opportunity to test them on HIV virus because of their risky way of life (own promiscuity 8, promiscuity of the partner 6, homosexuals 4,

64

prostitutes 3 and IV drug addicts). Out of 22 tested persons all of them have been HIV seronegative. The age of the people ranges from 17 to 74, average age: 29. By analysis of their risky way of life before consulations the following reasons has been found:

- 44% promiscuity
- 17% parents of adolescents(drug addicts, promiscuous, children that got trasfusion of blood and its products)
- 11% promiscous partners
- 10% homosexuals
- 8% prostitutes
- 7% receivers of blood transfusions
- 3% intravenous drug addicts.

For the time being we cannot be satisfied with the scope of population covered by the described way of counselling.

AIDS in Yugoslavia
/situation on the day March 31, 1990./
FEDERAL INSTITUTE FOR HEALTH CARE
April 1, 1990

Table 5.
Patients according to age and sex /cumulative/

Age	Male	Female	Total
5 - 19	2	/	2
10 - 12	1	/	1
13 - 14	2	/	2
15 - 19	5	/	5
20 - 24	7	/	7
25 - 29	19	6	25
30 - 34	16	5	21
35 - 39	17	1	18
40 - 44	12	1	13
45 - 49	5	/	5
50 - 54	8	/	8
55 - 59	7	1	8
60 - 64	/	/	/
65 and over	4	1	5
Total:	105	15	120

Per March 31, 90 there were 120 registered AIDS patients in Yugoslavia. Out of them more than 60% are at the age of 25 and 44. With respect to sex there are 7 times more males than females.

Table 6
Patients According to Transmission Groups

			EUROPE
Homo and bisexsuals	29	24.1%	46.9%
Heterosexsuals	14	11.6%	8%
Drug addicts	43	35.8%	31.7%
Haemophylics	25	20.8%	3.3%
Blood transfusion	2	1.6%	3.7%
Unknown	7	5.8%	6.5%

Among the patients there is the highest percentage of IV drug addicts (35.8%) followed by homosexuals and bisexuals (24%).

Table 7
Clinical Manifestation of The Illness

Opportune infection	80	66.6%	75.0%
Kaposzi's	1	0.8%	11.7%
Opport. + Kaposzi's	5	4.2%	4.2%
HIV Encephalophatia	9	7.5%	3.1%
Wasting syndroma	14	11.7%	3.1%
Lymphoma malignum	8	6.7%	2.4%
PIL	3	2.5%	0.5%

Table 8
Died Patients Until April 1, 1990

1985.	died	2
1986.	"	6
1987.	"	14
1988.	"	32
1989.	"	19
1990.	"	3

Out of the total number of the present patients in Yugoslavia 76 died. It makes 63% of all evidenced AIDS patients.

Table 9
Changes in AIDS 1985–1990

Year	Homo+ bisex.	Hetero sex.	Drug addicts.	Haemo philics.	Blood tran.	Unknown.	Total
1985.	1	-	-	-	1	1	2
1986.	4	1	-	1	-	-	6
1987.	5	-	7	3	-	3	18
1988.	10	5	14	7	2	1	39
1989.	8	6	19	9	-	2	44
until April 1, 1990.	1	2	3	5	-	-	11
Total	29	14	43	25	2	7	120

Number of the patients increasingly grows from year to year. In 1989 44 new cases were evidenced. Out of them the greatest number (19) were IV drug addicts.

Out of 120 patients, 7 do not live in our country. 113 patients are from 39 community from all republics, except Monte Negro in which there are no sick patients.

Out of 120 patients, until April 1, 1990. died 76 or 63.3%. In first three months 1989. the number of new sick patients was 14, and 1990. - 11 persons.

Table 10
Tested on HIV, Federal Institute of Health Care, March 14, 1990.
(comparative dates for SFRJ)

Grups	until 1987.		in 1987.		in 1988.		in 1989.	
	tested	HIV+	tested	HIV+	tested	HIV+	tested	HIV+
Homo and bisexuals	576	5%	601	2.49%	100	19%	84	19%
Heterosexuals	-	-	1085	0.27%	7941	0.51%	4804	0.60%
Drug addicts	1802	27.9%	1539	28.1%	1102	26%	891	32.3%
Haemophylics	632	22,9%	469	10.8%	336	28.5%	137	24.0%
Dyalised persons	1372	0-6%	1023	0.7%	1368	0.07%	2592	0.3%
Newb.from HIV+ mothers	-	-	-	-	-	-	14	14.2%
Sex.partner of HIV+ person	-	-	-	-	-	-	102	4.8%
Health service	-	-	-	-	-	-	742	-
Others	-	-	-	-	-	-	12696	0.08%

Table 11
Report of Tested Persons in HIV in 1989

	homo and bisex		hetero sex		drug addicts		haemo phyl		dieali sed		newb. of HIV+ moth.		sex partn. HIV+		health service		others		total HIV+
tested/HIV+ ->	t.	+	t	+	t.	+	t.	+	t	+	t.	+	t.	+	t.	+	t.	+	
B & H	2	–	2681	1	12	–	3	–	230	–	–	–	–	–	–	–	–	–	1
Monte Negro							there	were	no	tested	persons								
Croatia	9	3	1628	1	118	1	40	2	321	–	6	–	–	–	–	–	–	–	7
Macedonia	2	–	–	–	19	1	12	1	469	–	–	–	–	–	12	–	2030	–	2
Slovenia	7	3	110	2	4	1	–	–	–	–	–	–	–	–	–	–	82	–	6
Serbia	64	10	385	25	738	285	82	30	1572	8	7	2	102	5	730	–	9785	11	376
Centr. Serbia	46	9	385	25	725	285	72	30	1420	8	7	2	102	5	730	–	7737	11	375
Kosovo							there	were	no	tested	persons								
Vojvodina	18	1	–	–	13	–	10	–	152	–	–	–	–	–	–	–	1948	–	1
S F R J	84	16	4804	29	891	288	137	33	2592	8	14	2	102	5	742	–	12696	11	395

Table 11 shows HIV test results from some republics of Yugoslavia in 1989. Situation in individual republics is varying and it is not easy to explain the differences. First of all the level of health service and the approach to implementation of the prevention program are very different. In relation to the number of the inhabitants, as well as in all tested subgroups, the highest number of HIV sero-positive persons come from the region of Serbia, the provinces excluded. As far as the tested drug addicts are concerned, their number depends primarily on the number of the treated patients in individual republics. Only Serbia and Croatia have their programs for treatment of the addicts and that is the reason why higher number of the patients comes from these regions. However, out of 118 tested IV addicts from Croatia, only one patient was sero-positive, while out of 725 drug addicts from Serbia, the provinces excluded, not less than 285 patients (about 40%) were sero-positive. In the category of the haemophiliacs there are also significant differences and there were 41% infected patients in Serbia. The investigations, carried out in the world, also proved that great differences are possible in the epidemiological situation in connection with HIV infections in individual regions of the same state. However, some assuptions should be mentioned which would ensure answer to the question relating to so high difference between two republics (or between two largest cities in Yugoslavia far away only 400 km). It is more than evident that prevalence of HIV sero-positive patients in the total population greatly depends on prevalence of IV drug addicts as well as on approach to their treatment. As far as this is concerned, the basic strategy is described which was applied in treatment of addicts problem in Zagreb.

References

1. Burek V, Sakoman S, Hudolin V, Kovač D, Ficović P, Čepelja Z, Petričević I, Schonwald S, Soldo I, Borčić D. (1987),
   Analysis of Antibodies to Human T-Lymphotropic Virus Type III (Anti-HTLV III) among Populations at High Risk from AIDS in Yugoslavia, Liječnički Vjesnik,109: 216-9

2. Ćuk V, Hećimović H, Ćuk B, Hećimović A, (Vienna, 1991) Microcomputers Appliance in Dependence Disease Researching in Health Center "Novi Zagreb", 1st European Symposium on Drug Addiction and AIDS

3. Ćuk V, Starčević V, Hećimović A (Athens, 1989), An Example of the Informatcs Methods and Microcomputers Appliance in Dependency Disease Researching, VIII World Cogress of Psychiatry

4. Hećimović A, Sakoman S, Lang B, (Athens, 1989), Comprehensive Care about Drug Addicts in the Community of Novi Zagreb, VIII World Congress of Psychiatry

5. Hećimović A, Starčević V, Sakoman S, Ćuk V, Mikecin L, (Zagreb, 1990), Comprehensive Protection of Drug Addicts in the Municipality Novi Zagreb, III Congress of Health Centers of Yugoslavia

6. Hećimović A, Starčevi V, Hećimović Z, Ivanuša M, (Vienna 1991), The Role of Primary Health Care in Protection of Drug Addicts and AIDS in Novi Zagreb, 1st European Syposium on Drug Addiction and AIDS

7. Hudolin V, Sakoman S,(1984) Dependences Except Alcohohilism and Smoking Social Care

8. Hudolin V, Lang B, Sakoman S, Pehar M, Blažić-Čop N, Wolf-Nikoliš J, (Zagreb, 1988) Alcololism, Narcotic Addiction and Smoking as Family Problems, Woman 46

9. Hudolin V, Sakoman S, Lang B, Djordjević V, (Zagreb, 1982), Complex Treatment of Narcotic Addicts in SR Croatia Contributed Papers

10. Hudolin V, Budjanovac M, Lang B, Sakoman S, Dordjević V, Maras D, (San Daniele del Friuli, 1986) Our Experience in Treatment and Rehabilitation of Acoholics and Narcotic Addicts in Criminal Practice Le tossicodipendenze tra cura e repressione

11. Hudolin V, Djordjević V, Sakoman S, (Zagreb, 1982) Modern View of Narcotic Addiction in the book "Social Organization on Solving of Some Family Problems and Problems of Young People"

12. Sakoman S, Zagreb, 1986) Drugs. Alcohol, Tobacco in the Book "From Puberty to Maturity Mladost

13. Sakoman S, (Zagreb, 1988) Problems in Treatment of Drugs Addicts in Prisons Penologic Themes, Vol 3

14. Sakoman S, (Zagreb, 1988) Problems in Realization of Drug Addics Treatment in Prisons Penologic Themes, Vol. 3

15. Sakoman S, Djordjević V, Budjanovac M, Kova D, (Zagreb, 1982) Treatment and Rehabilitation of Drud Addicts in Prison Lepoglava Contributed Papers

16. Sakoman S, Srdar J, (Zagreb, 1984) Multidisciplinary Approach to Drug Abuse Control in Croatia Book: Interdisciplinarity in Science, Education and Inovation

17. Sakoman S, Hećimović A, Starčević V, (Vienna 1991) Drug Dependence and AIDS 1st European Symposium on Drug Addiction and AIDS

18. Starčević V, Hećimović A, Hećimović , (Viena 1991) AIDS in Federal Republics of Yugoslavia 1st European Symposium on Drug Addiction and AIDS

19. Contributed Papers (Zagreb 1987) 1st Yugoslav Symposium on AIDS

Drug Abuse in Spain: Epidemiology, Policy and Health Structure

F. J. ALVAREZ[1] and M. CARMEN DEL RIO

[1] Drugs and Alcohol Research Group, Department of Pharmacology and Therapeutics, Faculty of Medicine, University of Valladolid, E-47005 Valladolid, Spain

INTRODUCTION

In Spain, the problem of 'illegal' drug use and abuse is a relatively recent phenomenon, and it is in the eighties when the increase in the use and abuse of these substances became obvious. In our present study we show a general view of the problem of drug addiction in our country, making a special point of the epidemiology of use and abuse of these substances, the policy, legislatión and health structure related to 'illegal' drugs, and finally, we will show some comments regarding aids and drug addiction.

STATISTICS ON DRUG USE AND ABUSE IN SPAIN

The different sources of information on drug use and abuse available in our country show clearly that there has been a considerable increase in the consumption of 'illegal' drugs since the end of the seventies. Among these sources of information we can mention three important ones: (i) Epidemiological studies, (ii) the National Drug Dependence Information Network and (iii) other indirect indicators.

Epidemiological studies regarding the patterns of drug use and abuse are limited in our country, especially those cross national studies. The last one was carried out in 1984 (Navarro et al. 1985). Concerning specific target populations, like schools, university students and young adults the information available has widely increased (Queipo et al. 1988; Alvarez et al. 1989).

Figures for 'illegal' drug consumption by the general population (14-70 years old) of Castile and León (Spain) in 1989 (Alvarez et al. in press) are shown in Table 1. Cannabis was the most frequently consumed drug. During their 'lifetime' nearly one out of three people surveyed claimed to have taken cannabis. Stimulants were the favourite ones after cannabis: for instance, cocaine use was more frequently reported than amphetamines consumption. 'Past month' drug consumers were classified under 'regular' (those who take drugs at least twice per week) and 'occasional' (those who take drugs less than twice per week) drug users. Most of those surveyed were 'occasional' drug users (Table 1). Among 'regular' drug users, the greater prevalence was that of cannabis (2.8%), and less frequently that of cocaine, opiates and amphetamine users (0.3% of everyone of the substances mentioned above). Drug consumption was more frequent among males than among females (Table 1). 'Lifetime' drug consumption was more common among singles than among married people, those younger (17-29 years old) and those with work problems.

TABLE 1. DRUG CONSUMPTION IN CASTILE AND LEON (SPAIN)

| | 'Lifetime'(%) | | 'Past year'(%) | | 'Past month'(%) | | | |
| | | | | | 'Regular use' | | 'Occasional use' | |
	Male	Female	Male	Female	Male	Female	Male	Female
Amphetamines	7.4	2.9[c]	2.5	1.7	0.4	0.2	1.0	0.7
Cannabis	37.8	22.0[c]	18.1	8.9[c]	4.5	1.4[c]	6.2	3.8[b]
Cocaine	8.1	2.8[c]	4.3	1.4[c]	0.6	0.1	1.8	0.8
Inhalants	0.9	- [b]	0.5	-	-	-	0.2	-
Opiates	2.7	0.2[c]	0.9	0.1[b]	0.5	0.1	0.2	-
Psychedelic Drugs	4.1	0.6[c]	1.4	0.4[b]	0.1	0.1	0.6	0.2
Tranquillizers	2.0	0.2[c]	0.9	- [b]	0.2	-	0.6	-[a]

Chi-square males compared to female [a] $p < 0.05$, [b] $p < 0.01$, [c] $p < 0.001$. From Alvarez et al (in press).

Table 2 shows the figures concerning 'lifetime' drug use observed in some representative studies carried out in Spain. The comparison of drug use figures must be done with caution, as the studies cover different target populations, age ranges, and trends in drug use change throughout the years. In spite of these limitations, the comparison of the figures could reveal changes in the patterns of drug use. These figures shows the huge implementation of drug use in our country, mainly cannabis and stimulants (amphetamines and cocaine). As regards figures concerning Castile and León in 1987 (Alvarez et al. 1989) and 1989 (Alvarez et al. in press), the trends in drug use show an increase in cocaine consumption and, to a lesser extent, in cannabis, amphetamines and opiate use.

TABLE 2. 'LIFETIME' DRUG USE (%) IN SPAIN

	Cross National Studies				Castile and Leon			
Year of the study	1980	1984	1986	1984	1987	1989	1984	1990
Age range	> 15	> 12	16-65	15-29	14-30	14-70	Students	
References	1	2	3	4	5	6	7	8
Anphetamines	6.1	10.3	8.1	6.1	4.3	5.2	15.2	4.8
Cannabis	20.0	21.3	24.4	34.1	28.5	30.0	25.1	30.2
Cocaine	3.5	3.7	5.6	4.2	2.6	5.4	1.5	3.7
Inhalants	-	2.0	2.0	0.3	0.8	0.4	2.9	1.6
Opiates	2.0[a]	3.7	3.2	2.3	1.0	1.5	2.3	1.9
Psychedelic Drugs	5.3	4.4	4.8	4.8	2.6	2.4	1.3	0.3
Tranquillizers	13.5[b]	30.9[b]	15.2[b]	1.4	2.1	1.1	7.4	7.2

References, 1, Edis-Caritas Española. 1981; 2, Navarro et al. 1985; 3, Edis. 1987; 4, Zarraga. 1985; 5, Alvarez et al. 1989; 6, Alvarez et al. in press; 7. Queipo et al 1988.; 8. Alvarez et al. 1991.
[a] Heroin consumption; [b] included medical and non-medical consumption.

The National Drug Dependence Information Network (SEIT, Sistema Estatal de Información sobre Toxicomanias, Ministerio de Sanidad y Consumo 1990) implemented by the National Plan on Drugs is a continous notification system based on indirect indicators like those used in the United States of America by the Client Oriented Data Acquisition Process (CODAP) and the Drug Abuse Warning Network (DAWN). These indicators for epidemiological surveillance of drug dependence are (i) annual number of outpatient treatment requests for opiates and/or cocaine dependence, (ii) annual number of emergency room admissions related to or caused by immediate opiates and/or cocaine abuse, and (iii) annual number of acute deaths related to opiates and/or cocaine use.

Data of the first three years of the first two indicators are shown in Tables 3 and 4, and show an increase in the number of admission for treatment facilities and emergency room admission. These increases could be related both, to a real increase in the number of cases, as well as an increase in the number of centres included in the network and reporting to the National Drug dependence Information Network. In fact, one of the problems with the data offered by the National Drug Dependence Information Network is the coverage of the indicators, which is expected to be fully implemented in the next years. Treatment request rate by opiates and/or cocaine dependence was of 4.34 per 10.000 inhabitants in 1988 and 4.85 in 1989. Emergency room admission figures are obtained throughout both, the reporting hospital centres and the retrospective analyses of hospital emergency cards. Data about the third indicator, death related to drug abuse, are not available yet. A retrospective study concerning the six more populated cities in Spain, shows that death related to drugs has increased (1986= 163, 1987= 234, 1988= 237, 1989= 455, Ministerio de Sanidad y Consumo 1990).

TABLE 3. ANNUAL NUMBERS OF OUT-PATIENT TREATMENT REQUESTS FOR OPIATES AND/OR COCAINE DEPENDENCE IN SPAIN

	1987	1988	1989
ANNUAL NUMBERS OF OUTPATIENT TREATMENT REQUEST	10338	16481	18823
DRUG RELATED TREATMENT REQUEST			
- Heroin	97.1%	97.1%	96.5%
- Methadone	0.4%	0.1%	0.1%
- Other opiates	0.6%	1.1%	1.2%
- Cocaíne	1.9%	1.7%	2.2%
GENDER			
- Male	80.5%	81.0%	81.3%
- Female	19.5%	19.0%	18.7%
AVERAGE AGE	24.9	25.4	25.7
STARTING AGE OF DRUG CONSUMPTION	19.7	19.8	19.8

From Ministerio de Sanidad y Consumo (1990)

TABLE 4. ANNUAL NUMBERS OF EMERGENCY ROOM ADMISSIONS RELATED TO OPIATES AND/OR COCAINE ABUSE IN SPAIN

	1987	1988	1989
NUMBER OF EMERGENCY ROOM ADMISSIONS	3066	11737	15374
AVERAGE AGE	24.1	24.9	25.3
GENDER			
- Male	80.2%	79.0%	80.0%
- Female	19.8%	21.0%	20.0%
MAINLY CONSUMED DRUG			
- Heroin	98.7%	96.6%	95.6%
- Methadone	0.1%	0.1%	0.2%
- Other opiates	0.4%	2.0%	2.5%
- Cocaíne	0.8%	1.2%	1.7%
DRUG RELATED PROBLEM			
- Overdose	6.3%	6.7%	7.4%
- Side effects	3.9%	4.6%	4.2%
- Withdrawal	56.5%	31.3%	28.9%
- Organic problems	25.7%	36.0%	38.6%
- Psycopatologic problems	7.5%	5.8%	5.3%
- Others	0.1%	15.7%	15.6%
LEGAL STATUS			
- Non arrested	72.7%	77.9%	83.7%
- Arrested	27.3%	22.1%	16.3%

From Ministerio de Sanidad y Consumo (1990).

Other indicators, like market indicators and people arrested for drug offences have risen since early 1970s in Spain. The figures for 1980, 1985 and 1989 regarding opiates were 6.1, 253 and 712.9 kg of heroin confiscated, 58.1, 303 and 1852 kg of cocaine, and 11156, 47933 and 64225 kg of cannabis. The annual number of people arrested for suspected drug offences in Spain has risen to 9166 in 1980, 12863 in 1985 and 27404 in 1989.

All these data put together, show as pointed above, that drug use and abuse have increased in Spain since late 1970s, and that drug consumption is common in our country. However, in order to improve health planning, it is necesary to have better implementation and accuracy of indirect indicators as well as regular developments of epidemiological studies, mainly related to the general population. There are some European efforts made to improve the exchange and comparison of information on drug misuse within the Community, and develop an European network on health data on drug abuse, which Spanish authorities, health planners and researchers are paying special attention to.

SPANISH 'ILLEGAL' DRUG POLICY

Although Spanish authorities subscribed the United Nations conventions on narcotic drugs and psychotropic substances in 1961 and 1971, the National Plan on Drugs (Plan Nacional Sobre Drogas, Ministerio de Sanidad y Consumo, 1985) developed by the Spanish Governement in 1985 was the first serious attempt to establish a whole and rational policy against 'illegal' drugs in our country. The National Plan on Drugs has established the general guidelines to develop preventive activities, care structures and rehabilitation measures, joining and coordinating the actions carried out by the Central, Regional and Local administrations, as well as public and private activities. Although the National Plan on Drugs faces the overall phenomenon of drug abuse and dependence, the measures and policy are especially centred on the 'illegal' drugs field, forgotten smoking and alcohol, which are the main causes of death in Spain (smoking about 19% and alcohol about 6%). The guideliness established by the National Plan on Drugs are developed by the different Regional Plan on Drugs.

In the European context, Spain is an active member of the Pompidou Group (part of the Council of Europe, joining the group in 1984) and the Trevi Group, being the overall aim to reduce the demand for illicit drugs within the European Community, among other relationships with different European and American countries.

In addition, in 1990 two Spanish regions, Vasque Country and Castile and León, started a whole Health Policy under the criteria of WHO strategy 'Health For All'. Healthy lifestyles (targets 16 and 17) are of special interest to us, because of the huge consumption of alcohol (about 66% of the population are 'weekly' drinkers), smoking (about 49% of the population are current smokers) and drug consumption, as stated above. Concerning 'illegal' drugs, the policy under these strategies are related to the National Plan on Drugs activities.

SPANISH LEGISLATION ABOUT 'ILLEGAL' DRUGS

The legislation concerning 'illegal' drugs in the Spanish Penal Code is included in the article 344, in the general framework of health offences. The earlier reference to 'illegal' drugs was done in 1963 and lately in 1971. In 1983 there was an important modification in article 344, which meant giving a more lenient treatment of the offences against public health, an aspect which is criticised by certain groups. We have to point out that in the said reform drug consumption was not penalised and an explicit distinction between the 'hard' and 'soft' drugs was made, depending on the great or slight harm they can cause to our health.

In 1988 there was a new reform in the Penal Code, when an important increase in punishments was introduced, whit specific stronger penalties applied to the organizations dedicated to drug smuggling than those already existing, and which proposed a series of measures leading to the confiscation of all the earnings that the drug smugglers had been able to obtain in their illegal dealings. We must especially consider the introduction of a new rule, article 93 (bis) which gives the judge or the court the possibility to apply shorter terms of imprisonment for those facing sentences of less than two years and who had committed their offences due to their dependence on toxic drugs, narcotics or psychotropic substances (Alvarez, Queipo and Del Rio. in press).

SPANISH HEALTH STRUCTURE RELATED TO 'ILLEGAL' DRUGS

As regards in Spain, where the care system is public and covers almost the whole population, it has been established that it should be the public health care system, through its general network, which should give necessary care to the drug addict. To generalise, the Spanish 'illegal' drug care system proposed under the National and the different Regional Plan on Drugs, is implemented in the following therapeutic circuit which operates on three differente levels (Ministerio de Sanidad y Consumo. 1985; Junta de Castilla y León. 1989).

On the first level, the door of the public health care network and social services is open to the drug addict. This level is made up of primary care teams and basic social services, on these depend pinpointining the fundamental problem, initial evaluation and, finally, direct the addict to the mental health care team.

The second level is composed of means for specialized treatment facilities in which the mental health care team acts as the axis of the care system and as the group responsible for the formulation of a personal therapeutic programme, with effects on the drug addict and his environment. The mental health care team will look after the patients sent to them by the public services of the first level and the group will be responsible for directing the drug addict to the hospital level and the rest of the centres and services of the third level. Directing drug addicts to authorized disintoxication centres in hospitals and therapeutic communities will be suggested by the mental health care team.

The third level is made up of centres, services and programmes which are designed for the social rehabilitation of drug addicts. Therapeutic communities, day centres and the social services form part of these services.

In 1989 (Ministerio de Sanidad y Consumo. 1990) there were 49 general hospital disintoxication units, 369 out-patient treatment centres and 120 therapeutics communities (59 of them full private).

Clonidine and naltrexone are available without any restriction. However, maintenance treatments (over 21 days of treatment) with opiate agonist (ej. methadone) are under special regulation. The efficacy of clonidine, methadone (Camí et al. 1985) and naltrexone (García-Alonso et al. 1989) in Spanish drug abusers has been recently reported.

The multicentric study of the evaluation of treatment and folow-up of narcotic addicts (311 heroin addicts in 1985, Sanchez-Carbonell et al. 1988) followed by 6, 12 and 24 months, showed a decrease in the use of heroin (54% abstained from heroin use after 2 years), cannabis and tranquillizers, as well as an improved psychological status and decrease in illegal activities. In another study (298 heroin additcs, Muga et al. 1990), after an average of 25 months of follow-up, 40% of them were no longer intravenous drug users, the percentage of full-off was higher in those admitted for organic diseases (60%) than in those that had been treated for disintoxication (35%). Other serie of studies focussed on sociodemographic aspects and patterns of heroin users (Herrero and Baca. 1990).

AIDS AND DRUG ADDICTIONS IN SPAIN

Data for aids cases in Spain have increased since 1981. On 30 June 1990 (Plan Nacional sobre el SIDA, 1990), 6210 cases of aids were reported to WHO by the Spanish authorities (7047 cases on 30 September). This means 158.4 cases per million inhabitants, Spain being the third after Switzerland (205.2) and France (173.2) in the WHO European region. Male to female ratio was of five. For instance, 63% of aids cases were reported as being intravenous drug users, and 3% of intravenous drug users and homosexuals, second of the European region after Italy. Of those aids cases reported, 43.5% of them have been dead, 31.6% among intravenous drug users. Aids cases among intravenous drug users were mainly reported (45.3%) in those aged 25-29. Intravenous drug users with aids were in most of the cases heroin users. The HIV seroprevalence in intravenous drug users ranges between 50-70%.

We acknowledge the British Journal of Addiction for permission of use modified Tables 1 and 2 from Alvarez et al. (in press).

REFERENCES

Alvarez FJ, Queipo D, Del Rio MC, Garcia MC. (1989) Patterns of drug use by young people in the rural community of Spain. Br J Addict 84: 647-652.

Alvarez FJ, Queipo D, Del Rio MC, Garcia MC. (In press) Patterns of drug use in Castile and Leon (Spain). Br J Addict.

Alvarez FJ, Queipo D, Del Rio MC. (In press) Drogas de abuso: Epidemiología, legislación y políticas sobre drogas. In: Carvajal A (ed) Farmacoepidemiología. Universidad de Valladolid, Valladolid.

Alvarez FJ, Del Rio MC, Gomollon A, Queipo D (1991) Trends changes in substance use among university students in Spain. Wiener Zeitschrift (abstractband/kangrebheft). First European Symposium on Drug Addiction & Aids, 22-23 february 1991. Vienna.

Camí J, De Torres S, San L, Sole A, Guerra D, Ugena B (1985) Efficacy of clonidine and of methadone in the rapid detoxification of patients dependent on heroin. Clin Pharmacol Ther 38: 336-341.

Edis (1987) Drogodependencias. Servicios Generales de la Unión General de Trabajadores, Madrid.

Edis-Caritas Española (1981) La población Española ante las drogas. Documentación Social 42: 25-114.

Garcia-Alonso F, Gutierrez M, San L, Bedate J, Forteza J, Rodriguez-Artalejo F, Palop R, Lopez-Alvarez M, Perez-De-Los-Cobos JC, Camí J. (1989). A multicentre study to introduce naltrexone for opiate dependence in Spain. Drug Alcohol Depend 23: 117-121.

Herrero ME, Baca E. (1990) Specific treatment demand as a definitory trait of a typology in heroin addicts: differential profile of two subpopulations. Int J Addict 25: 65-79.

Junta de Castilla y León (1989) Plan regional sobre drogas. Junta de Castilla y León, Consejería de Cultura y Bienestar Social, Valladolid.

Ministerio de Sanidad y Consumo (1985) Plan nacional sobre drogas. Ministerio de Sanidad y Consumo, Madrid.

Ministerio de Sanidad y Consumo (1990). Sistema estatal de información sobre toxicomanias (SEIT), informe año 1989. Ministerio de Sanidad y Consumo, Delegación del Gobierno para el Plan Nacional Sobre Drogas, Madrid.

Muga R, Tor J, Ginesta C, Melus R, Jacas C, Rey-Joly C, Foz M. (1990) Natural history of parenteral drug addicts treated in a general hospital. Br J Addict 85: 775-778.

Navarro J, Lorente S, Varo J, Roiz M, Equipo de Investigación Sociológica. (1985) El consumo de drogas en España. Ministerio de Trabajo y Seguridad Social, Secretaría General para la Seguridad Social, Dirección General de Acción Social, Cruz Roja Española, Madrid.

Plan Nacional Sobre SIDA (1990). Casos declarados en la región européa de la OMS (32 paises) hasta la revisión del segundo trimestre de 1990, según criterios de definición de caso CDC 1987/OMS/1988. Publ Of Sesida 1: 264-267.

Queipo D, Alvarez FJ, Velasco A. (1988) Drug consumption among university students in Spain. Br J Addict 83: 91-98.

Sanchez-Carbonell J, Brigos B, Camí J (1988) Evolución de una muestra de heroinómanos dos años después del inicio del tratamiento (proyecto EMETYST). Med Clin (Barc) 92: 135-139.

Zarraga JL. (1985) Estudio sobre conocimiento y uso de drogas entre los jovenes. Revista de Estudios de Juventud 17: 249-283.

Drug Abuse and HIV-Infection in Poland

M. Staniaszek

Drug Dependence Committee of the Polish Psychiatric Association
Warsaw, 27 Nowowiejska Str., Poland

1. Characteristics of the population

Drug abuse appeard as a sociomedical problem in Poland in the beginning of the 1970's.

So far no representative study has been carried out on the drug abuse phenomenon. This makes it very difficult to estimate the real dimension of the problem.

The growth of drug abuse prevalence was observed in the beginning and in the second half of the '70s with the peak between 1982 and 1985, however a certain decrease has been noted since 1987 (Tables 1 and 2).

About 5 thousand drug abusers underwent therapy in 1990. In the general population the group of addicts requiring treatment is estimated to be 4-5 times higher. The number of people experimenting with psychoactive drugs (but without dependence symptoms) reaches about 200 thousand.

Certain features of the phenomenon have been altered with the passing time. In the 1970's psychoactive drug abuse among young people was usually connected with the philosophy of hippie -movement, i.e. searching for "new horizons" and new experiences.

In recent years the abuse of psychoactive drugs has rather been a sign of social maladjustment and personality disorders. Drug abusers come from various groups of the society, more frequently from working and lower classes (about 60%), from big cities, tourist centres and smaller towns.

Farmers children still belong to a smalll group (approx.6%).

Changes in patterns of drug use have also been observed. By the end of the 1960's and the beginning of the 1970's young people used various types of medicines: mainly psychotropic and atropinizing drugs or opiates (morphine, codeine).

At the end of 1970 production of a new kind of drug from poppy straw (called "kompot" or "Polish heroin") became wide-spread among drug addicts. They produced strong (hard) drugs at home utilizing easily accessible products.

Pure heroin, cocaine (crack) and LSD are not available in Poland.

The following data concern persons treated in in-patient clinics for drug abusers in 1989.

The number of opiate-users has grown very quickly since the second half of the 1970's. The opiate-dependents constituted 37,5% in 1976, 71,5% in 1979, and 82% in 1984. In 1989 they amounted to 79,2%.

Most of the addicts use opiates together with psychotropic drugs - mainly benzodiazepines (diazepam) or barbiturates.

In 1989 persons addicted to sedatives and hypnotic drugs (alone or mixed with alcohol) belonged to small group among the dependents (3,9%). Persons addicted to mixed drugs (without morphine group) made 8,8%. People using marihuana made 0,2% and those sniffing solvents 6,8%.

The majority of drug addicts are males and this predominance systematically increases. In 1989 they costituted over 77,4% of persons treated in in-patient services for drug users.

Persons aged from 20 to 29 make the most numerous group.

In 1989 they constituted 55% of the total in-patient population. The oldest group aged 30 years and more, is growing systematically (20% in 1985 and 30% in 1989).

According to Police Headquarter's data, 56% of drug users are neither employed nor do any studying. Among them the number of homeless and infected with HIV increases.

Almost all patients undertake treatment and rehabilitation voluntarily. In 1988 only 1,7% (54 persons) were sent by courts: 6 people were directed for observation and 48 for compulsory treatment or rehabilitation.

2. Treatment and rehabilitation

Treatment of addicts is organized by local health authorities while rehabilitation (social reintegration) network is run by health services, non-governmental organizations, Catholic Church and other religious groups.

In December 1990 there were:

28 specialized ut-patient units (first contact, after care) set up by health authorities.

16 consultative centres organized by the MONAR Associatrion,

12 "Poppy information telephones" managed by the "Powrot z U" Association,

7 prophylactic (part day) centres for young drug users belonging to the "Kuznia" Society,

11 detoxification wards (number of beds -110),

37 rehabilitation (social readaptation) centres - number of beds about 800.

The detoxification wards are usually located in psychiatric hospitals as separate units.

Withdrawal symptoms are treated by Clonidine or mild psychotropic drugs.

Substitute treatment or maintenance programmes with Methadone (or other substitutes from the Morphine group) are not practised in Poland but an experimental project on administration of Methadone to drug addicts with AIDS is anticipated.

Rehabilitation centres belong to:

-health services	-14 units, number of beds 270,	
-The MONAR association	-17	390,
-The "Kuznia" Society	-1	20,
-Catholic Church	-2	50,
-Protestant Church	-1	20.

Six centres are assigned for youth under 18 years of age who abuse mainly solvent substances.

Rehabilitation programmes applied by health and MONAR centres do not differ significantly from each other. They are run according to the principles of therapeutic communities.

Rehabilitation lasts about two years on average: for youth under 18 years of age the period is shorter and particular stress is laid on cooperation with the patient's parents.

Consumption of alcohol and other dependence-producing substances is forbidden in the centres, in some of them also smoking is banned. A breach of drug or alcohol abstinence results in expulsion from the centre.

Under the Law on Prevention of Drug Abuse, the treatment and resocialization of drug addicts are run also in prisons.

There are 7 detoxification wards in prison hospitals and 12 special resocialization divisions with about 200 beds. The therapy is focused on changing prisoners' life patterns. The drug users constitute about 1-3% of the total imprisoned population. In recent years, 300-500 prisoners have been subjected to the resocialization programmes.

3. Legislation and drug policy

On January 31, 1985 the Polish Parliament passed the Law on Prevention of Drug Abuse. It is the first act in our history which regulates all issues related to drug abuse.

The Law recommends a preventive-therapeutic strategy for drug abuse control. The Law also conforms to all international conventions on narcotic and psychotropic substances which have been signed by Poland.

It regulates measures to be applied in basic sectors:
- general and individual prevention,
- restrictions on the supply of dependence-producing substances (especially opium poppy and cannabis),
- preventive education for persons using drugs but still not drug-dependent,
- the provision of treatment, rehabilitation and social welfere for drug abusers,
- illicit traffic.

In the new Law the treatment and rehabilitation (social readaptation) are voluntary and free of charge.

The drug possesion and personal use are not punishable but drug-production and illicit drug trafficking are penalized.

On the basis of the new Law the Commission for Prevention of Drug Abuse has been grounded and it aims at indicating all kinds of problems connected with drug abuse as well as at inspiring and coordinating all activities in this field.

Each year the Commission prepares the National Programme of Drug Abuse Prevention that has to be approved by the Cabinet. The Programme comprises all activities within the framework of preventing, controlling and fighting drug abuse, organized by the government (ministries), local administration, non-governmental organizations, denominational associations etc.

It proceeds in 4 directions:
- reduction of the demand for psychoactive drugs,
- reduction of the supply of these drugs,
- modification of the attitudes of the society,
- fighting drug-related delinquencies.

On the basis of the Law a special Fund for Prevention of Drug Abuse has been set up. It was increased from 500 million zlotys in 1985 to 42 milliard zlotys (about 4,5 million US$) in 1990.

Most probably in 1991 this Fund will be dissolved. Following recommedations of the International Monetary Fund and the World Bank, the Government intends to stop financing special funds from its budget.

At present, changes in legislation are being discussed whether to introduce a new rule which would forbid and penalize the possession of drugs, especially those produced from poppy.

4. Staff

It is estimated that about 600 specialists (excluding administrative and technical staff) are employed in drug abuse treatment and rehabilitation facillities. The majority is employed in health service units, 150 people work for MONAR. In health services most of employees are university graduates (physicians, psychologists, pedagogists, etc.) and secondary school graduates (nursers, social workers etc.).Occasionally ex-drug addicts are employed if they completed their own therapy.

The Institute of Psychiatry and Neurology as well as the Drug Dependence Committee of the Polish Psychiatric Association organize systematically special training, coursers, workshops and other forms of education like lectures, conferences etc.

5. Non-governmental organizations

At present there exist 9 non-governmental (non-profit) organizations involved in the prevention of drug abuse. Through various activities they assist drug users.

These organizations operate all over Poland and they comprise 200 to 1000 members. Each of them is active in its own specific way. Their role, which systematically increases, is of great significance, especially nowadays when various aspects of social, political and economic situation in Poland constantly change.

All these organizations receive money from the Fund for Prevention of Drug Abuse in order to implement their activities.

Till now no organization of ex-drug addicts (e.g. Narcotics Anonymous) has been created in Poland.

6. Are there any specific conditions in Poland?

Causes of drug abuse among adolescents in Poland are similar to those in other countries. As far as the "demand" is concerned, the main reason is emotional and psychological immaturity and social maladjustment of young generation, which might result from educational insufficiency of family and school; it is rather regionally independent. However there are differences in the "supply" field.

Undoubtedly, an easy access to the poppy is a specifically Polish cause for drug abuse.

Why is the drug abuse situation so specifc in Poland?
1. Poland is self-sufficent.
   Raw materials used for the most popular drugs are cultiveded and also processed in Poland.
2. There exists no monopoly for illegal production and distribution of drugs, there is no organized drug-trafficking, either.
3. There is a black-market for individual producers and consumers.
4. The most dangerous drugs (opiates) are most easily accessible.
5. Sometimes Poland serves as a transit country and a production place for amphetamine which is distributed chiefly in nearby western and scandinavian countries.
6. Drug addiction is present chiefly in big cities and in tourist centres (about 95%), which might reflect a strong alcohol tradition in the countryside.

7. HIV/AIDS infection

In 1988 the new serious problem of the HIV-infection among drug users arose in Poland.

Since January 1986 drug addicts (IVDUs) have been tested for the presence of HIV antibodies. In 1986-87 all the tests were negative. The first positive HIV-tests were detected in August 1988 (after testing 2254 patients).

In the end of 1988 the total group of HIV-infected cases in Poland comprised 112 persons, among them 12 were addicts (11%).

In order to reduce the incidence of HIV-infections among drug users in March 1989 the Minister of Health set up a special preventive programme addressed to this group of population.

The Programme includes:
1. Education and training of medical workers.
2. Prophylactic activities for drug users:
    a/ information and education,
    b/ wide-spread HIV-testing,
    c/ needles and syringes exchange local schemes.
3. Medical care for HIV-carriers.
4. Special allowances for medical staff working with HIV-patients.

The proposal of condom distribution among drug users has not been accepted.

The serological testing of drug users for the presence of HIV-infection is voluntary and free of charge. Almost all the drug users have consented to these investigations. HIV-antibodies are detected by the ELISA method and the positive results are confirmed by the Western-blot technique.

The needles and syringes are of charge for drug addicts.

What are the results?

Until January 1, 1990 HIV-antibodies were found in 629 persons - among them 405 were IVDUs.

One year later the numbers were:

- 1435 registered HIV-carriers - among them 1026 were drug addicts (694 males and 332 females). This group makes about 70% of the total number of registered HIV-infected persons.

- among 50 cases of AIDS 16 persons were identified as drug addicts.

These figures indicate that HIV-infection is rapidly spreading among the population of drug users. It is estimated that among addicts registered in out-patient units, the percentage of HIV-carriers ranges from 15% to 20% and in some cities from 30% to 40% (Warsaw for example).

With the increasing prevalence of HIV-infection among drug users in recent years, a new social reactions have been noticed which considerably hinder the implementation of the Programme. Some of them are restricted to the milieu of drug addicts, some to workers of the health services and some to the society in general.

Here are some most characterstic examples:

- the society itself suffers from "fear of AIDS" epidemic, it is also afraid of people infected with AIDS.

- local communities very often demand the elimination of existing rehabilitation centres, they also are against setting up up new ones,

- it happens that society discriminates HIV-carriers and shows aggression towards them and occasionally towards people who work with drug addicts, too,

- drug addicts have not modified their health patterns (behaviours), especially they have not changed their sexual behaviour. They have neither altered their drug abuse model nor their life-styles. In addition, their weaker life instinct and psychological mechanisms of self-preservation are "out of order", it makes a bleak picture for the future,

- the level of knowledge about AIDS (ways of infection, ways of dealing with AIDS patient) among the health workers is low;

- the HIV-patients are frequently refused madical care (e.g. surgical or dentist), which results in their hiding the infection,

- the medical confidence is often not kept,

- there are many doubts expressed about and protests against free distribution of disposable equipment (needles and syringes) among drug addicts,

- also many parents protest against providing their addicted children with needles and syringes, as in their opinion such a possibility encourages drug addiction,

- many HIV-carriers cannot find a job for insurance reasons (disablity pension etc.),

- thefts and burglaries committed by drug addicts and especialy HIV-carriers have became much more frequent,
- female and male prostitution in order to earn their living is also on the rise.

Such kinds of behaviour - caused by various psychological backgrounds - generally express their protest against social rejection and condemnation.

During the implementation of the Programme some positive social activities in the HIV-infection field have also been started.

In the end of 1989, two new non-governmental organizations were established:

1. The Foundation "You are not alone",
2. The Association "Solidarity with AIDS-people PLUS".

The phenomenon of drug addiction is one of these difficult sociomedical issues which cannot be solved by one country alone. For this reason an international cooperation is indispensable.

Poland would also like to participate actively in the common effort to solve this urgent problem.

HIV-1-Prevalence Among Drug Deaths in Germany

K. PÜSCHEL[1] and F. MOHSENIAN[2]

[1] Institute for Legal Medicine, University of Essen, Hufelandstraße 55,
D-W-4300 Essen 1, Federal Republic of Germany
[2] Institute for Legal Medicine, University of Hamburg, Butenfeld 34,
D-W-2000 Hamburg 54, Federal Republic of Germany

Introduction

Death as fatal result of drug addiction is of enormous medical, legal and social significance.

Special attention is paid to the spread of HIV-infections and AIDS among the high-risk group of intravenous drug abusers (IVDA). Up to now there is a lack of reliable data concerning the incidence and prevalence of HIV-infections among IVDA. For prevention strategies and health policy a continuous monitoring of the development can be of great value. - We try to çain such data by means of scientific cooperation between the Institutes for Legal Medicine in the FRG. Data concerning the HIV-sero-status of drug deaths investigated by forensic scientists are sampled anonymously since 1985.

This study was supported by a grant from the Ministry for Research and Technology of the Federal Republic of Germany (FKZ Nr. I-077-89)

Definition of drug deaths

For epidemiological analysis a standardized definition of the term drug death is absolutely necessary. It is evident that it is difficult to distinguish between drug-induced deaths and other causes of death among drug addicts.

In the FRG the following definition has been worked out by the Bundeskriminalamt and is designed to record all deaths where causal connection to drug addiction (illicit drugs or substitutes) is evident:

- Death due to intentional or accidental overdose ("golden shot").

- Death due to long-term abuse of drugs (i.e. myocarditis, hepatitis, liver cirrhosis, AIDS).

- Suicides connected with drug addiction (i.e. hanging, shooting, jumping from the height).

- Fatal accidents influenced by drugs (i.e. traffic accidents, fall from the height, fire and carbon monoxide intoxication).

"Supply" with heroin has apparently become so plentiful that almost all drug deaths within the last 3 years were caused by intravenous heroin intoxication. - Other narcotics and other ways of application are of minor importance for the fatal outcome.

Statistics

It is estimated that about 100 000 people in Western Germany inject narcotics intravenously. Since 1970 drug deaths are centrally registered in the Bundeskriminalamt. The amount shows a steady increase until 1979, the year in which over 600 drug victims were counted. After 1979 the number of drug deaths de-

creased to 300-500 annually (Fig. 1). Since 1988 there was a
dramatic increase of drug deaths (991 in 1989, 1504 in 1990).

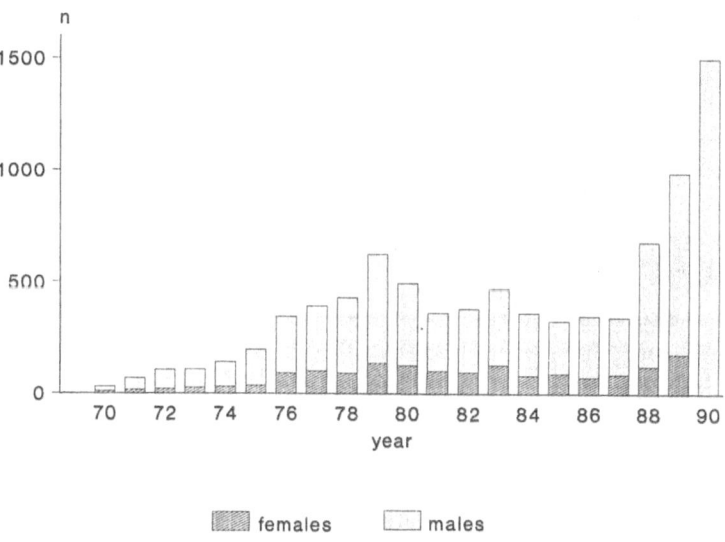

Fig. 1. Drug deaths in the FRG since 1970

Compared with other European countries the FRG has the highest
absolute number of drug deaths within the last decade, followed
by Italy, Great Britain and France. However, in Switzerland the
number of drug deaths per million inhabitants is much higher
than in the FRG (37 versus 16). 1989 this study included 542 of
991 drug deaths (54,7 %) registered in the FRG.

HIV-epidemiology

Monitoring of the HIV-1-seroprevalence of drug related fatalities was carried out in 14 German cities since 1985. Postmortem
testing proved to be a safe and reproducable procedure.
Positive results of the ELISA were confirmed by Westernblot.

In the first three years of the investigation period not all
drug deaths in all cities were tested. There might have been a

selection of certain cases with special anamneses or indicative
morphological findings. Since 1988 there is an unselected
testing of all drug related fatalities.

In Hamburg the HIV-1-prevalence among drug deaths has decreased
within the last years. In 1990 only 6 % were positive. - The
same tendency is observed in other big cities (i.e. Berlin,
Francfort and Munich).

Cumulated data of all 14 cities (n = 1358) also show a decreasing ratio of the HIV-1-prevalence between 1985 and 1989 (Fig.
2). The prevalence rate decreased from 29 % to 13 %.

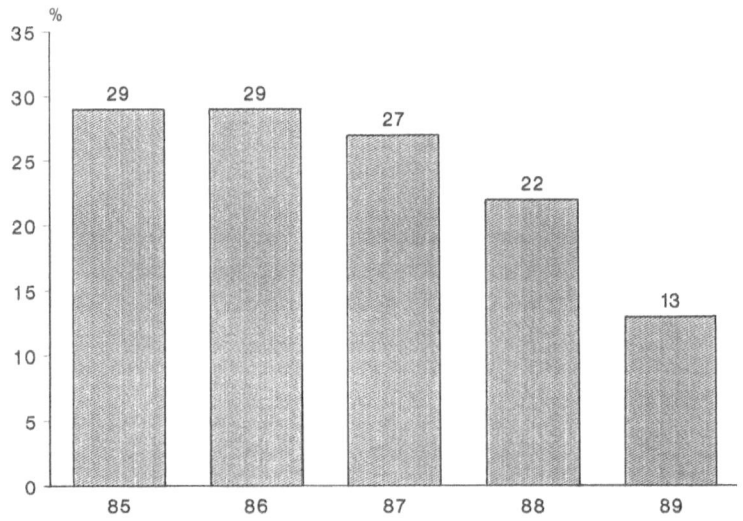

Fig. 2. HIV-1-prevalence among drug deaths in the FRG
1985 - 1989 (cumulated data of 14 cities, n = 1358)

Regional differences of HIV-1-prevalence are very obvious
(table 1). The highest HIV-1-prevalence was found in Berlin
(36 %), followed by Francfort (23 %) and Bremen (20%). In 1989
the HIV-1-prevalence rates in Berlin, Francfort, Munich and
Bremen seem to be equal (about 20 %) whereas Hamburg has a
comparably low prevalence rate.

Table 1. HIV-1-prevalence among drug deaths in different big
cities of the FRG 1985 - 1989 (n = 1358)

	n	HIV +
Francfort	293	66 (23 %)
Berlin	282	101 (36 %)
Hamburg	244	28 (11 %)
Munich	165	29 (18 %)
Bremen	95	19 (20 %)
Dortmund	71	7 (10 %)
Cologne	47	6 (13 %)
Duisburg	36	5 (14 %)
Hanover	32	3 (9 %)
Essen	26	2 (8 %)
Stuttgart	22	6 (27 %)
Düsseldorf	17	3 (18 %)
Munster	15	1 (7 %)
Bochum	13	0 (0 %)
	1358	276 (20 %)

Males dominated among drug related fatalities (sex ratio about
4 : 1). In contrast females were overrepresented in the group
of HIV-positives; the HIV-prevalence rate of female drug deaths
was 31 % compared to 17 % of men. The mean age of male drug
deaths was 29 years, that of women 27 years. On an average HIV-
positive male and female drug deaths were 2 years older than
HIV-negatives.

It has to be emphasized that the test rate of drug related
fatalities for HIV-antibodies at the institutes working together within this study today is 90-100 %. This means that our
data are at least representative for those drug deaths that are
investigated at Institutes for Legal Medicine.

From the point of view of forensic scientists it has to be
stated that within the last years HIV-1-prevalence among drug
deaths has by no means increased but has obviously decreased.

We tried to find out whether our data of drug deaths are representative for the situation of living IVDA. - Since 1985 all

patients admitted to withdrawal therapy to the General Hospital of Ochsenzoll in Hamburg were regularly tested for HIV-antibodies. The prevalence rate has slightly decreased from 14 % to 8 % (table 2). The prevalence rate of all IVDA tested since 1985 (10 %) equals the prevalence rate of drug deaths (10 %). Analogous prevalence rates in drug related fatalities and living IVDA were also found in Northrhine-Westfalia (table 3).

Table 2. IVDA (n = 879) and drug deaths (n = 370) in Hamburg tested for HIV-1-antibodies (1985 - 1990)

| | I V D A | | drug deaths | |
	n	HIV +	n	HIV +
1985	95	13 (14 %)	8	0
1986	147	16 (11 %)	22	5 (23%)
1987	169	18 (11 %)	51	8 (16%)
1988	134	15 (11 %)	75	11 (15%)
1989	163	11 (7 %)	88	4 (5%)
1990	171	13 (8 %)	126	8 (6%)
	879	86 (10 %)	370	36 (10%)

Table 3. HIV-1-prevalence rate among IVDA and drug deaths in Hamburg and in Northrhine-Westfalia (1985 - 1990)

| region | I V D A | | drug deaths | |
	n	HIV +	n	HIV +
Hamburg	879	86 (10 %)	370	36 (10 %)
Northrhine-Westfalia	330	33 (10 %)	316	33 (10 %)

Conclusions

1. Drug deaths are - to a certain extent - a parameter of the
    effectivity of the control programs for drugs, for
    measures of therapy and preventive prescribing of drugs.

2. Serological screening of drug deaths is very useful for
    the epidemiology of HIV-infections. - Continuous moni-
    toring of the HIV-1-status of drug deaths shows the spread
    of this disease among the risk group of intravenous drug
    addicts.

3. The data of drug deaths concerning HIV-1-epidemiology are
    representative for the situation of living intravenous
    drug abusers.

4. Former prognoses about an enormous increase of HIV-1-serc-
    prevalence in i.v. drug abusers have not come true.

5. From the statistical point of view our data concerning the
    spread of HIV-infection within the high-risk group of drug
    addicts and about regional differences are not yet compre-
    hensive enough.

6. Of course, the number of HIV-1-infected drug addicts can-
    not undergo a real reduction. The only way to get rid of
    HIV-seropositivity is to die.
    The following explanations may be given for the diminished
    prevalence rate:

    - Selection mechanisms of testing in former years.
    - Increasing number of new consumers during the last 3
    years with a diminished risk of acquiring HIV-infection
    because of prevention strategies.
    - Increasing number of IVDA who have developed full-blown
    AIDS. Many of them are hospitalized or get substitution
    therapies. When they die they are not registered as drug
    related fatalities because the manner of death is classi-
    fied as "natural" on the death certificate.

96

Literature

Janssen, W., Trübner, K., Püschel, K.: Death caused by drug
  addiction: a review of the experiences in Hamburg and the
  situation in the Federal Republic of Germany in comparison
  with the literature. Forensic Sci. Int. 43, 223-237 (1989).

Püschel, K., Trübner, K., Klöppel, A., Gesemann, M., Heintschel
  von Heinegg, E., Thraenhart, O., Hummelsheim, G., Springer,
  E., Bonte, W., Madea, B., Bajanowski, T., Brkanovic, M.: HIV-
  1-Prävalenz bei Drogentoten in Nordrhein-Westfalen. Rhein.
  Ärztebl. 45 (Heft 2), 47-54 (1991).

Hepatitis B, Hepatitis C and AIDS in Drug Deaths

K. Trübner[1], S. Polywka[2], K. Püschel[1], and R. Laufs[2]

[1] Institut für Rechtsmedizin der Universität, Gesamthochschule Essen,
Hufelandstraße 55, D-W-4300 Essen, Federal Republic of Germany
[2] Institut für Medizinische Mikrobiologie und Immunologie, Universitätskrankenhaus
Eppendorf, Martinistraße 52, D-W-2000 Hamburg, Federal Republic of Germany

Introduction

Needle sharing among drug addicts leads to the transmission of infectious
diseases such as hepatitis B and AIDS. Since the identification of the
hepatitis C virus (HCV) drug addicts have been regarded as an important
reservoir for hepatitis C. The hepatitis C virus is a major cause of
the chronic non-A, non-B hepatitis. HCV is a single stranded encapsula-
ted RNA virus probably belonging to the flaviviruses with a diameter
of 50 - 60 nm (Grob and Joller-Gemelka 1990). However, until now
only one HCV associated antigen is available for detection of specific
antibodies in infected patients. Seroconversion may take 3 to 6 months
or more and may occur after onset of clinical symptoms. We have little
knowledge about the persistence of HCV antibodies in cases of chronic
or resolved non-A, non-B hepatitis. A negative test result therefore
does not exclude HCV infection as the patient may have antibodies against
other antigen determinants of the virus. Confirmatory tests are necessary
to give further information on infectiosity and clinical outcome of
patients with antibodies against HCV (anti-HCV) (Marwick and Skolnick
1990).

As HCV is obviously transmitted parentally, groups at risk resemble
those at risk for hepatitis B virus (HBV) or human immunodeficiency virus
(HIV), i. e. intravenous drug addicts, hemophiliacs, homosexuals and
patients receiving blood transfusions (Stevens et al. 1990; Laufs et al.
1990; Mosley et al. 1990). However, in about 40 % of sero-positive patients the route of transmission remains unknown (Marwick and Skolnick
1990).

Real epidemiogical data about the drug scene is not readily available
because of the criminal and subculture milieu in which drug addicts pur-
chase and consume drugs. This data is available during a stay in hospital,
in prison or in penal clinic or in case of the death of a drug addict.
So it makes sense to carry out post mortem serological investigations of
drug deceased to obtain prevalence rates of the HIV infection or other
infectious diseases such as hepatitis B and hepatitis C to obtain epidemiological data of the spread of these infections among drug addicts.

Material and methods

Autopsies were carried out on 297 drug addicts (245 male, 52 female) and
blood samples were taken within 24 hours after admission of the corpses
to the Institute for Forensic Medicine at the University Hospital Ham -
burg–Eppendorf and stored at 4 $^\circ$C,
Sera were tested for anti–HBc using the commercially available test kit
of Abbott Diagnostica (Chicago, Illinois, Corzyme^R). Anti–HCV was detected
with an ELISA system that used recombinant HCV C 100–3 antigen on the
solid Phase (Ortho, Raritan, New Jersey). Testing for HIV 1 was performed
by ELISA (VIRONOSTIKA II^R, Organon Teknika, Eppelheim, FRG) as a screening method; those testing positively were confirmed by an immnunofluores-
cence test (self-production) and by Western blot (HIV-1 Biotech Western
Blot^R Kit, DuPont Company, Wilmington, Delaware).
Statistical methods used in this study included chi–square–test and
Fisher's exact test where appropriate.

Results and Discussion

In our study we compared rates of addicts showing seropositivity to
HCV with those positive for HBV and HIV 1. Out of 282 drug victims
113 showed anti-bodies against hepatitis C virus, i.e.
40.1 %. Rates of anti–HCV did not differ significantly
between males and females (39.9 % vs. 40.9%). Regarding the
years 1988, 1989 and 1990 there is a slight decrease from 43.2 % to
37.2 % in 1990 (table 1).
The marker that shows previous hepatitis B is the anti-HBc – the antibody against hepatitis B core antigen. This antibody persists lifelong
and is therefore a good indicator for hepatitis B.

This marker was detected in 95 cases – i.e. a percentage of 33.8 %.
So every third drug death has had hepatitis B during his life. There
is a marked decrease from 44.6 % in 1988 to 27.6 % in 1990 (table 1).
The reasons for this decrease could be that the period of drug abuse
of the deceased becomes shorter, and or that the knowledge about AIDS
and its prevention – the relatively more frequent usage of sterile
needles is practised.
This trend is visible too regarding the development of the HIV–antibody
in the last three years. 23 sera were positive for anti–HIV, i.e. 8 %.
There was a decrease from 14.9 % in 1988 to 4.6 % in 1989 and a slight
increase to 6.3 % in 1990 (table 1).

Table 1

Prevalence of anti–HCV, anti–HBc and anti–HIV 1
in drug victims

	1988		1989		1990		Total	
	n	%	n	%	n	%	n	%
anti–HCV	32	43.2	36	41.4	45	37.2	113	40.1
anti–HBc	33	44.6	29	33.3	33	27.6	95	33.8
anti–HIV 1	11	14.9	4	4.6	8	6.3	23	8.0

We were especially interested to see what and how many coinfections
were detectable. Coinfections with HCV and HBV were seen in 57 cases –
compared with the 56 drug deaths with a hepatitis C infection without
hepatitis B, that means that 50 % of all drug deaths with hepatitis C
have caught hepatitis B too in their lifetime. This association between antibodies against HCV and markers for an HBV infection was highly significant. A similar correlation between both infections was
found by Stevens et al. (1990) in volunteer blood donors. This strong
association was not discovered in other risk groups, e.g. haemophiliacs
or patients on haemodyalysis as a study carried out by Polywka et al.
(1990) showed. In contrast to the strong association of hepatitis B and
hepatitis C in our study, no association was able to be found between
hepatitis C and HIV infection. Only 8 drug deaths with hepatitis C were
HIV positive but 105 were HIV negative. On the other hand, HIV–sero-

positivity is not necessarily connected with hepatitis C as the 15 HIV-positive but hepatitis C negative prove. In many sera we found markers for one infection only (table 2).

It has been suggested that infectivity is highest in acute or chronic hepatitis B infection followed by HIV 1, whereas it is lower in HCV. Therefore, rates for HCV should be lowest. However, mortality among persons who are already HIV 1 positive is highest followed by HBV and HCV, this accounts for the high prevalence of anti-HCV in drug addicts who do not die from infection.

Table 2

Association between HCV and HBV or HIV 1

	HBV		HIV 1	
	+	−	+	−
HCV +	57	56	8	105
HCV −	39	130	15	154

With increasing age the rate of HCV infected persons among deceased drug addicts rose. We found the highest prevalence of HCV positivity in the age-group 30 – 34 years. 57 % of all deceased were HCV positive. Drug addicts younger than 30 were less frequently positive than those older than 30 years (31 % versus 54 %).

The mean age of HCV negatives (27 years) was lower than that of HCV-positives (31 years). In all age groups with the exception of those older than   39 years, the prevalence of HCV among female addicts was higher than that of male addicts.

A similar dependency upon age is found in hepatitis B infection. Because of the fact that the antibody against the hepatitis core-antigen is persisting lifelong it is logical the prevalence of anti-HBc is increasing with age.

Epidemiological investigations concerning post mortal serological findings for antibodies to hepatitis B, hepatitis C and the HIV infection can contribute to our knowledge about the spread of these infectious diseases in the risk group of intravenous drug addicts. It is useful to continue monitoring examinations of these antibodies to see how the epidemic will develop with regard to the group of drug addicts in the course of the next years.

Literature

1) Grob PJ, Joller-Jemelka HJ (1990)
   Hepatitis-C-Virus (HCV), Anti-HCV and Non-A,
   Non-B-Hepatitis.
   Schweiz Med Wschr 120:117-124

2) Laufs R, Polywka S, Krüger W, Nolte H, Friedrich K,
   Hening H (1989)
   Hepatitis-C-Virus-Antikörper bei Hapatitis-Patienten
   und Risikogruppen.
   Dt Ärztebl 86(50):2273-2274

3) Marwick C, Skolnick A (1990)
   Research seems to be gaining upper hand on what's
   been called non-A, non-B hepatitis.
   JAMA 263(1):14-17

4) Mosley JW, Aach RD, Hollinger FB, Stevens CE,
   Barbosa LH, Nemo GJ, Holland PV, Bancroft WH,
   Zimmermann HJ, Kuo G, Choo Q-L, Houghton M (1990)
   Non-A, non-B hepatitis and antibody to hepatitis
   C virus
   JAMA 263(1): 77-78

5) Polywka S, Laufs R (1991)
   Hepatitis C virus antibody among different groups
   at risk and patients with suspected non-A, non-B
   hepatitis
   Infection: in press

6) Stevens CE, Taylor TE, Pindyck J, Choo Q-L, Bradley DW,
   Kuo G, Houghton M (1990)
   Epidemiology of hepatitis C virus. A preliminary study
   in volunteer blood donors.
   JAMA 263(1):49-53

Monitoring of HIV-Spread in Regional Populations of Injecting Drug Users – the Berlin Experience

F. Bschor[1], R. Bornemann[2], Ch. Borowski[3], and V. Schneider[1]

[1] Institut für Rechtsmedizin der Freien Universität Berlin, Hittorfstraße 18, D-W-1000 Berlin 33, Federal Republic of Germany
[2] I. Medizinische Klinik der Krankenanstalten Bielefeld Mitte, Federal Republic of Germany
[3] General Practioner, Berlin-Charlottenburg, Federal Republic of Germany

Introduction

The epidemiological WHO-data for AIDS show, as we all know, that the increase of AIDS cases from the group of intravenous drug users (IVDU) is higher than in the other risk groups, and has reached a total of about one third of all cumulative reported AIDS cases in Europe (4). The vertical Virus transfer to the next generation is mainly caused by infected mothers from the group of drug users or by mothers with sexual contact to drug users. Regarding the horizontal virus transfer from the population at risk to the general population in the pattern-1-countries there is little doubt that the IVDU population is of great importance (3,7,13).

Therefore, drug users become a major target for AIDS prevention. This is clearly seen everywhere, but the scientific base for the prevention strategy is not yet satisfying. AIDS prevention strategy has to consider the regional HIV-spread in the drug area, firstly by continuous regional monitoring of HIV-spread among this risk group and secondly by long-term cohort studies on the effect of different intervention measures. Here, we will discuss HIV-monitoring only.

In the last few years, there could be seen remarkable differences in HIV-prevalence between European countries, even between cities, as we know for example from the neighbouring Scottish cities of Glasgow and Edinburgh (11). In Germany we made the same experience. These differen-

ces urge us to concentrate on local conditions, leading to such differences. Our findings may lead to prevention measures basing on such
results of an scientifically adequate surveillance strategy.

Aspects of HIV-monitoring

We will now focus on the different methods to gather such data. Our
question is: which possibilities for the estimation of HIV-spread among
injecting drug users are at hand? Table 1 gives a survey of such sources, as well as the obstacles coming along with them.

Table 1: **Sources to find out HIV-1-spread in the
IVDU-population of the region**

SOURCE	HANDICAPS
AIDS data	"10 years after"
field research	selection bias
HIV-1-serodiagnostic data from laboratories	reporting problems
special IVDU admissions	selection bias
indicator mosaic from several admission groups	depends on test willing-ness and test rate

Best known and most used are the AIDS-statistics from WHO or from
the national collaborating centers for data-collection. In Germany this
is the National AIDS Center at the Federal Health Bureau in Berlin
(AIDS-Zentrum beim Bundesgesundheitsamt). For example, in our country,
until October 1990 from the City of Hamburg only 18 AIDS cases from the
IVDU group were cumulatively reported, compared to 131 AIDS cases in
Berlin from this group. These data are useful mainly for Health Service
planning and for retrospective studies. They show, how the regional HIV
spread looked like ten years ago, or, in which areas the infection risk
then was high or low, respectively. For monitoring purposes they are
not helpful.

Another source for the estimation of HIV-spread could be laboratory
data, the gathering of serodiagnostically discovered HIV-positives. In
some countries, for instance in the UK or in Germany, positive HIV-tests

have to be reported anonymously by the laboratory to a national center.
Now, in relation to the respective population number, these data might
serve as a measure for HIV/AIDs monitoring. If we take, for example,
data from the Drugs & HIV monitoring unit of the Mersey Regional Health
Authority, 1989 we find only six HIV-infection reports per one million
inhabitants from the IVDU group, whereas in London there were 31, and
in Edinburgh 171 respectively (7,8). For comparison some German data:
in Hamburg there have been reported 48 HIV-infections from the IVDU
group per one million inhabitants, and in Berlin 278 respectively
(Bundesgesundheitsamt). Such laboratory data could be helpful for monitoring purposes in case that the reporting system works precisely. But
does it? How many double reportings are included? What is about positive
findings when the risk group of the tested person is unknown or not
registered? Considering these handicaps, the use of the laboratory data
for monitoring seems not to be reliable enough.

In Germany there have been efforts to get knowledge about the HIV
epidemiology bei means of field research with volunteers in the drug
scene. This epidemiological approach was explained on the same congress
(6), and so details can be neglected here. Nevertheless, one point
should be mentioned. This type of field research is highly subjected to
selection biases and, on the other hand, is not reproducible in continuous monitoring and therefore not really satisfying.

Methods and results

May we now propose an approach which may be able to cope with these obstacles:
The starting point for the idea of an indicator mosaic, initiated 1988
by Bschor et al.(2), was the experience that all institutions, which
have to deal with drug users, get in contact with special subgroups,
for instance those, who ask for advice, others, who wish to check their
serostatus, others, who want to get in drug free stationary treatment,
or, in Germany only recently, who wish to come into methadone maintenance treatment. Furtheron drug addicts are often admitted into prison.
Such different admission circumstances lead inevitably to a selection
bias, if we check the HIV-serostatus in single settings only.

Considering this situation, our intention was to initiate the cooperation of different institutions which get in contact with drug users

and which are willing and able to check the serostatus of their clients.
Surely you know that in the first years, since 1985, when the HIV-antibody test was available, a longlasting debate about HIV-testing began.
Some experts recommended strong reserve against testing (12). It was
therefore not astonishing, that in the first years of the epidemic
there was a reserve, too, against gathering surveillance data about the
HIV-prevalence of admission groups in treatment institutions.

In consequence of this longlasting reserve against testing in treatment
units, firstly we investigated in Berlin and, cooperating with Püschel,
in Hamburg as well, the seroprevalence in drug related deaths (9). The
development of HIV-prevalence rates in death cases in Berlin since 1985
is shown in the left columns of table 2. Significant differences between
Berlin and Hamburg were found. In Berlin, the HIV-prevalence in the
death cases in the first years of the epidemic was as high as about
50%, decreasing since 1988 to now 20-25%. The rates in Hamburg were
much lower and decreased from 23% 1987 to 6% in 1990. In Germany,
today, the scientists of the forensic institutes are convinced, that
the serodiagnostic investigation has to be part of a regular forensic
autopsy. By this, pieces for a regional HIV-monitoring-mosaic become
available in most German cities. But it remains questionable if these
death cases rates reflect the regional trends of the HIV-spread in the
IVDU population (10).

Table 2: **HIV-1-SEROPREVALENCE IN IVDU, BERLIN WEST**

Year	DRUG RELATED DEATHS		LIVING IVDU POPULATION	
	N*tested	HIV-pos	N**tested	HIV-pos
1985	36	30%	n.a.	n.a.
1986	51	49%	124	32%
1987	37	49%	195	27%
1988	78	38%	195	28%
1989	77	21%	208	26%
1990	132	23%	241	24%

Test ratio *) in deaths 90-95%, **) in livings about 80%
n.a.= non available

Therefore, it was naturally our objective to complete the indicator mosaic by gathering data from yearly admissions in treatment units, in the same way as in the forensic institutes. But the success was up to now only partial. In most cooperating units, in the medical ones as well as in the psychosocial ones, the test rate was low and therefore the HIV-prevalence data not reliable enough, particularly a double selection bias was involved: selection by the different admission motivation and selection by differences in test willingness. Merely from one admission group the test rate was about 80% and these HIV-prevalence data of 963 IVDU patients, treatment seeking IVDUs admitted between 1986 and 1990 (right columns of table 2), can be estimated as a relatively reliable piece of a regional indicator mosaic.

Comparing the data development over the years one can see in the two data rows of table 2, that there is a common decreasing trend in both rows, in the death cases as well as in the living. Besides this decreasing trend there is to be seen a clear trend of prevalence convergence. During 1989 and 1990, the prevalence rates were nearly equal in the row of the death cases and the row of the living IVDU. It seems quite possible, that in the beginning of the epidemic the lifestyle of those who were HIV-infected could have been more chaotic and influenced by panic reactions and therefore this subgroup was in a greater death risk than the noninfected ones.

It is necessary to analyze these data in detail, for instance with respect to gender differences. Considering the situation with respect to gender, we find that the seroprevalence in the female group is considerably higher than in the male group, in the death cases in nearly all past years, as well as in the living. Such details are going to be analyzed and published in near future. The recent trend of decreasing HIV-rates is supported by our investigations in inpatient detoxification patients and IVDU prison admissions, coming down from approximately 25% in 1988 to about 15% in 1990 (1). But the test rate in these groups is still too low, compared with our other mosaic pieces.

Discussion

It is only recently that a remarkable change in the approach to the HIV-antibody-test has occured. Nowadays the majority of helpseeking drug patients has knowledge of his/her serostatus or wishes to check it up, naturally only if confidentiality is guaranteed and this is above all to be mentioned: In former years, with less knowledge about the HIV/-AIDS-disease, a positive test result was coming along with the perspective of incurability and short life expectance. Today the chances for longer and better life are higher, connecting the knowledge about a positive HIV-serostatus with earlier diagnosis and the chance of more efficient treatment in case of HIV-linked opportunistic diseases. So, the motivation of the patients to accept HIV-testing is nowadays widespread and therefore gathering of comprehensive prevalence data in the institutions is less difficult and less problematic. Indeed, the composition of a scientifically satisfying surveillance strategy by means of the proposed indicator-mosaic is no longer utopically.

If such an indicator mosaic is composed and is going to be applied year by year in the respective region, obviously the work in the difficult field of drug addiction and AIDS would come to a more effective standard. It seems reasonable, that such a sensitive gathering of confidential data should not be centralized in official state institutions, but should rather be achieved in the framework of research activities realized by cooperation of those physicians, who are in direct responsible contact with the patients.

Conclusions

It is quite clear that this presentation of the indicator-mosaic-approach is only a beginning and not yet a firm basis for strategic conclusions. By means of an intensive further development of this approach we would be able to assess more precisely the regional risk situation in total as well as in separate groups. It seems necessary and possible in view of the globalwide HIV/AIDS-problem in the IVDA risk group to define international guidelines for a satisfying surveillance strategy, like the Australian guidelines (5), by paying attention to these aspects:
- defined sampling frame for continuous monitoring,
- providing major demographic data (age, gender) for tested and untested IVDU,
- testrate related to the total of the yearly admissions,
- broad variety of admission settings for gathering a comprehensive overview of the local IVDU population and to reduce selection biases.

108

In combination with a profound knowledge of local variables possibly influencing HIV-spread in the IVDU population, a comprehensive indicator-mosaic would allow targeting prevention measures on special issues und would help to compare the effects of different local intervention systems and through such comparison contribute to the transfer of effective treatment and prevention measures.

As shown in this paper, a decreasing trend in HIV-prevalence was found in the Berlin region. By means of a continuous monitoring it is possible to demonstrate clearly, that the predicted apocalyptic extent of the HIV-spread is missing even in the high-risk group of the IVDU population of Berlin, but that further efforts are necessary and controllable in their effects.

Literature
1) Bornemann R, Bschor F, Platz W, Rex R, Püschel K, Schneider V (1990) Rückgang der HIV-1-Prävalenz bei i.v.-Drogenabhängigen in Berlin W und Hamburg: Erfolg der Prävention? 3. Deutscher AIDS-Kongreß Hamburg 24.-27.11.1990
2) Bschor F, Schneider V, Bornemann R, Püschel K (1988) Dynamics of HIV-spread amongst iv-drug addicts. Proceedings of the 35th International Congress on Alcoholism and Drug Dependence. Oslo Vol I:378-386
3) Des Jarlais DC, Friedman SR, Stoneburger RL (1988) HIV Infection and Intravenous Drug Use: Critical Issues in Transmission Dynamics, Infection Outcomes, and Prevention. Reviews of Infectious Diseases 10:151-158
4) European Centre for the Epidemiological Monitoring of AIDS. AIDS Surveillance in Europe. Quarterly Report Nr 28 from 31st Dec 1990
5) Kaldor J (1990) Review of Australian HIV Seroprevalence Studies among Intravenous Drug Users (IVDU) DRAFT National Centre in HIV Epidemiology and Clin. Research, Faculty of Medicine, The University of New South Wales
6) Kleiber D (1991) Drug Addiction and AIDS in Germany. First European Symposium on Drug Addiction and AIDS, Vienna Feb 21-23 1991
7) Mersey Regional Health Authority Drugs and HIV Monitoring Unit (1990) HIV infection among drug injectors in England. Internat. J. Drug Policy I/4:15-15
8) Newcombe R (1989) Preventing the spread of HIV infection. Internat.J Drug Policy I/2: 20-27

9) Püschel K, Lieske K, Laufs R, Bschor F, Schneider V, Marcus U
   (1988) Entwicklung der HIV-1-Antikörperprävalenz bei Rauschgift-
   toten in Berlin und Hamburg. AIFO 3: 452-454

10) Püschel K, Mohsenian F, Bornemann R, Bschor F, Schneider V,
    Penning R, Spann W, von Karger J, Madea B, Metter D: HIV-1-Prä-
    valenz bei Drogentoten in verschiedenen Großstädten der Bundesre-
    publik Deutschland und in Westberlin zwischen 1985 und 1988.
    Z Rechtsmed 103:407-414

11) Robertson JR, Bucknall ABV, Welsby PD, Roberts JJK, Inglis JM,
    Peutherer JF, Brettle RP (1986) Epidemic of AIDS related virus
    infection among intravenous drug users. Br Med J 292:527-529

12) Rosenbrock R (1986) AIDS kann schneller besiegt werden. Gesundheits-
    politik am Beispiel einer Infektionskrankheit. VSA Verlag Hamburg

13) Velimirowicz B (1987) AIDS und Drogenabhängigkeit aus der Sicht
    des Epidemiologen. AIFO 2:323-334

5 Years Follow-up on Viennese Heroin Addicts

A. Uhl[1], A. Springer[1], F. Maritsch[1], and V. Pfersmann[2]

[1] Ludwig Boltzmann Institut für Suchtforschung, Mackgasse 3, A-1230 Wien, Austria
[2] Anton Proksch Institut, Kalksburg, Mackgasse 3, A-1230 Wien, Austria

In 1986/87 we did a followup study on all opiate addicted patients who were admitted to the intensive care unit of the Viennese University Clinic in the years 1980 and 1981 (Uhl A, Springer A, Maritsch F, Pfersmann V, Presslich O, Mayer, A, 1980). The followup periode was 5 years. Out of the wealth of data, that we collected, we will for this presentation focus on issues related to the health state of the patients and on conclusions about an adequat care and treatment system for the addicted population. Let us discribe first the site of our study and the Viennese care system.

This intensive care unit is only one link in a network of a variety of corresponding inpatient and outpatient facilities for drug users and drug addicts in and around Vienna. These facilities range from counseling and crisis intervention to long-term inpatient therapy and aftercare. Allmost all patients in our sample had been in contact with several different institutions before admission to the intensive care unit and/or in the followup periode, depending on their specific needs at the point of time as well as on legal requirements. In this non-experimental situation the treatment effects of the different institutions are confounded and it is not possible to attribute any changes in the studied patients simply to one specific institution. The goal of the project therefore could not be an isolated evalution of the intensive care unit, who's patients we followed up, but rather a broad evaluation of the whole therapy network. The primary aim was to get an overview over the specific problems and needs of the study population and to see to what degree these needs were met in the existing institutions.

223 patients had been admitted to the intensive care unit in the years 1980 and 1981. Since the total sample-size was not too large for our project capacities, we decided to followup the total population rather than a sub-sample. Out of the 223 patients 25 patients (11%) had died in the 5 year followup periode. Within the surviving cases we could achieve 100 (45%) extensive followup interviews and in 36 cases (16%), we were at least able to get satisfactory information on some major issues, including their present drug consumption behavior. The later information was either based on a telefone contact with the patient himself or on information from parents, relatives or friends. In other words we had usable information on 161 patients out of 223 (72%) - a rate, that was only possible with intensive and persisting attempts through all possible strategies ("Fig. 1").

Followup Rates for all Patients (n = 223) and all Surviving Patients (n = 199)

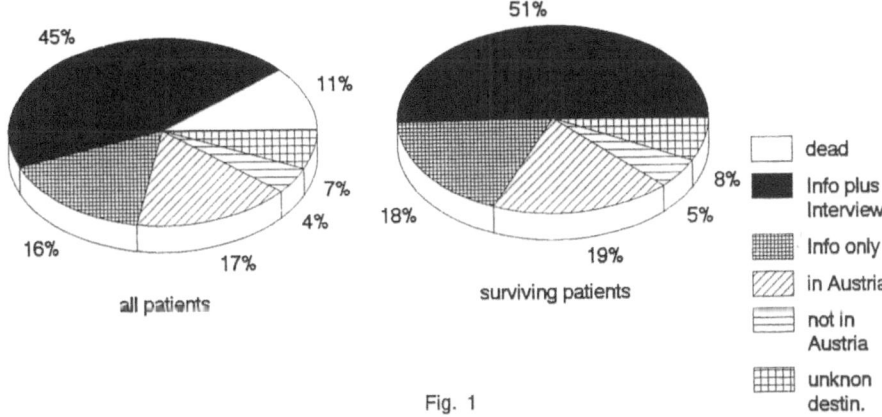

Fig. 1

About the remaining 62 patients (28%) we could find out that 10 had lived outside of Austria in the followup year, 37 had lived at an Austrian address, but didn't respond and 15 persons could not be traced at all.

Now some informations on the structure of the total sample at the relevant admission to the intensive care unit:

- the median age was 24 years (ranging from 15 through 38 years).

- 14% had been diagnosed as "Polydrug Abusers". "Polydrug Abuse" as understood here in correspondence to the clinic's diagnostic scheme, is not simply any multi-substance abuse, but restricted to a specific consumption pattern, where medical drugs play a central role to the patient's abuse pattern ("Fig. 4").

Diagnosis of all Patients (n = 223) in 1980/81

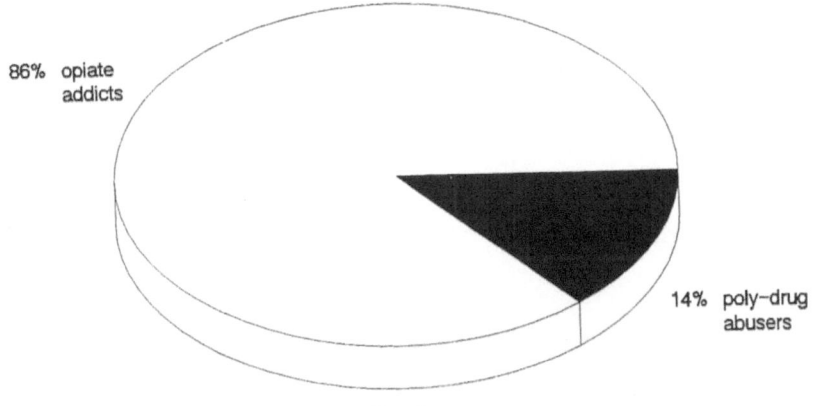

Fig. 4

The drug consumption pattern of the actually followed up population, excluding the patients who had died, five years after the admission to the intensive care unit (n=135) was as follows:

- 50 patients (37%) were classified as "drug-problem free" (at least for 3 month no misuse of medical drugs and no consumption of any other drugs eccept in some cases moderate alcohol consumption and/or sporadic cannabis consumption.

- 12 patients (9%) were inpatients in a longtime drug-therapy center.

- 11 patients (8%) were in an oral substituion therapy with Methadone.

- 10 patients (7%) were in prison.

- 35% were female ("Fig. 2").

Sex Ratio of all Patients (n = 223)

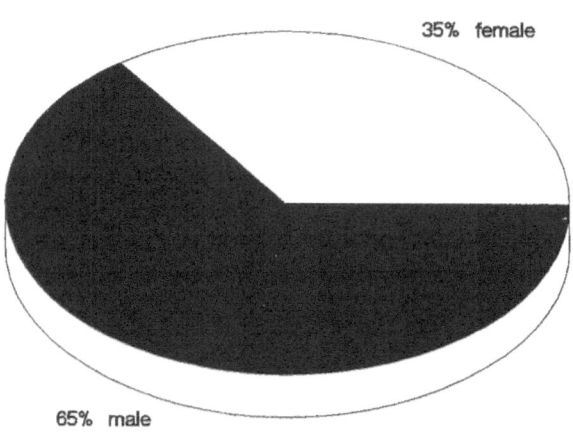

35% female

65% male

Fig. 2

- 42% had had a career of more than 4 years of opiate addiction ("Fig. 3").

Time of Opiate Addiction of all Patients (n = 223) till 1980/81

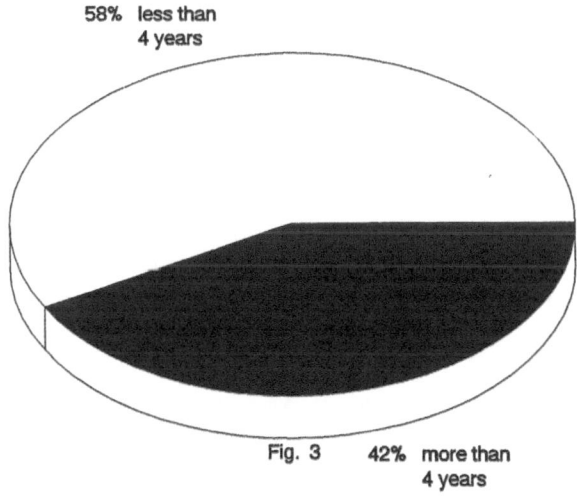

58% less than
4 years

Fig. 3   42% more than
4 years

- 14 patients (10%) had been misusing alcohol and/or medical drugs but no illicit drugs within the last three month prior to the followup interview.

- 38 patients (28%) had been using illicit drugs within the last three month prior to the followup interview. In case the only illicit drug was Cannabis, it had to be more than sporadious consumption to qualify for this category ("Fig. 5").

Outcome of all Patients (n = 223) and Followed Up Survivors (n = 135) in 1986/87

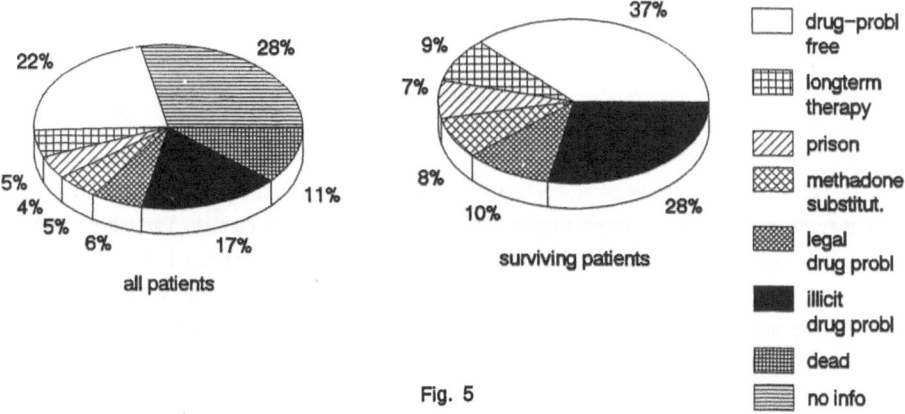

all patients

surviving patients

drug–probl free
longterm therapy
prison
methadone substitut.
legal drug probl
illicit drug probl
dead
no info

Fig. 5

These results show, that more than a third (37%) of the followed up survivors managed to be drug-free 5 years after admission to the intensive care unit and 9% were in a long-time drug therapy center. In other words roughly half of the patients were drug-free or attempting to reach freedom of drugs.

There can be no doubt that drug abstinence is a desireable goal for any addict. Our data suggest that patients with a strong inclination to abstinence achieve this goal much easier if their drug career is relatively short. Otherwise there can be no doubt, that a large number of addicts are not at all motivated towards abstinence. It makes little sense to force them into an abstinence oriented therapy trying to shorten their time of drug abuse. As time passes and circumstances change a relevant portion of them may mature out. Some of them will need and seek the help of an abstinence oriented therapy. Some addicts of course will never become motivated to quit drug consumption totally, but they will accept a substitution offer within a rather resticted setting. Some finally will want too keep up their drug habit and even reject maintainance with methadon.

The popular contraversy between the "early intervention approach" and the "maturing out approach" makes no sense, because both positions are right. They are based on data which are found in different sub-populations:

In therapy institutions with extensive motivation checking preparation you will find highly motivated patients and their prognoses is better if their drug career is short. If otherwise you do research on unselected addicts who showed no abstinece motivation for a long periode you will find that more individuals will become fed up with their state of life and for them in the long run abstinence becomes an increasingly desirable goal; they mature out.

If one exepts, that there are different subpopulations of addicts with different perspectives and possiblities, drug policy has to take care of all of them and not sacrifice one group for the sake of the other group or for professional interests.

For the highly motivated group it is essential to have enough capacities in abstinence oriented therapy facilities to treat them without a long delay and enough diversity to be ready for different needs and problem structures.

For patients, not ready to go for abstinence yet, but who might mature out, it is essential to offer counselling, medical advice and basic medical help, without stressing the abstinence goal. For these cases the goal has to be a different one: To minimize the damage to their health as long as they do not qualify for an abstinence approach and to forward them to the proper facilities once their motivation towards abstinence rises. If the pressure on the patients is too high they will stay away, with negative consequences to their physical state. In this general health approach methadone maintanance can play an important role, keeping the addicts in close contact to the health-care system. Patients have to show up regularly in order to get their methadone supply and therefore can be checked and advised physically, socially and psychologically. Problems arising out of relapses, - consumption of bad quality drugs, intravenous injections etc. - cannot be ruled out, but their impact can be reduced.

This general health approach takes also care of patients who will never mature out and stay either on methadone maintainance or their original drug consumption pattern for the rest of their lives.

We came to these postulations for a realistic and diversified care approach for all different subtypes of addicts looking into the health state of our study population.

Concerning the AIDS issue, it has to be understood, that our followup interviews took place 1986 or 1987 shortly after HIV-testing had come in use.

59% of the interviewed individuals (n = 100) had undergone an HIV-test before the followup interview. A differential look at the data shows that only 19% of the patients who were "drug-problem free" at the followup time had undergone an HIV-test, - understandable enough -, while 82% of the patients who had not given up their drug abuse had undergone testing. 12% of the tested patients turned out to be HIV-infected.

The studied population overall was found to be in a rather bad state of health, including hepatitis or other disturbancies of the hepatic system (78-85%), gastric troubles, mostly gastric ulcers (48%), infections or diseases of the skin (up to 40%), lymphatic edema (10%), etc. ("Fig. 6").

State of Health of Interviewed Patients (n = 100) in 1986/87

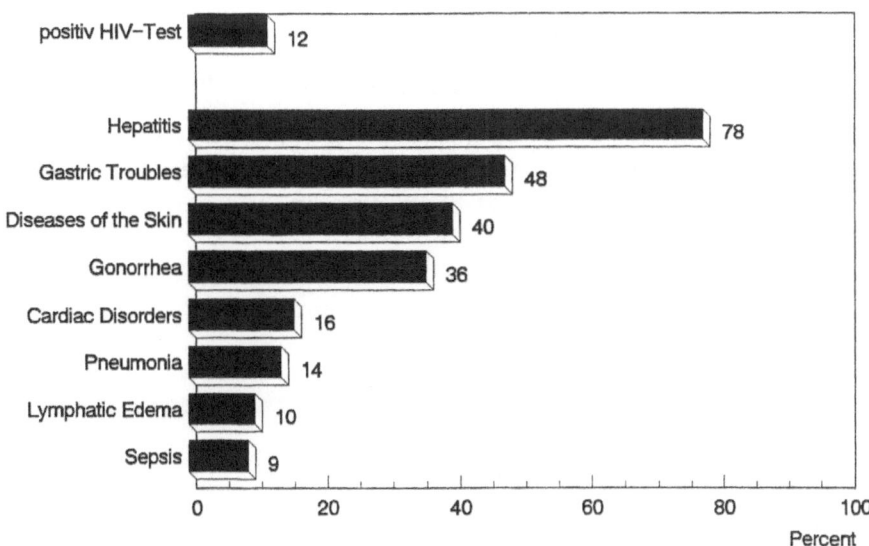

Fig. 6

As can be seen, it is not the AIDS virus alone, that endangers the health of the drug addicts, but that there is a whole variety of well-known medical complications connected with drug abuse and with specific patterns of abuse. AIDS is only new, sensational and seen as a risk for the general population coming from the addicted sub-culture. But even without AIDS the live-span of a heroin addict has to be expected to be reduced markedly under the now existing social and political circumstances.

The bad health state of opiate addict is partly dependent from their drug abuse but also from variables of their life style. Traditionally it has been rather difficult to bring an addicted individual in contact with the medical care system. The renewed interest in the medical aspects of drug abuse and of course the necessity to know about AIDS/HIV prevalence rates leads away to a more medicalised attitude in the treatment of the addictions. Among these medical facilities Methadone-treatment stands out. All these new developments have made it easier to bring opiate addicts in contact with the medical care and to hold them in the care system for the time of their drug abuse. Therefore it is possible to improve the state of health of these individuals and to give them the opportunity to live a less risky life even if staying addicted. Close contact to medical care can also reduce the damage that may develop after a relaps into a more risky pattern of abuse.

All these issues are very important not only for improvement of the health state of the opiate addicts, but also for the minimization of risks for the general population.

We hope that this attitude on drug abuse will stay with us and will not only be concerned with the linkage between drug abuse and AIDS. Some medical problems of drug abuse will linger even if medical science will develop new possibilities to combat the spread of the AIDS-virus or the illness itself in a more efficient way.

Literature:

Uhl A, Springer A, Maritsch F, Pfersmann V, Presslich O, Mayer, A (1988) Opiatabhängigkeit: Eine katamnestische Untersuchung an opiatabhängigen Patienten nach stationärer Entzugsbehandlung über den Zeitraum 1980/81 bis 1986/87. Bundeskanzleramt. Wien (Originalarbeiten, Studien, Forschungsberichte, Vol. 2/88)

Antibody Prevalence of Parenterally Transmitted Viruses (HIV-1, HTLV-I, HBV, HCV) in Austrian Intravenous Drug Users

J. Pont, C. Neuwald, and G. Salzner

Sonderanstalt Wien-Favoriten, Hardtmuthgasse 42, A-1100 Wien, Austria

Abstract

From 1985 to 1990 the sera of 372 recently imprisoned intravenous drug users (IDU) were tested for HIV-1 antibodies. The seroprevalence was 18 %, males 16 % and females 31 %. HIV-1 seroprevalence in Austrian IDU has not increased since 1986. All sera tested for HTLV-I-antibodies were negative. The majority of the HIV-1 seropositive drug users had been infected before 1985. The reported frequency of needle sharing has decreased since 1986. Of 151 IDU tested for HCV antibodies 75 % were positive for anti-HCV, 68 % were positive for hepatitis B markers, 59 % were positive both for HBV and HCV markers, and 13 % were positive for HIV-1 antibodies. In conclusion: In Austrian IDU HIV-1 seroprevalence has not increased since 1986; HTLV-I infection has not yet entered; HCV seems to be the most frequent parenterally transmitted virus.

Introduction

The purpose of this study was 1.) to examine the course of HIV-1 antibody prevalence since 1985 in Austrian intravenous drug users (IDU) 2.) to find out whether human T-cell leukemia virus type I (HTLV-I) has entered the population of Austrian IDU and 3.) to test the prevalence of antibodies against hepatitis C virus (HCV) in comparison with hepatitis B markers and anti-HIV-1 in IDU. In addition we intended to

118

collect data on risk behaviour of imprisoned IDU and on possible exposure to infection with these viruses during detention.

Materials and Methods

In the Sonderanstalt Wien-Favoriten, a penal institution with therapeutic facilities for male drug addicts, from 1985 to 1990 all newly admitted prisoners were offered blood tests for markers of hepatitis B (HBs-antigen., anti-HBc, anti-HBs), anti-HIV-1 and alanin aminotransferase (ALAT). From 1986 to 1988 the same blood tests were offered to female prisoners in the penal institution Schwarzau. 97 % of all male prisoners and 98 % of male IDU and 98 % of female prisoners underwent the offered blood tests. Medical history was focussed on drug use and risk behaviour for parenteral virus infection. 661 prisoners, 419 men and 242 women, were examined, 327 of the men and 45 of the women had a history of intravenous drug use. Median age was 27 years (18 to 44 years) and 25 years (19 to 35) for male and female IDU respectively. The sera of 270 male prisoners, 151 of them intravenous drug users, were tested for anti-HTLV-I (Serodia ATLA, Fujirebio Inc., Tokyo, Japan) and anti-HCV (Ortho HCV antibody ELISA system) as well. Anti-HIV-1 was assayed with the Abbot Recombinant HIV-1 EIA, the confirmation test was Western blot (Institute of Virology Vienna).

Results

HIV-1 antibody prevalence: None of the 289 prisoners who never had used drugs intravenously and also none of the female prisoners who had been engaged in prostitution and never had injected drugs were positive for HIV-1 antibodies. HIV-1 antibody prevalence data of newly imprisoned IDU from 1985 to 1990 is shown in table 1. The overall prevalence is 18 %, 16 % for male and 31 % for female IDU. Since 1986 there has been no increase of anti-HIV-1 prevalence rates in this population.

Table 1
HIV-1 antibody prevalence of
newly imprisoned IDU from 1985 to 1990

		1985	1986	1987	1988	1989	1990	1985–1990
IDU tested	n	76	101	71	45	49	30	372
	male	76	78	58	36	49	30	327
	female	-	23	13	9	-	-	45
anti HIV-1 pos	n	12(16%)	25(25%)	17(24%)	2(4%)	6(12%)	5(17%)	67(18%)
	male	12(16%)	16(21%)	12(21%)	2(6%)	6(12%)	5(17%)	53(16%)
	female	-	9(39%)	5(38%)	0	-	-	14(31%)

Anti-HTLV-I prevalence: in none of 270 sera, 151 of which
being sera of IDU, were anti HTLV-I antibodies present.
Hepatitis B and hepatitis C markers: 114 of 151 (75 %) sera
of IDU were positive for anti-HCV, whereas 9 of 119 (8 %) of
non-IDU were positive. Prevalence of anti-HCV, hepatitis B
markers, anti HIV-1 and anti-HTLV-I in IDU reveal HCV to be
the most frequent parenterally transmitted virus in IDU, as
shown in table 2.

Table 2
Prevalence of anti-HCV, any HB marker
anti-HIV-1 and anti-HTLV-I in IDU

	IDU n=151
Anti-HCV positive	114 (75 %)
Any HB marker pos.	102 (68 %)
Anti-HIV-1 positive	20 (13 %)
Anti-HTLV-I positive	0

19 of 20 anti-HIV-1 positive IDU were positive for anti-HCV
(95 %), 17 were positive for any hepatitis B marker and 16
were positive both for anti-HCV and hepatitis B markers. The
frequency of multiple infections with HCV, HBV and HIV-1 is
demonstrated in table 3.

Table 3
Frequency of multiple infections
with HCV, HBV and HIV-1 in IDU

			IDU n=151
HCV + HBV + HIV-1	16 (11 %)
HCV + HBV -	89 (59 %)
HCV - + HIV-1	3 (2 %)
- HBV + HIV-1	1 (0,7 %)
HCV - -	21 (14 %)
- HBV + -	12 (8 %)
- - -	23 (15 %)

Chronic hepatitis: Chronic liver disease was assumed in case
of an increase of alanin aminotransferase (ALAT) by more
than 50 U/l for at least 6 months. Hepatitis B marker and
anti-HCV of these patients are listed in table 4. In IDU
with probable hepatitis B as well as hepatitis Non A Non B
the prevalence of HCV was higher than 80 %.

Table 4
IDU with chronic hepatitis
(ALAT >50 U/l for at least 6 months)

		Anti HCV pos
HBsAG positive	8	7 (88 %)
Anti-HBc positive anti HBs negative	19	16 (84 %)
Non A Non B hepatitis (=negative HB markers or anti-HBs pos)	32	26 (81 %)
	59	49 (83 %)

History of intravenous drug use and risk behaviour
The average duration of intravenous drug use was 7 years
(0 to 22 years). Frequent needle sharing was admitted by
92 % of IDU; by 95 % and 80 % of IDU examined before and
after the end of 1987, respectively. The last instance of
needle sharing was dated back an average of 8 months (2 to
17 months) by the IDU admitted before the end of 1987 and 34
months (4 to 40 months) by the IDU imprisoned since 1988. In
retrospect exposure to HIV-infection by needle sharing
and/or sexual contact with HIV-seropositive partners was
reported by 79 of 327 (24 %) of male IDU and by 39 of 52

(75 %) male HIV-seropositive IDU. 92 of 327 (28 %) male IDU and 16 of 52 male HIV seropositive male IDU had a history of other sexually transmitted diseases.

21 prisoners asked for retesting their HIV-1 antibody serostatus because of putative or real exposure to HIV infection during detention. 9 of 21 did not want to comment on the kind of exposure, 6 admitted needle sharing, one had shared the tatooing instrument with a HIV-seropositive IDU, one reported both homosexual contact and needle sharing and one had pricked his finger with an injection needle which had been hidden in potting earth. 3 prisoners felt exposed after having come to blows with bleeding injuries and bites. Up to now in non of these cases a seroconversion was assessed.

Discussion

The prevalence of both parenterally and sexually transmissible viruses in IDU is of particular epidemiological importance for the spreading of these viruses beyond the classical risk populations. (Velimirovic 1987). The majority of epidemiological data on IDU comes from detention centers as detailed examination of IDU is often difficult in outpatient wards or guidance centers for drug addicts due to the irregular life style of these patients. (Köhler 1986, Krasser 1986, Pont 1986, 1989, Fuchs 1988, Sauer 1987). According to Zoulek (1986) there are no differences in HIV-1 prevalence of IDU from prisons, guidance centers and treatment institutions. Our data is collected from the two Austrian detention institutions with the highest concentration of IDU: Sonderanstalt Wien-Favoriten is the Austrian penal institution with treatment facilities for male drug addicts and Strafvollzugsanstalt Schwarzau is the detention center for female prisoners. Both prisons serve all Austrian provinces and thus represent the Austrian average in respect to prevalence data of imprisoned IDU.

HIV-1 antibody prevalence in female IDU exceeds that in male IDU in this study as well as in reports by others (Köhler 1986, Krasser 1986, Zoulek 1986, Harms 1987, Heckmann 1987). This may be due to the lower information level of female IDU resulting in less careful handling of contaminated needles and syringes (Arnold 1987) and/or the higher probability of infection in heterosexual intercourse.

The majority of studies in HIV-1 antibody prevalence in IDU in Europe reported a steady annual increase. In Italy the HIV-1 antibody prevalence in IDU rose between 1980 and 1985 from 0 to 53 % (Ferroni 1985); in Spain 1983-1985 from 11 % to 48 % (Rodrigo 1985), in Barcelona 1984-1987 from 62 % to 78 % (Tor 1987). In Switzerland there was an increase of anti-HIV-1 in IDU between 1982 and 1985 from 16 % to 32 % (Mortimer 1985); in Germany 1983 to 1985 from 10 % to 24 % (Zoulek 1986) and in Berlin 1982-1986 from 18 % to 68 % (Harms 1987). According to our data in Austrian IDU there has been no increase of anti-HIV-1 seroprevalence since 1986 just as in studies from the Austrian Tyrol (Fuchs 1988) and from Berlin (Püschel 1988). The possible reasons for this might be: a) A change of behaviour concerning the use of contaminated injection utensils and a decrease of the frequency of needle sharing. Purchasing needles and syringes in pharmacies and whole sale stores has been remarkably facilitated in Austria. b) Drug addicts of younger age and newcomers in the drug scene in Austria and Germany incline towards non-intravenous drug use and non-opioid drugs (Reuband 1987).

In the USA antibodies against HTLV-I, which is associated with adult T-cell leukemia and tropical spastic paraparesis, have prevalences up to 9 % in white IDU and up to 49 % in black IDU (Mildvan 1988, Weiss 1987). In Italian IDU HTLV-I seroprevalences up to 5 % (Gradilone 1986) and 27 % (De Rossi 1986) have been observed. Both in the USA and Italy endemic HTLV-I clusters have been recognized, but endemic prevalence rates were exceeded by prevalence rates in IDU. In spite of rather frequent tourist traffic of Austrian IDU to Italy (Pont 1986), so far there has been no detectable invasion of HTLV-I into Austrian and German IDU (Pont 1989, Fuchs 1988, Krämer 1988).

The 30 % incidence of other sexually transmitted diseases in IDU gives rise to fears that sexual transmission of retroviruses might become as important as needle sharing in the drug using population and that HIV-infection will continue to spread from IDU to non-drug-users by sexual transmission.

In addition to the wellknown frequency of hepatitis B virus infections in IDU, parenterally transmitted Non A Non B virus infections have been postulated for a long time (Mosley 1977) and their importance for chronicity in hepatitis of IDU has been emphasized (Pont 1983), The recently developed recombinant-based immunoassay for serum anti-HCV (Kuo 1989) revealed HCV to be the major causal agent of Non A Non B hepatitis in IDU as well as in other patients with parenteral exposure (Esteban 1989). The seroprevalence of anti-HCV in this study ranges among the highest reported prevalences of HCV in IDU. In Austrian IDU HCV seems to be the most frequent parenterally transmitted virus.

REFERENCES

Arnold Th, Frietsch R: Zur AIDS-Problematik in der Drogen-
    arbeit (1987). Suchtgefahren 4, 237-247

De Rossi A, Dalla Gassa O, Del Mistro A: HTLV-III and
    HTLV-I infection in populations at risk in the Veneto
    region of Italy (1986). Eur J Cancer Clin Oncol. 36,
    557-559

Esteban JI, Esteban R, Viladomin L et al: Hepatitis C
    virus antibodies among risk groups in Spain (1989)
    Lancet ii: 294-296

Ferroni P, Geroldi D, Galli C, Zanetti AR, Carguel A:
    HTLV-III antibodies among Italien drug addicts.
    (1985) Lancet ii: 52-53

Fuchs D, Unterweger B, Hausen A et al: Anti-HIV-1 antibodies, anti-HTLV-I antibodies and Neopterin levels in parenteral drug addicts in the Austrian Tyrol. Journal of Acquired Immune Deficiency Syndromes (1988) 1: 65-66

Gradilone A, Zani G, Barillari G et al: HTLV-I and HIV infection in drug addicts in Italy. Lancet (1986) ii: 753-754

Harms G, Bienzle U, Schneider V, Bschor F: HIV-Antikörperprävalenz bei Berliner Drogenabhängigen AIFO (1987) 2: 392-393

Heckmann W, Seyrer Y: AIDS und Drogenabhängigkeit: Stand der Dinge. Suchtgefahren (1987) 33: 337-345

Köhler H, Lange W, Rex W, Koch MA, L'age-Stehr J: Antibodies to LAV/HTLV-III in Berlin prison inmates with risk factors for hepatitis B from 1980-1985. Proceedings of the II. International Conference on AIDS (1986) 121

Krämer A, Goedert JJ, Blattner WA, Marcus U: No evidence of HTLV-I infection in intravenous drug abusers in West-Germany. Journal of Acquired Immunodeficiency Syndromes (1988) 1: 163-164

Krasser C et al: Bundesgesundheitsblatt (1986) 26: 343

Kuo G, Choo QL, Alter HJ et al: An assay for circulating antibodies to a major etiologic virus of human non-A, non-B hepatitis. Science (1989) 244: 362-364

Mildvan D, Des Jarlais D, Sotheran J et al: Prevalence and significance of HTLV-I in a cohort of intravenous drug users in New York. Proceedings IV. International Conference on AIDS, Stockholm (1988) abstr. 4517

Mortimer PP, Vandervelde EM, Jesson WJ, Pereira MS, Burkhardt F: HTLV-III antibody in Swiss and English intravenous drug abusers. Lancet (1985) ii: 449-450

Mosley JW, Redeker AG, Feinstone SM, Purcell RH: Multiple hepatitis viruses in multiple attacks of acute viral hepatitis. N Engl J Med (1977) 296: 75-78

Pont J: Untersuchungen an alkohol- und drogenabhängigen Untergebrachten hinsichtlich chronischer Lebererkrankungen. Wien Zschr Suchtforsch (1983) 6: 55-57

Pont J, Neuwald Ch, Kunz Ch, Werdenich W:HTLV-III-Sero-
    logie, Epidemiologie und Klinik inhaftierter i.v. drogen-
    abhängiger Männer in Österreich. Wien Klin Wochenschr
    (1986) 98: 454-457

Pont J, Neuwald Ch, Lichtenauer B, Salzner G: Keine
    Prävalenzzunahme von HIV-1 und HTLV-I-Antikörpern bei
    i.v.-Drogenabhängigen in Österreich während 1985-1988
    AIFO (1989) 4: 198-201

Püschel K, Liske K, Laufs R: Entwicklung der HIV-1-Anti-
    körperprävalenz bei Rauschgifttoten in Berlin und Hamburg.
    AIFO (1988) 3: 452-454

Reuband KH: Drogenstatistik 1986. Informationsdienst der
    Deutschen Hauptstelle gegen die Suchtgefahren (1987)
    40-70

Rodrigo JM, Serra MA, Aquilar E:HTLV-III antibodies in drug
    addicts in Spain. Lancet (1985) ii:156-157

Sauer A, Behnken LJ, Rübsamen-Waigmann H, Brede HD,
    Helm EB: HIV-Infektion in der Justizvollzugsanstalt 1
    Frankfurt am Main. AIFO (1987) 2: 502-507

Tor J, Muga R, Melus R, Ginesta C, Ribera A, Foz M: HIV
    infection prevalence in intravenous drug abusers in
    Barcelona 1984-1987. European Conference on Clinical
    Aspects of HIV Infection, Brussels (1987) abstr. 23

Velimirovic B: AIDS und Drogenabhängigkeit aus der Sicht
    des Epidemidogen. AIFO (1987) 2: 323-334

Weiss SH, Ginzburg HM, Saxinger WC: Emerging high rates of
    human T-cell Lymphotropic virus type I and HIV infection
    among U.S. drug abusers. III. International Conference
    on AIDS. Washington D.C. (1987) abstr. F6.5.

Zoulek G, Gürtler L, Eberle J, Lorbeer B, Deinhardt F:
    Zunahme der Prävalenz von Antikörpern gegen LAV/ HTLV III
    bei Drogenabhängigen in der Bundesrepublik Deutschland.
    DMW (1986) 111: 567-570

Statistical Investigation on the Relation of Intravenous Drug Addiction and HIV-Infection. A Survey of the Years 1985 to 1989 by the Institute of Forensic Medicine in Vienna

D. Risser, W. Vycudilik, G. Bauer, and Ch. Reiter

Institute of Forensic Medicine, University of Vienna, Sensengasse 2,
A-1090 Wien, Austria

Introduction

About ten years ago the first cases of AIDS (acquired immune deficiency syndrome) were reported to the Centers for Diseases Control (CDC), and about seven years ago the etiological agent, HIV-1 (human immunodeficiency virus type 1), was discovered (Anderson 1988). HIV infection is spread by sexual contact, by infected blood or blood products, and perinatally by mother to infant. Regardless of the portal entry of the virus, the common denominator of HIV infection is a selective tropism of the virus for certain cells of the immune system and the central nervous system. It results in immunosuppression and neuropsychiatric abnormalities (Fauci 1988). Transmission of AIDS by intravenous drug users (IVDUs) became apparent early in the AIDS epidemic when increasing numbers of heterosexual drug addicts in New York and New Jersey were diagnosed with opportunistic infections. As the AIDS epidemic has progressed, IVDUs have consistently comprised the second largest risk group among AIDS patients reported to the Centers for Diseases Control (Chaisson 1987). Forensic implications due to this risk group are increasing, and therefore postmortem HIV-antibody testing is performed when dead IVDUs have to be examined at the Institute of Forensic Medicine in Vienna.

Methods

At the Institute of Forensic Medicine in Vienna 149 corpses of drug addicts were examined between 1985 and 1989. Their addiction was proved either by their history or by the final autopsy report. Blood samples have been drawn whenever possible to carry out serological investigations. In most cases the post-mortem examination was postponed for 24 hours. If an infection by the HI-virus was ascertained, an autopsy could be made under essentially improved hygienic care. Furthermore the possibility that the deceased might just have been in the phase of seroconversion can never been excluded. To minimize the risk of infection protecting glasses, masks and chain-gloves are used whenever corpses are examined that belong to this risky group.

But not all corpses could be subjected to the tests. In some cases no blood could be taken because of considerable changes due to decay.

Age and sex distribution of IVDUs were analysed.

When determining their cause of death all investigated corpses were also tested by gas chromatography in respect to blood alcohol, as alcohol might increase the effect of centrally acting drugs.

To provide information on the intervall between drug adminstration and death, the morphine concentrations in the medullla oblongata and the cerebellum have been determined (Vycudilik 1988). If this period had been short, the ratio of $C_{med}:C_{cer}$ was below 1. The ratio exceeded 1 if at least a number of hours had passed. The data referred to were found by means of gas chromatography/mass spectrometry.

Results

Considering that in Vienna the total number of post-mortem examinations for legal proceedings between 1985 and 1989 mounts to 2750, the number of examined drug addicts represents a share of 5,4 per cent (n = 149). During the same period 295 people died on drugs in Austria; this means that about 50 per cent of them were examined at the

Viennese institute. Among these 149 drug addicts there were
91 intravenous drug users (IVDUs) whose parenteral drug
abuse was confirmed by their history and/or needle marks -
revealed at the autopsy.

69 IVDUs have been tested for HIV-antibodies. In 22 cases a
HIV-infection could be proved, indicating a HIV-prevalence
of 32 per cent. The ratio men:women among parenteral drug
users was 4:1. Female IVDUs showed a far higher HIV-
prevalence - about 45 per cent - than male drug addicts
with 29 per cent.

In 21 examined IVDUs an ethanol concentrations between 0,3
and 2,33 mg/g could be found. In respect to its
distribution peak alcohol concentration significantly
accumulates at 1,2 mg/g.

Only 1 female, a HIV-positive iv-drug addict showed an
elevated ethanol concentration of 0,65 mg/g. Among the
males one HIV-infected IVDU showed 0,85 mg/g.

Though the alcohol concentration is rather low it must be
taken into consideration that even a low concentration,
combined with centrally acting drugs, may increase the
effect and thus become a root cause for death. A longer
survival period leads to a decrease of an originally higher
blood alcohol concentration with an average rate of 0,1 mg
per hour.

As syringes near the body and/or histologically fresh
needle marks were found at the autopsy, intravenous drug
administration was evident in 47 cases. 12 other persons,
known as predominant IVDUs, had orally taken the drug,
whereas the last mode of application could not be
ascertained in further 30 cases. In order to prove oral
consumption, relatively high amounts in the range of
milligrams of opiates must be detected in the stomach and
intestine lumen. But as these alkaloids are reabsorbed into
the stomach the interpretation of results meets with
difficulties.

In two cases the drug could be detected in the mucous
membrane of the nose, which proved that the drug was
sniffed.

48 per cent of the IVDUs died from an overdose of morphine/heroine. 26 per cent of the deaths were caused by abuse of barbiturates and 14 per cent by a combination of both, opiates and barbiturates. A variety of drug combinations, such as opiates with codeine and/or cocaine was found in 9 per cent of the cases. In a single case the stimulant fencamphamine could be verified among this group of polytoxicomanic drug mortalities. 3 per cent did not show a basic relationship between death and intravenous consumption of drugs. Deaths were caused by natural illnesses, such as pneumonia and heart-diseases. One person had committed suicide by slashing his wrists.

In 36 cases of death caused by intravenous application of morphine/heroine, a determination of the cerebral distribution was available. 31 per cent showed the ratio below 1, with an average concentration of 435+/-698 Ng/g in the medulla oblongata; in contrast to this cases with the ratio above 1 revealed a average drug concentration of 315+/-438 Ng/g. Due to the small number of investigated cases, it is impossible to interpret the differences between HIV-positive and HIV-negative intravenous drug cases.

Discussion

Parallel to a significant increase of drug mortalities in Vienna within the years 1985 to 1989 the number of HIV-infections increased continually. This growing tendency could be traced with males as well as with females (Table 1). This is in contrast to the findings of Püschel et. al. (1990), who showed a slight decrease of the HIV-prevalence in 1988 in several German cities. Loimer et al. (1990) investigated injecting drug users at the drug addiction outpatient ward of the Psychiatric University Clinic of Vienna. HIV-antibodies were found up to 29.7 per cent in 1989, similar to our findings with 32 per cent among dead IVDUs. These data corresponds to the results of several recent studies on HIV-infection among IVDUs rating from 18.9 per cent (Koblin 1990) to 46.5 per cent (Page 1990).

The far higher HIV-prevalence among female IVDUs -
comparable to the results of Püschel - may be ascribed to
prostitution. Chandrasekar et al. (1990) found among
parenteral drug abusers (PDAs), hospitalized at Detroit
Receiving Hospital that older drug addicts mainly comprise
men, similar to our group of examined drug deaths. The
average male intravenous drug addict dies at the age of 27.
In contrast to women's life expectancy, which is usually by
far higher, the average female intravenous drug addict dies
at about 23. A correlation between HIV-infection on one
hand and alcohol comsuption, concentration of used drug or
drug type on the other could not be established in our
study.

Table 1. Prevalence of HIV antibodies among dead intravenous drug users in Vienna 1985-1990

IVDUs	1985	1986	1987	1988	1989
total #	16	15	15	23	22
tested for HIV	4	12	12	21	20
females tested	0	3	3	3	2
females infected	0	0	2	3	0
males tested	4	9	9	18	18
males infected	3	2	2	5	5

HIV-testing in the course of autopsies of drug deaths are,
for two reasons, necessary: first, to minimize the risk of
infection, second to check the spreading of the HI-virus
within the population.

References

Anderson RM, Robert MM (1988) Epidemiological parameters of
HIV transmission. Nature 333:514-519

Chaisson RE, Onishi R, Moss AR, et al. (1987) Human
immunodeficiency virus infection in heterosexual

intravenous drug users in San Francisco. Am. J. Public Health 77:169-72

Chandrasekar PH, Chitwood DD, Klimas NG, Smith PC, Fletcher MA (1990) Risk Factors for HIV-Infection Among Parenteral Drug Abusers in a Low-Prevalence Area. Souther Medical Journal 9:996-1001

Fauci AS (1988) The Human Immunodeficiency Virus: Infectivity and Mechanisms of Pathogenesis. Science 239:617-622

Koblin BA, McCusker J, Lewis BF and Sullivan JL (1990) Racial/Ethnic differences in HIV-1 seroprevalence and risky behavior among intravenous drug users in a multisite study. American Journal of Epidemiology 5:837-846

Loimer N, Presslich O, Hollerer E, Pakesch G, Pfersman V & Werner E (1990) Monitoring HIV-1 infection prevalence among intravenous drug users in Vienna 1986-1990. AIDS CARE 3:281-286

Page JB, Lai S, Chitwood DD, Klimas NG, Smith PC, Fletcher MA (1990) HTLV-I/II seropositivity and death from AIDS among HIV-1 seropositive intravenous drug users. Lancet 335:1439-1441

Püschel K, Mohsenian F, Bornemann R, Bschor F, Schneider V, Penning R, Spann W, von Karger J, Madea B, Metter D (1990) Prevalence of HIV-1 infection among deaths connected with drug abuse in various West German cities an in West Berlin between 1985 and 1988. Z Rechtsmedizin 103:407-414

Vycudilik W (1988) Comparative Morphine Determination in Brain Segments by GC/MC. A Means of Determining the Survivel Time. Z Rechtsmedizin 99:263-272

HIV-1 Infection Among Intravenous Drug Users in Vienna 1986–1991

N. Loimer, O. Presslich, E. Werner, G. Pakesch, E. Hollerer,
V. Pfersmann, and H. Vedovelli

University of Vienna, Department of Psychiatry, Waehringer Guertel 18–20,
A-1090 Wien, Austria

INTRODUCTION

Current research and clinical experience with AIDS in the population of intravenous drug users demonstrates that members of this group have multiple opportunities for exposure to HIV (Friedland & Klein 1987). Following the introduction of HIV into a community of intravenous drug users (IVDUs), it may infect over 50% of individuals within three to four years (Des Jarlais et al. 1988), the potential for a major heterosexual epidemic remains a subject of speculation (Johnson, 1988). The time until AIDS diagnosis after infection is estimated with a mean of 9.8 years (Bacchetti & Moss 1990). The second wave of HIV epidemic in Europe has already formed the injecting drug users into the major component of this epidemic. There has been a dramatic increase in the incidence of AIDS among IVDUs in Europe (Ferroni et al.1985; Fuchs et al. 1985; Ancelle-Park et al. 1987; Robertson et al. 1986, Harms et al. 1987; France et al. 1988; Loimer et al. 1990a) and in the United States (Chamberland et al. 1984; Des Jarlais et al. 1987; Drucker 1987; Allen et al. 1988; Hahn et al. 1989). In Europe higher though less than exponential rates of growth are observed among intravenous drug users. Projections of total cumulated cases to the end of 1991 lie in the range of 23,000 - 33,000 cases among this group (Downs et al. 1990).

It is a characteristic feature of the epidemiology of HIV-1 and AIDS among injecting drug users that there are very marked geographical variations in levels of infection. In Europe, there is a noticable north to south division in the rates of seropositivity, with higher rates occurring in the south (Ancelle-Park et al. 1987; Robertson et al. 1986; France et al. 1988). Transmission of HIV-1 can occur when IVDUs share syringes and needles that contain blood from other IVDUs already HIV-1 infected (Marmor et al. 1987; Wodak et al. 1987; Schoenbaum et al. 1989) or other injection equipment (Loimer et al. 1991). Traditional efforts to clean syringes between uses showed only slight evidence of being protective (Chaisson et al. 1987). Ghodse et al. (1986) described the marked changes in self-reported sharing of needles and syringes after the awareness of the risks became more widespread. Syringe exchange has been a cornerstone of HIV prevention strategies for people who inject drugs. They reach many of those taking risks, but they do not attract all those drug users who engage in the most risky activities (Stimson et al. 1988; Hart et al. 1989). These results suggested that educational information and dissemination of knowledge and facts concerning the high risk involved, prevented parts of the injecting population from further harm, but focussed mainly on the use of sterile needles and syringes (Robertson et al. 1988).

With the emergence of AIDS, effective treatment of IVDUs has become even more crucial. For opiate abuse, however, methadone treatment represents a widely offered and extensively accepted modality (Bschor, 1986; Ball et al. 1988; Cooper 1989; Dole 1989; Selwyn et al. 1989; Sorensen et al. 1989; Novick et al. 1990). In consideration of the spread of HIV-1 infection through the heterosexual population, it must be pointed out that sexual contact among drug injectors and others plays an all important role, because IVDUs represent a possible source of danger in being sexual partners of healthy people (Brown et al. 1987; Moss, 1987; Johnson 1988; France et al. 1988, Donoghoe et al. 1989; Battjes et al. 1990; Loimer et al. 1990c). Sexual partners of IVDUs who themselves do not inject, risk infection through sexual contact. This may be an important route of transmission or bridge between HIV-positive injecting drug users and the non injecting population (Donoghoe et al. 1989).

The current knowledge of the dynamics of transmission among drug injectors and their sexual partners is incomplete. The data collected and presented here however should help to increase the understanding of risks for HIV-1 infection and transmission in a European city. Statistics on current numbers of diagnosed AIDS cases reflect patterns of infection some 8 to 10 years earlier. At present, AIDS remains a disease for which there is neither a cure nor an effective treatment. Therefore, prevention measures are the only actions which offer real hope for at-risk populations (Peterson & Marin 1988). Today intravenous drug users comprise the largest at-risk group for AIDS and HIV-1 infection in Austria. The human immunodeficiency virus is forcing a fundamental re-examination of our models for understanding drug misuse and, in particular, a reappraisal of the aims and methods of responding to the drug taker.

OPIATES AND THE AUSTRIAN LAW

In Austria, the First Opium Act (1928) drew heavily from international conventions and proceedings. During the Nazi occupation their laws regulated drug affairs. After the liberation of Austria in 1945, a new opium act was passed in 1946, amended in 1948 and 1951. The most recent amendment was made in 1985. Austria signed the Single Convention on Narcotic Drugs of New York in the revised version. The advent of AIDS in Austria provided a spur to the development of new strategies for drug users.

On September 25th, 1987, methadone was legalized for therapeutic use in case of:

1.) long-term drug addiction with intravenous application of the drug, and several unsuccessful withdrawal therapies and/or

2.) opiate addiction through intravenous application of the drug along with an existing HIV-1 infection.

The criteria for methadone maintenance are as followed:

- the application mode is obligatory
- the patient is under the supervision of his doctor
  (urine analyses for all drugs of abuse)
- the patient is not allowed to refuse additional treatments
  (for example psychotherapy)
- the patient has to avoid any use of narcotic drugs
- the treatment has to be reported to the authorities

On January 8th, 1991, the "methadone act" was ammended according to the experiences obtained during the last four years. At present the entire treatment is regulated unfortunately the daily oral dose was fixed in a range between 40 to 150 mg on a once a day basis. No emphasis was given to therapeutic drug monitoring and to individual differences in metabolism. The main problem with this new regulation is that there are no therapeutic communities or other settings available for patients under methadone treatment.

OPIATE ABUSE IN AUSTRIA

After the Second World War, only several hundred morphine addicts, mainly doctors, nurses and war disabled, were registered and their illness was dealt with by prescribing a long - term treatment of morphine. In the mid-sixties, this situation changed rapidly. In 1970, the number of drug users was estimated at 10, 000; about 500 injected raw opium. Until today, the number of illegal drug users has constantly been increasing. In 1980, the number of registered heroin addicts was 1, 230. In regard to an important estimated number of unknown cases, there must have been 8, 000 to 10, 000 heroin addicts. Today the estimated number of heroin addicts varies from 10, 000 - 20, 000. In addition to heroin, "opiumtea" is consumed by some Austrian opiate addicts exclusively, or when heroin is difficult to obtain. This opiumtea is extracted from dried poppy-heads. Depending on the country of origin, they contain a considerable amount of substances that can be found in raw opium.

METHOD AND SAMPLE

Beginning in December 1985, a standardized method to monitor HIV-1 infection levels and trends among injecting drug users (IVDUs) has periodically been administered at the drug dependence outpatient ward of the Psychiatric University Clinic of Vienna. This has helped to develop an effective program to reduce the further spread of HIV-1 among drug users. A climate in which there is no stigma attached to HIV testing was created at our outpatient clinic, and this made this study possible. All IVDUs treated at the clinic in December 1985/January 1986, December 1986/January 1987, April 1988, February 1989, February 1990 and February 1991 were asked to be tested anonymously for HIV-1 antibodies by means of a screening test (ELISA) and a supplemental test (Westernblot). However, some patients refused to be tested. Adhering to the policy of anonymity, some patients were retested and reinterviewed. All the patients were clinically examined and a standardized questionnaire about their drug use history and their drug use behavior was administered. (Table 1).

TABLE 1. MONITORING DRUG USERS AT THE PSYCHIATRIC CLINIC OF THE UNIVERSITY OF VIENNA 1985/86 - 1991

	1986	1987	1988	1989	1990	1991
Patients (total)	107	194	144	233	175	138
IVDUs (total)	82	159	129	208	162	124
IVDUs (HIV tested)	82	159	119	195	156	123
IVDUs (Females tested)	25	42	37	47	47	32
IVDUs (Males tested)	57	117	82	148	109	91
IVDUs mean age (yrs)	26.5	26.2	27.2	28.3	28.7	30.7

RESULTS

PREVALENCE OF HIV-1 1986-1991

Table 2 gives an overview of HIV-1 prevalence among Viennese IVDUs: In the first sample, HIV-1 antibodies were found in 8.5% (7); in the second sample in 14.5% (23); in the third in 27,7% (36), in 1989, the HIV-1 prevalence was 29,7% (58); and in 1990, the HIV-1 prevalence was 26.9% (42) and in 1991, 28.5% (35). Attention should be drawn to the fact that HIV prevalence has increased year by year among females. This reflects the likely emergence of the AIDS epidemic as a predominantly heterosexual disease in the near future.

Between 1988 and 1989, HIV-1 seroprevalence increased dramatically. The frequency of HIV-1 seroprevalence among IVDUs remained nearly stable between 1988 and 1989 and showed even a mild decline in 1990.

A key characteristic of this infected population is their age, with most reporting that they first used intravenous drugs in the late 1970s. This is, by large, a population of middle aged, long term, chronic heroin injectors. However, there is also a remarkable group of drug HIV infected users under 25.

TABLE 2. PREVALENCE OF HIV-1 ANTIBODIES AMONG INTRAVENOUS
DRUG USERS IN VIENNA 1985 - 1991

IVDUs	1986	1987	1988	1989	1990	1991
tested	82	159	119	195	156	123
HIV-1 infected	8.5%	14.5%	27.7%	29.7%	26.9%	28.5%
Females tested	25	42	37	47	47	32
Females infected	12.0%	21.4%	18.9%	28.8%	34.0%	31.2%
Males tested	57	117	82	148	109	91
Males infected	7.0%	11.9%	29.9%	28.1%	23.8%	27.2%

SHARING

Several explanations are offered for the marked geographical variations in the number of HIV-1 infected drug users in different parts of Europe. Cultural divergencies, particularly attitudes to the sharing of injection equipment, might explain the differences when considering cities in Austria (Innsbruck, Vienna). Gatherings of 5 to 10 drug injectors are not uncommon in Vienna while shooting galleries are totally unknown.

About 30% of the infected IVDUs interviewed already knew they were HIV-1-positive at the time of the first interview. In spite of this, 45% answered that they had previously shared needles. This figure dropped dramatically in the following investigations. Interestingly, an increase of drug users who never shared needles for drug application was observed. (Table 3) Educational interventions should also address users of sterile equipment in order to inform the injecting population of risks of infection through the simultaneous filling of the syringe, which can also cause an HIV-1 infection even in case of using sterile equipment (Loimer et al.1991). In 1989, 65% of those not HIV-1 infected continued to fill their syringes together with other IVDUs.

Table 3. REPORTED INCIDENCE OF NEEDLE SHARING (%) AMONG
INTRAVENOUS DRUG USERS IN VIENNA 1985-1991

	1986	1987	1988	1989	1990	1991
IVDUs (total)	82	159	129	208	162	124
Never	23.1%	38.3%	28.6%	31.7%	27.7%	26.8%
Previously	45%	26.5%	28.8%	29.9%	43.2%	55.4%
Always	32.9%	35.2%	42.6%	38.4%	29.1%	17.8%

INTRAVENOUS DRUG USE IN FOREIGN COUNTRIES

In 1987/1988, 69% of the IVDUs with HIV-1 infection reported intravenous drug use in foreign countries. This figure dropped to 50% in 1989 and 38% in 1990, indicating that the spread of HIV-1 infection in Vienna no longer depends on the mobility of the drug users. The number of IVDUs reporting IV use abroad remained constant. (Table 4) This trend continued in 1991.

Table 4. REPORTED INTRAVENOUS DRUG USE IN FOREIGN COUNTRIES WITHIN THE LAST FIVE YEARS PRIOR TO THE INVESTIGATION

	1987/88	1988	1989	1990	1991
IVDUs (total)	159	129	208	162	124
% i.v. abroad	39.6%	54.3%	45.2%	40.1%	35.7%
% HIV-1 infected who injected abroad	69%	63%	50%	38%	27.3%

METHADONE MAINTENANCE

Drug users enrolled in a methadone treatment system for heroin addiction tend to stop or decrease their use of heroin. The relatively low level (around 8.5%) of HIV-1 seroprevalence among IVDUs in 1986 provided an opportunity for an intervention to slow the spread of HIV-1 infection via needle use. In late 1987, a methadone maintenance program primarily addressing HIV-1 infected drug users was introduced in Austria. The high attraction of the clinic for IIIV-1 infected drug users increased the number of patients seeking treatment (Table 1).

Information collected by testing 92 HIV-1 negative patients during methadone maintenance therapy each year at the drug dependency outpatient clinic of the Psychiatric University Clinic of Vienna has been used to calculate seroconversion rates. Even in the light, that all patients had occasionally engaged in additional high risk practices for HIV-1 infection, as was seen from the regular urine samples taken, only three patients seroconverted during the course of the methadone treatment. All three had HIV-1 infected sexpartners and showed an extremely bad compliance. Sexual transmission of HIV is now thought to be as important as needle sharing in the drug using population. There are fears that infection spreads from the older cohort of long-term heroin users to the younger, more sexually active drug users. Table 5 shows in 1988, 75.7%; in 1989, 84.4%; in 1990, 88%, and in 1991, 94.9% of HIV-1 infected IVDUs were treated with methadone.

Table 5. METHADONE MAINTENANCE FOR HIV-1 INFECTED
INTRAVENOUS DRUG USERS

	1988	1989	1990	1991
IVDUs tested for HIV-1	119	195	156	123
Patients in M M P	53	111	99	78
% MMT (IVDUs)	44.5%	53.3%	62.8%	63.4%
% MMT and HIV-1 infected	75.7%	84.4%	88%	94.3%

To control illegal drug use during the methadone maintenance treatment, more
than 7, 000 urine samples were taken until February 1991 at our outpatient ward.
Between July 1990, and December 1990 all urine samples of methadone patients
were additionally screened for ethanol using TDx^{R}REA^R (Abbott). In total 168
different patients were tested; in 25.6% of the tests, the result for ethanol was
positive. The mean total ethanol concentration in urine was 62.9 mg/dl for females
and for 46 mg/dl males .

DEVELOPMENT OF DISEASE

The injecting drug addicts being treated at the Psychiatric University Clinic of
Vienna first came into contact with the HIV-1 infection in or about the year 1982.
The onset of symptoms appears to be closely followed by the development of
AIDS and an explosion of new cases is predicted in the very near future. (Table 6)

Table 6. YEAR OF FIRST REPORTED POSITIVE HIV-1 TEST

	1989	1990	1991
1983:	1.7%	2.4%	2.8%
1984:	8.6%	4.8%	2.8%
1985:	27.6%	28.6%	25.7%
1986:	22.5%	19%	14.3%
1987:	15.5%	19%	20%
1988:	20.7%	11.9%	11.5%
1989:	3.4%*	11.9%	11.5%
1990:		2.4%*	8.6%
1991:			2.8%*

* new cases

DISCUSSION

Drug users represent a high risk group of persons who are in danger of acquiring HIV infection. They are now recognized as contributing greatly to the spread of the infection into the heterosexual population. In Vienna, however an explosive spread of HIV-1 infection among IVDUs was not observed. In fact, the frequency of HIV-1 penetration remained low compared with figures from the Austrian state of the Tyrol (Fuchs et al.1985) or Italy (Ferroni et al.1985). This might be due to the high proportion of IVDUs using sterile needles and syringes exclusively, or to an abuse behavior described as typically "Austrian": Poppy-heads (sold in florist shops to make dried bouquets) are extracted by boiling, and this "opium tea" is drunk whenever heroin is hard to obtain. Its use, however, is not related to risk-laden practices.

It should be noted that in Austria, up to now, only opiates are taken intravenously. The increase of HIV-1 seroprevalence from 1986 to 1988 might be attributed to the introduction of a methadone maintenance program (late 1987) primarily addressing HIV-1 infected drug users. Many IVDUs underwent HIV-1 tests to get, if infected, the benefits of methadone maintenance. The high attraction of the clinic for HIV-1 infected drug users increased the number of patients seeking treatment but the frequency of HIV-1 prevalence remained low compared with figures from Brooklyn or Puerto Rico (Hahn et al.1989). These data suggest the notion that the rapid HIV-1 penetration through an injecting population can be stopped by keeping the drug user away from risk laden practices (Robertson et al.1988; Bschor, 1986; Allen & Curran 1988). The introduction of methadone maintenance had a major effect in reaching more IVDUs for educational interventions. Antibodies to HIV-1 in needles and syringes used by IVDUs (Wodak et al.1987; Stimson et al.1988) led to the implementation of needle exchange programs (Hart et al.1989).

Further educational interventions should address even IVDUs who do not share needles in order to inform them of all the possible risks associated with some needle habits and sex practices. As the tendency to view the condom primarily as a contraceptive device rather than a means of prophylaxis against HIV infection and the belief that condom use is unnatural prevail (Siegel & Gibson 1988), the low level of acceptance among no-infected drug users could be demonstrated.

Drug users are accused of being responsible for a possible explosion of AIDS in the general population. Brown et al.(1987) talk of the "potential bridge of infectivity".

A climate in which there is no stigma attached to HIV testing was created at the Psychiatric University Clinic of Vienna. This fact might provide insight into how to prevent further harm for the injecting population, but similar long-term studies are necessary to gain a better understanding of the AIDS epidemic, so that the risks the injecting population takes can be reduced. Sucessful results during methadone maintenance treatment with regard to the reduction of the spread of HIV-1 were substantiated and well documented. This means a challenge to all programs with high rejection rates and abstinence philosophy. Methadone maintenance is one of the most helpful means available for reducing the risks of HIV-1, provided that programems of low threshold and high quality are expanded.

If the HIV-1 infection-rate continues to increase among IVDUs, this is a sign of an abstinent-orientated, conservative policy. The drug users should be helped to keep away from risk-laden practices in order to protect themselves from further harm. Yet HIV-1 infection is being increasingly criminalized. Victimization may drive at-risk individuals underground. Discrimination can augment public anxiety and lead to distrust of official pronouncements.

Summing up, the only possibility to prevent fatal HIV infections among drug addicts seems to be in the initiation and continuation of contact with the drug using population and in the decriminalizion of the use of drugs. The implementation of methadone maintenance should be introduced on a national level as early as possible.

REFERENCES

ALLEN JR, CURRAN JW (1988) Prevention of AIDS and HIV infection: needs and priorities for epidemiologic research. Am J Public Health 78:381-386.

ANCELLE-PARK R, BRUNET JP, DOWNS AM (1987) AIDS and drug addicts in Europe. Lancet 12:626-627.

BACCHETTI P, MOSS AR (1990) Incubation period of AIDS in San Francisco. Nature 338:251-253.

BALL JC, LANGE WR, MYERS CP, FRIEDMAN SR (1988) Reducing the risk of AIDS through methadone maintenance treatment. J Health Social Behav 29:214-226.

BATTJES RJ, PICKENS RW, AMSEL Z, BROWN LS. (1990) Heterosexual transmission of human immunodeficiency virus among intravenous drug users. J Infect Dis 162(5):1007-1011.

BROWN LS, MURPHY DL, PRIMM BJ (1987) Sex partners of intravenous drug abusers: implications for the next spread of the AIDS epidemic, Paper presented at the 49th Annual Scientific Meeting of the Problems of Drug Dependence.

BSCHOR F (1986) Drug replacement treatment of drug addicts. Deut Med Woschr 111:1658-1659.

CHAISSON RE, OSMOND D, MOSS AR, FELDMAN HW, BERNACKI, P (1987) HIV, Bleach, and needle sharing. Lancet 1430.

CHAMBERLAND ME, CASTRO KG, HAVERKOS HW, MILLER BI (1984) Acquired immmunodeficiency syndrome in the United States:an analysis of cases outside high-incidence groups. An Intern Medicine 101:617-623.

COOPER JR (1989) Methadone treatment and acquired immunodefiency syndrome. JAMA 262:1664-1668.

DES JARLAIS DC, FRIEDMAN SR, STONEBURNER RL (1988) HIV infection and intravenous drug abuse: Critical issues in transmission dynamics, infection outcomes and prevention. Rev Inf Dis 10:151-158.

DES JARLAIS DC, WISH E, FRIEDMAN SR, STONEBURNER R, YANCOWITZ SR, MILDVAN D, EL-SADR W, BARDY E, CUARDRADO M (1987) Intravenous drug use and the heterosexual transmission of the Humane Immunodefiency Virus: current trends in New York City, NY State J Med 238-286.

DRUCKER E (1986) AIDS and addiction in New York City. Am J Drug Alcohol Abuse 12, 1&2:165-181.

DOLE V (1989) Methadone treatment and the aquired immunodefiency syndrome epidemic. JAMA 262:1681-1682.

DONOGHOE MC, STIMSON GV, DOLAN KA (1989) Sexual behavior of injecting drug users and associated risks of HIV infection for non injecting sexual partners. AIDS CARE 1:51-58.

DOWNS AM, ANCELLE-PARK RA, BRUNET JB (1990) Surveillance of AIDS in the European Community: recent trends and predictions to 1991. AIDS 4, 11:1117-1124.

FERRONI P, GEROLDI D, GALLI C, ZANETTI AR, CARGNEL A (1985) HTLV-III antibody among Italian drug addicts. Lancet 52.

FRANCE AJ, SKIDMORE CA, ROBERTSON JR, BRETTLE RP, ROBERTS JJJ, BURNS SM, FOSTER CA, INGLIS JM, GALLOWAY WBF, DAVIDSON SJ (1988) Heterosexual spread of immunodeficiency virus in Edinburgh. Brit Med J 296:526-529.

FRIEDLAND GH, KLEIN RS (1987) Transmission of human immunodeficiency virus. N England J Med 317:1125-1135.

FUCHS D, BLECHA HG, DEINHARDT F, DIERICH P, GOEBEL FD, HENGSTER P, HINTERHUBER H, SCHÖNITZER D, TRAILL K, WACHTER H (1985) High frequency of HTLV-III antibodies among heterosexual intravenous drug abusers in the Austian Tyrol. Lancet 1506.

GHODSE AH, TREGANZA G, LI M (1986) Effect of AIDS on sharing of eqipment among drug abusers. Brit Med J. 295:698-699.

HAHN RA, ONORATO IM, JONES TS, DOUGHERTY J (1989) Prevalence of HIV infection among intravenous drug users in the United States. JAMA. 261:2677-2684.

HART GM, CARVEL ALM, WOODWARD N, JOHNSON AM, Williams P, Parry JV (1989) Evaluation of needle exchange in central London: behavior change and anti-HIV status over one year. AIDS. 3:261-265.

HARMS G, LAUKAMM-JOSTEN U, BIENZLE U, GUGGENMOOS-HOLZMANN I (1987) Risk factors for HIV infection in German i.v. drug abusers. Klin Wochenschr 65:376-379.

JOHNSON AM (1988) Heterosexual transmission of humane immunodeficiency virus. Brit Med J. 296:1017-1020.

LOIMER N, PRESSLICH O, HOLLERER E, PAKESCH G, PFERSMANN V, WERNER E (1990a) Monitoring HIV-1 infection prevalence among intravenous drug users in Vienna 1986-1990. AIDS CARE. 2,3:281-286.

142

LOIMER N, PRESSLICH O, HOLLERER E, WERNER E, PAKESCH G, PFERSMANN V, SCHMID-SIEGEL B (1990b) Prävalenz von HIV-Infektion bei intravenös Drogenabhängigen 1986 bis 1989 in Wien. Wi Kli Woschrift 102, 4:106-110.

LOIMER N, PRESSLICH O, HOLLERER E, PAKESCH G, PFERSMANN V, WERNER E (1990c) Sexual behavior and prevalence of HIV-1 infection among intravenous drug users in Vienna 1986-1989. J Sex Educat Therap 16, 4:242-250.

LOIMER N, WERNER E, PRESSLICH O (1991) Sharing spoons: A risk factor for HIV-1 infection in Vienna. Brit J Addict 86:775-778.

MARMOR M, DES JARLAIS DC, COHEN H, FRIEDMAN SR, BEATRICE ST, DUBIN N, EL-SADR W, MILDVAN D, YANCOVITS S, MATHUR U, HOLZMAN R. (1987) Risk factors for infection with human immunodeficiency virus among intravenous drug abusers in New York City. AIDS. 39-44.

MOSS AR (1987) AIDS and IV drug use the real heterosexual epidemic, Brit Med J 294:389-390.

NOVICK DM, JOSEPH H, CROXSON TS, SALSITZ EA, WANG G, RICHMAN BL, PORETSKY L, KEEFE JB, WHIMBEY E (1990) Absence of antibody to human immunodefiency virus in long term, socially rehabilitated methadone maintenance patients. Arch Intern Med 150:97-99.

PETERSON JL, MARIN G (1988) Issues in the prevention of AIDS among black and hispanic men. Am Psychol 43:11,871-877.

ROBERTSON JR, BUCKNALL ABV, WIGGINS P (1986) Regional variations in HIV antibody seropositivity in british intravenous drug users. Lancet 4435-1436.

ROBERTSON JR, SKIDMORE CA, ROBERTS JJK (1988) HIV infection in intravenous drug users: a follow-up study indicating changes in risk-taking behavior. Brit J Addict 83:387-391.

SCHOENBAUM EE, HARTEL D, SELWYN PA, KLEIN RS, DAVENNY K, ROGERS M, FEINER C, FRIEDLAND G. (1989) Risk factors for human immunodeficiency virus infection in intravenous drug users. N England J Med 321:874-879.

SELWYN PA, FEINGOLG AR, IEZZA A, SATYADEO M, COLLY J, TORRES R, SHAW JF. (1989) Primary care for patients with HIV infection in a methadone maintenance program. Ann Intern Med 111, 9:761-763.

SIEGEL K, GIBSON WC. (1988) Barrriers to the modification of sexual behavior among heterosexuals at risk for acquired immunodefiency syndrome. NY State J Medi 2:66-70.

SORENSEN JL, BAKTI SL, GOOD P, WILKINSON K (1989) Methadone maintenance program for AIDS-affected opiate addicts. J Substance Abuse Treatment 6:87-94.

STIMSON GV, ALLDRITT L, DOLAN K, DONOGHOE M, LART RA (1988) Injecting equipment exchange schemes: Final report. London, Goldsmiths'College.

WODAK A, DOLAN K, IMRIE AA, GOLD J, WOLK J, WHYTE BM, COOPER D (1987) Antibodies to the human immunodefiency virus in needles and syringes used by intravenous drug abusers. Med J Australia 147:275-276.

Opioid Receptors

H. SCHMIDHAMMER

Institute of Organic and Pharmaceutical Chemistry, University of Innsbruck,
Innrain 52a, A-6020 Innsbruck, Austria

The pharmacological concept of receptors, based upon the observation of rigid structure-activity relationships, stereospecificity, and the observation of maximal pharmacological responses goes back to the turn of the century. Almost hundred years ago, Fischer (1894) proposed the lock - key - model for the system enzyme - glycoside. Later, Langley (1909) and Ehrlich (1913) further developed this model which can be applied for receptors as well.

In the early nineteenfifties, the determination of structural requirements of semisynthetic and synthetic opioids led to the hypothesis of Beckett and Casy (1954a, b) that they interacted with specific binding sites. Opioid structure-activity relationships established for literally thousands of compounds (de Stevens 1965; Jacobson et al. 1970; Janssen et al. 1960, 1966) revealed very rigid requirements for activity, including strict stereospecificity (Portoghese 1966, 1970). Furthermore, both in vivo testing and bioassays clearly fulfilled the other criteria expected of a receptor-mediated action, including cross tolerance and dependence. The synthesis of the pure opioid antagonist naloxone as well as the mixed agonist-antagonist nalorphine, and their ability to reverse opioid analgesia and respiration depression, also provided strong evidence for a receptor-mediated inter-action. With such strong pharmacological evidence in favor of a receptor mechanism of action, it is was not surprising that many groups attempted to label it biochemically. In 1973, three laboratories reported the biochemical demonstration of opioid binding sites using tritium labeled naloxone (Pert and Snyder 1973), tritium labeled dihydromorphine (Terenius 1973), and tritium labeled etorphine (Simon et al. 1973).

Martin (1967) first proposed the existence of multiple types of opioid receptors on the basis of interactions of morphine and nalorphine, as well as detailed structure-activity relationship studies which had been carried out by Portoghese (1965, 1966).

Nowadays the existence of at least three major types of opioid receptors - μ, κ, and δ - is generally recognized.

The demonstration of specific opioid binding sites in many species suggested the existence of endogenous substances for these binding sites. Hughes and Kosterlitz first described such endogenous substances, peptides containing five amino acids, and called them enkephalins (for "in the head").

Subsequently, numerous peptides with opioid-like effects have been found in the central nervous system and in peripheral tissues. These endogenous opioid peptides vary in seize, but their amino terminals most share a similar enkephalin sequence of amino acids. Currently, three separate, individually gene-derived families of endogenous opioid peptides are recognized: the endorphins, the enkephalins, and the dynorphins. ß-Endorphin interacts predominantly with the μ and δ receptors, Leu-enkephalin and Met-enkephalin interact predominantly with the δ receptors and dynorphin shows preference for κ receptors.

Under normal circumstances, most cells that contain endogenous opoid peptides do not appear to release them continuously. Instead, endogenous opioids are released when homeostasis is disrupted following the imposition of stress. Once released, they act upon specific opioid receptors that generally directly inhibit secondary systems. For example, endogenous opioids appear to inhibit pain, respiratory function, cardiovascular performance, gastrointestinal transit, and several other physiological functions as well as certain behaviors.

To define the distinct physiological and pharmacological roles of the various opioid receptor types, a number of highly potent and receptor selective peptide ligands - particularly of the agonist series - were prepared and studied. Since these peptides are not stable against peptidases and are not able to pass the blood-brain-barrier, such compounds are not useful as drugs. For the same reasons, the utility of such ligands as pharmacological and biological tools is limited. This fact has created a need for highly selective opioids which are stable against peptidases and are capable of entering the CNS easily. a number of non-peptide, selective μ and κ agonists have been known already for several years, but there is no selective non-peptide delta agonist described so far. Recently non-peptide, competitive, highly selective antagonists have been developed, since particularly antagonists are useful tools in opioid research. For κ and δ receptors nor-BNI (norbinaltorphimine) and naltrindole, respectively have been reported by Portoghese et al. (1987, 1988). The highly selective μ antagonist cyprodime has been developed by Schmidhammer et al. (1989). Until then, naloxone was the only non-peptide, competitive μ antagonist available. But naloxone is not a very selective compound, it shows considerable κ and δ receptor affinity. These new selective antagonists are used as pharmacological tools and further pharmacological and biological studies with them are presently in progress.

With the μ receptor a high-affinity and a low-affinity site was found. These sites were called μ_1 and μ_2. Naloxonazine, a μ_1 selective non-equilibrium antagonist developed by Pasternak and Hahn (1980), greatly facilitated the studies of these binding sites. Treatment of animals with naloxonazine eliminated the high-affinity binding of a series of μ-selective opioid agonists. This loss of binding was associated with a dramatic shift of the analgesic dose-response curve to the right, implying that μ_1 sites mediated analgesia. On the other hand, μ_1 blockade did not alter the respiratory depression of morphine or most of the signs associated with morphine dependence (Goodman et al. 1988). These findings would imply that a selective μ_1 opioid analgesic could exhibit less side effects than morphine. Very recently these types of compounds have been developed by Hungarian scientists (Krizsan et al. 1991). These ligands are codeinone derivatives which are obviously μ_1-agonists and at the same time μ_2-antagonists. Further pharmacological studies with these compounds are in progress.

There is some evidence that also κ and δ subtypes are subdivided. But is seems too early to draw conclusions out of these studies.

Attempts to purify all types of opioid receptors to homogeneity have been in progress for about a decade, with the ultimate aim of determining the full amino acid sequence and sugar composition of these macromolecules. Key steps in the purification procedure are solubilzation and fractionation. Viability of isolated material is monitored by comparing binding activities before and after fractionation. Affinity chromatography for fractionation became very popular in accomplishing this task. Recently, purification of μ, κ, and δ binding proteins to apparent homogeneity has been achieved by several groups (Gioannini et al. 1985, Simonds et al. 1985, Cho et al. 1986, Demoliou-Mason et al. 1986, Simon et al. 1987).

In the last few years a number of laboratories succeeded in scaling up their purification procedures. The amino terminals for all three major subtypes were found to be blocked. This means that relatively large amounts of the protein are needed for microsequencing purposes. Recently, several laboratories were able to produce monoclonal and polyclonal antibodies directed against opioid receptors. These preparations might provide good tools for isolation, identification, and expression cloning. At this moment only preliminary reports of these studies are known.

It is to hope that complete structural information will be available in the near future, and that this information will lead to a better understanding of the functional relevance of opioid receptors. And it is quite feasible that these informations could lead to the discovery of analgesics without the undesireable side effects and also to drugs with alternative therapeutic potential, which for instance could include effects on food intake, mood, seizures, shock, and immune function.

146

References

Beckett AH and Casy AF (1954a) Stereochemistry of certain analgesics. Nature
173: 1231-1232.

Beckett AH and Casy AF (1954b) Synthetic analgesics: stereochemical
considerations. J. Pharm. Pharmacol. 6: 986-1001.

Cho TM, Hasegawa JI, Ge BL, Loh HH (1986) Purification to apparent homogeneity
of a μ-type opioid receptor from frog brain. Proc. Natl. Acad. Sci. USA 83: 4138-
4151.

Demoliou-Mason CD and Barnard EA (1986) Purification and characterization of rat
brain opiate receptors. British Opioid Colloquium, Nottingham, abstr. 04.

de Stevens G (1965) In: Analgetics vol. 5, Academic, New York p 475.

Ehrlich P (1913) Chemotherapeutics: scientific principles, methods and results.
Lancet 2: 445-451.

Fischer E (1894) Einfluss der Configuration auf die Wirkung der Enzyme. Chem.
Ber. 27: 2985-2993.

Gioannini TL, Howard A, Hiller JM, Simon EJ (1985) Purification of an active opioid-
binding protein from bovine striatum. J. Biolog. Chem. 260: 15117-15121.

Goodman RR, Adler BA, Pasternak GW (1988) Regional distribution of opioid
receptors. In: Pasternak GW (ed) The opiate receptors, The Humana Press,
Clifton, New Jersey, pp 197-228.

Holaday JW (1985) Endogenous opioids and their receptors. In: Current concepts,
The Upjohn Company, Kalmazoo, Michigan.

Hughes J, Smith TH, Kosterlitz JW, Fothergill LA, Morgan BA, Morris HR (1975)
Identification of two related pentapeptides from the brain with potent opiate
agonist activity. Nature 258: 577-579.

Jacobson AE, May EL, Sargent LJ (1970) Analgetics. In: Burger A (ed) Medicinal
Chemistry part II, 3rd, Wiley Interscience, New York.

Janssen PAJ, Hellerbach J, Schnider O, Besendorf LT, Pellmont B (1960)
Diphenylpropylamines, Morphinans. In: Synthetic analgesics part I, Pergamon,
New York.

Janssen PAJ, Hellerbach J, Schnider O, Besendorf LT, Pellmont B (1960) Diphenylpropylamines, Morphinans. In: Synthetic analgesics part II, Pergamon, New York.

Krizsan D, Varga E, Hosztafi S, Benyhe S, Szücs M, Borsodi A (1991) Irreversible binding of C-6 derivatives of morphinan-6-ones to rat brain opioid receptors. Life Sci 48: 439-451.

Langley JN (1909) On the contraction of muscle, chiefly in relation to the presence of "receptive" substances. IV. The effect of curare and of some other substances on the nicotine response of the sartorius and gastrocnemius muscles of the frog. J. Physiolog. 39: 235-295.

Martin WR (1967) Opioid antagonists. Pharmacol. Rev. 19: 463-521.

Pasternak GW and Hahn EF (1980) Long-acting opiate agonists and antagonists: 14-hydroxydihydromorphinone hydrazones. J. Med. Chem. 23: 674-676.

Pert CB and Snyder SH (1973) Opiate receptor: demonstration in nervous tissue. Science 179: 1011-1014.

Portoghese PS (1965) A new concept on the mode of interaction of narcotic analgesics with receptors. J. Med. Chem. 8: 609.

Portoghese PS (1966) Stereochemical factors and receptor interactions associated with narcotic analgesics. J. Pharm. Sci. 55: 865-887.

Portoghese PS (1970) Relationships between stereostructure and pharmacological activity. Ann. Rev. Pharmacol. 10: 51-76.

Portoghese PS, Sultana M, Nagase H, Takemori AE (1988) Application of the message-address concept in the design of highly potent and selective non-peptide δ opioid receptor antagonists. J. Med. Chem. 31: 281-282.

Portoghese PS, Nagase H, Lipkowski AW, Larson DL, Takemori AE (1987) Bimorphinans as highly selective, potent κ opioid receptor antagonists. J. Med. Chem. 30: 238-239.

Schmidhammer H, Burkard WP, Eggstein-Aeppli L, Smith CFC (1989) Synthesis and biological evaluation of 14-alkoxymorphinans. 2. (-)-N-(cyclopropylmethyl)-

4,14-dimethoxymorphinan-6-one, a selective μ opioid receptor antagonist. J. Med. Chem. 32: 418-421.

Simon EJ, Hiller JM, Edelmand I (1973) Stereospecific binding of the potent narcotic analgesic ^{3}H-etorphine to rat brain homogenates. Proc. Natl. Acad. Sci. USA 70: 1947-1949.

Simon J, Benyhe S, Hepp J, Khan A, Borsodi A, Szücs M, Medzihradsky K, Wollemann M (1987) Purification of a κ-opioid receptor subtype from frog brain. Neuropeptides 10: 19-28.

Simonds WF, Burke TR Jr., Rice KC, Jacobson AE, Klee WA (1985) Purification of the opiate receptor of NG108-15 neuroblastoma-glioma hybrid cells. Proc. Natl. Acad. Sci. USA 82: 4974-4978.

Terenius L (1973) Characteristics of the "receptor" for narcotic analgesics in synaptic plasma membrane fractions from rat brain. Acta Pharmacol. Toxicol. 33: 377-384.

Addiction Potential of Opiates in Medical Use

E. BEUBLER

Department of Experimental and Clinical Pharmacology,
Universitätsplatz 4, A-8010 Graz, Austria

Today, opiates are the most important drugs in the treatment of severe, exspecially severe chronic pain. Already in 1680, Thomas Sydenham, the so called English Hippocrates told us: "Among the remedies which it had pleased Almighty God to give to man to relieve his sufferings, none is so universal and so efficacions as opium" and only recently P. D. Wall has written in "Pain": "A real triumph of medicine in the past 50 years has been to re-establish a proper place for the ancient therapy of narcotics in the treatment of pain. Pioneers as Dame Cicely Saunders, have played a crucial role in that victory. It is a disgraceful episode in the history of medicine that doctors and scientists allowed themselves to join a mass hysteria which confused the tremendous benefits of narcotics for the patient in pain with the social abuse of the same compounds. Any number of completely irrelevant aspects of narcotics were introduced to the utter confusion of good people including doctors, clerics, politicians and patients. It was commonly suspected that the prescription of narcotics was a polite way of killing patients under the guise of treating their pain." (End of citation) (1)

Actually, many physicians, exspecially in Austria, are still reluctant to use morphine because they believe that the drug rapidly becomes ineffective due to tolerance and that morphine causes drug dependence or addiction, respectively.

The consumption of opiates for the treatment of severe pain in Austria and Germany is still far below other countries like Canada, England or the Scandinavian countries (2). We know, e.g. that Sweden increased the consumption of opiates for medical use 5-fold in seven years, the number of opiate addicts on the street, however, remained unchanged. This proves that increase of opiates in medical use does not increase opiates on the black market.

Addiction is the compulsion to take a drug in order to experience its psychological effects and, according to the WHO, addiction is accompanied by tolerance

> physical dependence and
> psychological dependence

Tolerance is feared by many, forgetting that dose increase is necessitated more by excalating pain from disease progression than from true pharmacological tolerance. Tolerance appears sometimes when morphine or other opiates are repeatedly injected. A recent study has shown that even intravenous administration does not result in tolerance if the so called PCA (= patient controlled analgesia) method is used. Continuous infusion increases the amount of morphin to cope with pain. With the PCA-method, the needed amount of morphine is stable and patients stop themselves when pain is over (3).

Tolerance rarely occurs to any significant extent with chronic oral morphine administration when used for treatment of severe chronic pain. In fact, if the dosage is optimized, it may even be possible to reduce the dose from time to time.

There is no doubt that many patients on opiates have a physical dependence. Withdrawal of opiate medication must be gradual and well supervised. Withdrawal of opiate is possible when pain is relieved, even after several month of intake.

For the treatment of severe pain opiates have to be given orally. Further, opiates have to be administered by the clock, four hourly the morphine solution and 12 hourly the new slow release preparation, with the aim that no pain occurs inbetween administration periods. This, as we know, reduces tolerance and it was siceley Saunders, who introduced this scheme of administration.

The choice of the opiate depends on the degree of pain - after non opiates one gives weak opiates and, if not appropriate, strong opiates. The opiates currently used in the treatment of pain are: codein and dihydrocodein (weak opiates) and pethidin piritramid, morphine and fentanyl (strong opiates).

To evaluate the addiction potential of strong opiates in medical use we have to compare the opiates with other pharmacological groups:

Table 1

Frequency of drug dependence of different pharmacological groups, reported spontaneously by physicians in 1984.

benzodiazepines	50 %
hypnotics	21 %
weak opiates	12 %
stimulants	8 %
weak analgesics	4 %
laxatives	1 %
strong opiates	0.1 %
	= 765 cases reported

Table 1 shows the frequency of drug dependence of different pharmacological groups, reported spontaneously by physicians in 1984 in Germany (4). 765 cases of drug dependence were reported alltogether. 50 % of the cases showed drug dependence due to the intake of benzodiazepines, 21 % due to hypotics; 12 % due to weak opiate, mostly codein used as a private maintenance-programme. Only one case was reported concerning strong opiates and this was dicotide, an antitussive drug.

Table 2

Frequency of drug dependence

benzodiazepines (related to all patients taking those)	25 %
Weak analgesics (related to all patients suffering of chronic headache)	60-70 %
strong opiates (related to all patients with severe pain)	0.03 %

Table 2 shows a different view on the matter of drug dependence.

Looking on all patients receiving benzodiazepines, 25 % develop drug dependence. Taking all patients with chronic headache, 60-70 % develop drug dependence on weak analgesics. The development of drug dependence to strong opiates, on the other hand, is neglectable.

As a conclusion, a sentence out of the textbook in pharmacology, should be cept in mind: "no patient should ever wish for death because of his physicians reluctance to use adequate amounts of effective opiates" (5).

References

Wall PD (1990) Neuropathic pain, Editorial. Pain 43: 267-268

International narcotic control board-Vienna. Narcotic Drugs. Estimated world requirements for 1989, United Nations, New York 1988

Hill NF, Chapamn CR, Kornell JA (1990) Self administration of morphine in bone marrow transplant patients reduces drug requirement. Pain 40: 121-129

Keup W (1986) Arzneimittel-Mißbrauch. Arzneiverordnung in der Praxis 1: 1-8

Jaffe JH (1985) Drug addiction and drug abuse. In: Goodman and Gilman: The Pharmacological Basis of Therapeutics Macmillan Publishing Co. Inc. New York, S32-S82

Methadone Maintenance Treatment for Harm Reduction Approach to Heroin Addiction

M. J. KREEK

The Rockefeller University NY, New York 10021, USA

It is estimated that there are now over one million persons who have used heroin regularly in the United States and possibly two million that have used heroin at some time. Of these, it is estimated that at least 500,000 are "hard-core" heroin addicts, defined as users of multiple, regular self-administered doses of short-acting opiates such as heroin each day for one year or more, with the development of tolerance, physical dependence and drug seeking behavior, thus, addiction. (42,43,54)

In 1981, AIDS disease was first recognized. In our laboratory we were able to unbank and uncode sera which had been banked prospectively from studies carried out in the late 1960s forward. (11,79,81) Based on the findings from our laboratory, and to some extent later confirmed by others, it was found that heroin addicts in New York City seeking entry into methadone maintenance treatment showed evidence of HIV-1 positivity from 1978 onwards. (11,79,81) From 1978 to 1983 there was a rapid escalation of the prevalence of HIV-1 positivity. Since 1983 this prevalence has plateaued at a level of 50% to 60%. (11,42,54,58,77,78,79,81,85) Further studies by our group, in collaboration with the group of Des Jarlais, showed that the first entry of HIV infection into the parenteral drug abusing population in New York City was probably around 1975. (10,68) This estimate is based on the later identification of a small number of infants who were HIV-1 infected by 1977; thus their mothers must have been HIV-1 infected prior to that time. The prevalence of intravenous heroin use and the fact that the second, and in some regions, the first risk group for becoming infected with HIV virus with progression to AIDS, are intravenous drug abusers, has led to increased concern with respect to the management of opiate addiction, an area which we have been involved in studying since 1964. (13,42,49,54)

After initiation of narcotic use, chronic repeated opiate use will lead to the development of tolerance, that is, the need for increasing doses to achieve any given effect, followed by the development of physical dependence, best demonstrated by the appearance of the abstinence syndrome on abrupt opiate withdrawal. (13,26,27,42,43,93) A cascade of physiological signs and symptoms may be seen when an opiate drug is suddenly removed from either a laboratory animal model or a human who has developed tolerance and physical dependence (26,43,93). In clinical studies, a protracted abstinence syndrome has also been defined. Since first observed by clinical research workers at the United States Public Health Services facility for addiction in Lexington, Kentucky, many other groups have added on to the list of signs and symptoms of atypical or abnormal physiology which may be observed in opiate-free, former heroin addicts for more than six months following cessation of opiate use. (26,42,43,) Also drug craving, that is, a very specific hunger or desire to self-administer .opiate drugs, accompanies the protracted abstinence syndrome and contributes to the relapse of drug-free former heroin addicts to use of narcotic drugs, frequently preceded by heavy licit or illicit use of alcohol and other prescription medications.

Although no biochemical or molecular definitions for opiate tolerance or physical dependence have yet been elucidated, nevertheless these are phenomena which can be easily documented either in the laboratory or the clinical setting. (27,43) Similarly there are to date, no biochemical or molecular definitions of "drug hunger" or "drug craving", although the sequence of physiological events which may be involved have been in part elucidated. It is appreciated that conditioned responses, that is, response to environmental cues, and according to some recent work from our laboratory, also internal cues, may contribute to the intensity of drug craving and thus relapse to opiate drug use. (8,17,18,19,20,22, 23,24,25,26,27,31,43,64,70,73,74,90,93,102) However attempts to manage opiate dependency exclusively by classical methods of de-conditioning to achieve extinction, have proven not to be effective.

In 1964, I had the privilege of joining Dr. Vincent Dole at The Rockefeller University who had just been joined by a psychiatrist with years of working with addicts, Dr. Marie Nyswander, and to participate as part of the original recent research team organized to determine whether or not chronic pharmacotherapy could be used for the management of addiction. (13) At that time, we postulated that there was a metabolic basis for addiction. (13,25,31)

Most of the studies in my own independent laboratory organized in 1974-75, over the last 17 years have been focused on various aspects of determining the biological or metabolic basis of addiction. These studies include molecular studies of the nature of the endogenous opioid system and how it may relate to addictive diseases. (1,2,3,4,6,7,17,18,19,20,22,23,24,29,31,34,41,42,43,47,51, 52,64,70,73,74,90,96,97,98,99,102)

We have postulated that although there may be intrinsic genetic factors which make some individuals more vulnerable, or at greater risk, for developing opiate addiction than others, multiple genes and not a single gene, are probably involved, (such as been postulated to be the case for the majority of alcoholics). Pharmacological factors alone do not seem to be of fundamental and sole importance in opiate addiction; even after the opiate drug has been completely withdrawn, and has been eliminated from the body for weeks, months or even years, the vulnerability for relapse persists. There is increasing evidence that there may be a physiological basis for this addiction. Thus we have postulated that chronic use of an opiate drug may impact upon normal physiology and cause very persistent, long-term alterations in normal physiological responses, some of which may in fact be permanent. Host response variability, as well as genetic predisposition, may play a very important role in effecting these changes.

Having postulated a metabolic basis of addiction, then a pharmacotherapeutic approach would seem to be most appropriate.(13,42,43,48,54,92) The goals of pharmacotherapy should include prevention of withdrawal symptoms, prevention or reduction of drug craving, and finally restoration towards normalcy of any

156

physiological functions which become disrupted by drug use.
Multiple daily self-administrations of heroin are needed by the
heroin addict first to achieve a euphoria or so-called "high", but
later simply to attempt to prevent withdrawal symptoms and to have a
brief period of feeling and being "normal" or "straight". (13) If
no opiate is self-administered, withdrawal symptoms or "sickness"
will ensue.

In our early studies in 1964, we addressed the question of
whether the synthetic opiate methadone, which seemed, from early
limited clinical studies of its potential use in pain management, to
be possibly longer acting other than available opiate drugs, could
be used in the chronic pharmacotherapy of heroin addiction. At that
time, there were no analytical techniques such as gas chromatography
to measure plasma levels of methadone, or of morphine or heroin.
(12,27,28) Therefore clinical observations solely had to be used in
determining the pharmacokinetic properties, as well as
pharmacodynamic effects of methadone at that time.

Our early studies at The Rockefeller University Hospital showed
that: 1) whereas heroin had to be administered intravenously to
have any substantial effect, methadone could be administered orally;
2) whereas the onset of action of heroin was immediate after
intravenous administration, approximately 30 minutes was required
for the onset of methadone effects after oral administration; 3) We
also found that the duration of action of methadone, both with
respect to preventing withdrawal symptoms and also with respect to
preventing drug hunger was approximately 24 to 36 hours as
contrasted to only 4 to 6 hours for heroin. Of greatest importance,
we early on documented that (4) if the dose of methadone was
selected appropriately to be less than the degree of tolerance that
had been developed by that individual, there was no euphoria or no
"high" resulting from methadone administration, as contrasted with
heroin, which, when used in doses which, by intent, usually exceed
the degree of tolerance of the individual, produce a profound
euphoria described as a "rush" followed frequently by a feeling of
"warmth" and "high" persisting for up to 30 minutes or more.
Finally, we find that (5) whereas withdrawal symptoms ensue within 3
to 4 hours after last dose of heroin is administered in a tolerant
and dependent individual, the effectiveness of methadone in

preventing withdrawal symptoms persist for over 24 hours. (13,42,43, 54)

During single, daily, oral dosing of former heroin addicts with methadone, there is a sustained "straight" or normal state with no "high" or euphoria and with no opiate withdrawal symptoms for the 24 hour dosing interval. (13) In a series of double-blinded random-order, design studies, in which short-acting opiates such as heroin were injected against the background of daily oral dosing of methadone, it was shown that the high degree of opioid tolerance developed by chronic methadone dosing provided a "blockade" of any euphoric effects of superimposed short-acting narcotics, due to the high degree of opioid and cross-tolerance which have been developed by the methadone treatment. (13) Thus any illicit use of heroin or other short-acting opiates superimposed against the background of methadone would result in euphoric effects. This phenomenon has been proven to be of great importance in methadone maintenance treatment. (13,42,43,48,52) If an adequate dose of methadone is used, it is financially essentially impossible for a former heroin addict so treated to obtain a sufficiently large amount of heroin to exceed the degree of tolerance which is developed and sustained during chronic methadone maintenance treatment. Thus the individual must make a decision either to give up the euphoric "high" of heroin use and accept the physological and behavioral normalization provided methadone or to leave treatment.

Later when analytical techniques were developed for the measurement of methadone and similar drugs in plasma we were able to show that indeed the pharmacokinetic profile was very similar to that which had been described much earlier by our clinical observations. (12,13,28) The methadone plasma was sustained over a period of 24 hour dosing interval, the peak methadone levels occur approximately 2 to 4 hours after last dose administration. The peak levels represent a bare doubling of the native or sustained levels. (28)

It is the profound differences in the pharmacokinetic profile of methadone in humans as contrasted to the pharmacokinetic profile of heroin or other short-acting opiates in humans that allow methadone to be effectively used in the maintenance treatment of addiction. Methadone has a 24 hour half-life as contrasted to the one hour half-life of heroin in humans, coupled with the four to six hour half-life of its major metabolite, morphine. (5,9,12,14,15,16, 21,28,30,32,33,35,36,37,38,39,40,44,46,55,56,57,60,61,62,63,65,69,7-1,72,75,76,80,82,89,91,94,95,100,101)

Therefore, methadone satisfies our proposed profile for any potential pharmacotherapeutic agent for use in chronic treatment of an addiction. It is effective after oral administration, with systemic bioavailability that exceeds 70%. Also it has a long biological half-life in humans. There are minimal side effects during chronic administration. Prospective studies performed by my group initially from 1964 and reported in 1973 of patients maintained for three years or more on high doses of methadone and many subsequent studies, including a current study by my group of patients in treatment for ten years or more (Novick et al work in progress) have shown that methadone is safe when used in former opiate addicts with no two toxicity or serious adverse affects. It has also been shown based on prospective studies, that methadone maintenance treatment is effective for a substantial number of persons with opiate addiction. (42,54)

At this time over 150,000 persons have been treated with methadone maintenance treatment in the United States; approximately 100,000 are currently in treatment. (42,48,54) The voluntary retention in treatment varies enormously, from 50% to over 80%. In programs where adequate doses of methadone, usually 60 to 100 mg/day, are used for most subjects, and which are well-constructed programs with appropriately trained and diverse staff, less than 10% of the individuals continue to use illicit opiates such as heroin. However it should be underscored that when patients leave methadone maintenance treatment, whether voluntarily or involuntarily, and are followed prospectively, several studies have shown that more than 70% will relapse back to illicit opiate use with two years. (42,48,54) The beneficial actions of methadone are that it prevents opiate withdrawal symptoms and drug hunger, and it also blocks any euphoric effect following any self-administration of short-acting, illicit narcotics. The mechanism of action of methadone is by providing a steady state profusion of opioid at critical opiate receptor sites.

We have also shown that methadone maintenance treatment has profound public health implications with respect to the prevention of HIV-1 infection and AIDS. (11,42,48,49,54,79,81) In 1984, the study which we carried out to identify the time of entry into HIV-1 infection in the parenteral drug abusing population in New York City revealed another extremely important finding. It was found that less than 10% of the hard-core heroin addicts who had both entered an effective methadone maintenance program prior to the HIV-1 epidemic hitting New York City in 1978 and had remained in continuous treatment, were anti-HIV-1 positive in 1984, a time when more than 50 to 60% of street addicts and addicts entering methadone maintenance treatment were shown to be anti-HIV-1 positive. (11,79,81) Subsequent findings have been made by other groups in the United States as well as the groups of Blix and Gunne in Sweden. Thus methadone maintenance treatment, by virtue of preventing drug craving and abstinent symptoms, thus reducing or eliminating any continued use of illicit drugs, usually self-administered with unsterile equipment, prevents exposure to HIV-1 infection. (2,13,42,54) Also host defenses may be markedly improved since studies from our group have shown that immune function becomes normalized during chronic methadone maintenance treatment. (26,27,31,42,45,49,53,54,58,59,67,79,83,84,87,88)

The long-term effects or sequelae of heroin addiction that are deleterious include profound abnormalities in neuroendocrine and neurotransmitter function, profound abnormalities in immune function, as well as the sequelae of progression of hepatitis B virus infection, hepatitis delta agent infection and human immunodeficiency virus infection as well as other infectious diseases. (11,26,27,31,42,45,49,50,53,54,58,59,66,67,77,78,79,81,83, 84,85,86,87,88)

Many research groups have shown that in humans, acute administration of opiates and also chronic administration of short-acting opiates such as heroin, have profound effects on neuroendocrine function. (8,26,27,31,42,43) These effects include inhibition of release of ACTH from the anterior pituitary and inhibition of release of beta-endorphin which comes from the same gene product, proopiomelanocortin. Also, altered release of cortisol from the adrenal center occurs with resultant lowered levels of cortisol and abnormal circadian rhythm of its release during cycles of heroin addiction. Short-acting opiates also inhibit release of LH; the lower levels of LH which result in lower levels of testosterone. Acutely, opiates also effect increase in release of vasopressin and increase in release of prolactin.

A variety of endocrine studies have shown that during chronic, steady dose methadone maintenance treatment, there is complete normalization of the hypothalamic-pituitary-adrenal axis, as reflected by normal levels and normal circadian rhythm of levels of beta-endorphin, ACTH and cortisol, along with normalization of responses to the chemically-induced stress of the metyrapone test. (20,24,25,26,31,42,43,54,64,70,73,74)

Several groups have shown that the important hypothalamic-pitiuitary-gonadal axis is profoundly disrupted by heroin addiction, with reduction of the pulsatile release of LH, coupled with abnormal circadian rhythms and tonic levels of steadily released LH. (8,26,27,31,42,43) These abnormalities are frequently accompanied by abnormalities of secondary amenorrhea in females and with a decreased conception rate for the amount of unprotected sexual exposure. These changes also may lead to relative hypogonadalism with decreased libido and often decreased sexual performance in males.

It has been shown that during chronic methadone maintenance treatment, normal pulsatile release of LH returns to normal, with the normal preovulatory surge in females. This leads to return to normal measures ??? in most females former heroin addicts in methadone maintenance treatment within six months to one year. It has been shown also that circadian rhythm of LH release and tonic levels of LH become normal; thus in male subjects gonadal function returns to normalcy. (26,27,31,42,43,54,64) All aspects of reproductive biology return to normal in both male and female former heroin addicts during chronic methadone maintenance treatment.

Thus two of the most important neuroendocrine mechanisms related to survival, as well as to normal physiological functioning, and which have been shown to be profoundly disrupted by cycles of heroin addiction, become normalized during steady dose long-term methadone maintenance treatment.

In addition, many studies have been performed by our laboratory and others to define the immune status of intravenous drug users who are not in treatment, as well as to define the immune status of those who are in various treatments, including methadone maintenance treatment. (26,31,42,45,49,53,54,59,67,79,83,84,87) Many groups including our own also performed various laboratory and in vitro studies of immune function to determine what the role of both of exogenous opiate drugs, as well as other potential drugs of abuse may be on immune function; to determine what may be the effects of treatment agents; and finally to determine what may be the role of the endogenous opioid system, or the endorphins, on the various specific indicies on immune function. (3,4,86,88) These will not be discussed in detail. However it should be mentioned that recent studies from many groups have shown that classical neuroendocrine function plays a very important role in modulating normal immune function. Therefore, disruption of neuroendocrine function may be anticipated to contribute to disruption of the immune function. Thus, although our group and others have shown that there are very few direct in vitro effects of opiates, such as heroin, or morphine, on specific indicies of immune function, in both animal models and in humans, profound disruption of immune function may be found after administration of such a short-acting opiate. There is increasing evidence that these alterations are due to an indirect opiate effect by virtue of altering neuroendocrine function.

We have performed a sequence of studies to determine immune function in both active heroin addicts and in methadone maintained patients. In one highly controlled study, three groups of subjects were examined. (83) First, a group of "hard-core" active heroin addicts who were found on testing to be HIV-1 negative, second a group of very long-term methadone maintenance patients who had been in continuous methadone maintenance treatment for eleven to twenty-one years, most receiving high doses of methadone and all of whom were found to be free from HIV-1 infection on testing, and finally a group of normal volunteer subjects were included. The heroin addict group and the methadone maintained group had a similar number of years of intravenous drug abuse and a similar prevalence of exposure to hepatitis B virus, which may also alter immune function.

In this group it was shown that whereas the absolute numbers of CD4 cells and absolute numbers of CD8 cells are highly significantly abnormal in active heroin addicts, the absolute numbers of these cell types became normal in the long-term methadone maintenance patients. It was also shown that the immunoglobulin IgM levels, reflecting B cell function, which were significantly elevated in heroin addicts became normal in the methadone maintained patients. Studies of natural killer cell activity have been of especial interest for study in my laboratory. Natural killer cells provide the first line of defense against many viral infections as well as against progression of tumors of various types. Natural killer cells do not demand prior sensitization before they can carry out their cytotoxic action. Our group and others have found that natural killer cell activity is highly significantly reduced in heroin addicts. As we showed in this highly controlled study, it was found that long-term, high dose methadone maintained patients had absolutely normal natural killer cell cytotoxicity activity.

In summary, we found that chronic stable dose maintenance treatment with the long-acting opioid methadone allows a former heroin addict to become both normal behaviorally and normal functionally. We have shown that drug-craving and drug-seeking behavior disappears and that narcotic abstinence symptoms are prevented. We have also shown as very important physiological functions which are profoundly disrupted during cycles of heroin addiction, including the hypothalamic-pituitary-gonadal axis and hypothalamic-pituitary-adrenal axis, become normalized during methadone maintenance treatment. Finally we and others have found that many indicies of immune function are abnormal in heroin addicts, primarily probably because of frequent use of unsterile needles and concomitant diseases which are common and are no longer a problem during methadone maintenance treatment, but also possibly in part due to the fact that short-acting opiates such as heroin, disrupt immune function indirectly possibly by the documented disruption of normal neuroendocrine function. We have found that in long-term methadone maintenance patients in whom neuroendocrine function has become normalized, specific indicies of both cellular and humoral or immune function become normal. Implications of the normalization of immune function as well as neuroendocrine function, for the initial infection with and progression of HIV-1 infection to AIDS have yet to be fully elucidated. However, clearly for a variety of diseases, normal physiological function including immune function, is desirable and potentially protective.

Acknowledgements

The work of Dr. M.J. Kreek and her laboratory, as reported in this paper, was supported in part by the ADAMHA National Institute for Drug Abuse Research Center Grant P50-05130; the ADAMHA-NIDA Research Scientist K05-00049 to Dr. Kreek; a contract from the New York State Division of Substance Abuse Services; the Herbert and Nell Singer Foundation; the Alfed Nogi Memorial Fund, and two grants for the Aaron Diamond Foundation in New York City.

References

1. Albeck, H., Woodfield, S., Kreek, M.J.: Quantitative and pharmacokinetic analysis of naloxone in plasma using high performance liquid chromatography with electrochemical detection and solid phase extraction. J. Chromatog. 488:435-445, 1989.

2. Albeck, H., Woodfield, S., Wahlstrom, A., Kreek, M.J.: Naloxone pharmacokinetics in man following an intravenous dose. In: Problems of Drug Dependence, 1990: Proceedings of the 52nd Annual Scientific Meeting of the Committee on Problems of Drug Dependence. Harris, L.S. ed., NIDA Research Monograph Series. Rockville, MD, in press 1991.

3. Bodner, G., Albeck, H., Soda, K.M., Kreek, M.J.: Modulation of natural killer cell activity: Possible role of hypothalamic-pituitary-adrenal hormones. In: New Leads in Opioid Research. Eds. Van Ree, J.M., Mulder, A.H., Wiegant, V.M., and Van Wimersma Greulanus, T.B., Excerpta Medica, Amsterdam 330-331, 1990.

4. Bodner, G., Soda, K.M., Kennedy, J., Kreek, M.J.: Modulation of NK Activity: role of neuroendocrine status. In: Problems of Drug Dependence, 1990: Proceedings of the 52nd Annual Scientific Meeting of the Committee on Problems of Drug Dependence. Harris, L.S. ed., NIDA Research Monograph Series. Rockville, MD, in press 1991.

164

5. Bowen, D.V., Smit, A.L.C. and Kreek, M.J.: Fecal excretion of methadone and its metabolites in man: Application of GC-MS. In: <u>Advances in Mass Spectrometry</u>, N.R. Daly, ed., Philadelphia, PA: Heyden & Son, Inc., <u>7B</u>:1634-1639, 1978.

6. Culpepper-Morgan, J.A., Holt, P.R., Kreek, M.J.: Colonic opiate receptors change with age: Preliminary data. In: <u>Problems of Drug Dependence, 1987: Proceedings of the 49th Annual Scientific Meeting of the Committee on Problems of Drug Dependence</u>. Harris, L.S. ed., <u>NIDA Research Monograph Series</u>, Rockville, MD DHHS Publications No. (ADM)88-1564 81:267, 1988.

7. Culpepper-Morgan, J., Kreek, M.J., Holt, P.R., La Roche, D., Zhang, J., O'Bryan, L.: Orally administered kappa as well as mu opiate delay gastrointestinal transit time in the guinea pig. <u>Life Sciences, 42:</u> 2073-2077, 1988.

8. Cushman, P. and Kreek, M.J.: Some endocrinologic observations in narcotic addicts. In: <u>Narcotic and the Hypothalamus</u>, E. Zimmerman and R. George, eds., New York, NY: Raven Press, 161-173, 1974.

9. Cushman, P., Kreek, M.J. and Gordis, E.: Ethanol and methadone in man: A possible drug interaction. <u>Drug and Alc. Dep.</u>, <u>3</u>:35-42, 1978.

10. Des Jarlais, D.C., Friedman, S.R., Novick, D.M., Sotheran, J.L., Thomas, P., Yancovitz, S.R., Mildvan, D., Weber, J. Kreek, M.J., Maslansky, R., Bartelme, S.,Spira, T. Marmor, M. HIV I Infection among intravenous drug users in Manhattan, New York City 1977 to 1987. <u>JAMA</u> 261:1008-1012, 1989.

11. Des Jarlais, D.C., Marmor, M., Cohen, H., Yancovitz, S., Garber, J., Friedman, S., Kreek, M.J., Miescher, A., Khuri, E., Friedman, S.M., Rothenberg, R., Echenberg, D., O'Malley, P.O., Braff, E., Chin, J., Burtenol, P., Sikes, R.K.: Antibodies to a retrovirus etiologically associated with Acquired Immunodeficiency Syndrome (AIDS) in populations with increased incidences

of the syndrome. <u>Morbidity and Mortality Weekly Report</u>, <u>33</u>:377-379, 1984.

12. Dole, V.P. and Kreek, M.J.: Methadone plasma level: Sustained by a reservoir of drug in tissue. <u>Proc. Natl. Acad. Sci.</u>, <u>70</u>:10, 1973.

13. Dole, V.P., Nyswander, M.E. and Kreek, M.J.: Narcotic blockade. <u>Arch. Intern. Med.</u>, <u>118</u>:304-309, 1966.

14. Hachey, D.L., Kreek, M.J. and Mattson, D.H.: Quantitative analysis of methadone in biological fluids using deuterium-labeled methadone and GLC-chemical-ionization mass spectrometry. <u>J. Pharm. Sci.</u>, <u>66</u>:1579-1582, 1977.

15. Hachey, D.L., Mattson, D.H. and Kreek, M.J.: Quantitation of methadone in biological fluids using deuterium labeled internal standards. In: <u>Proceedings of the Second International Conference on Stable Isotopes</u>, E.R. Klein and P.D. Klein, eds., ERDA-CONF-751027, Springfield, VA: National Technical Information Source, U.S. Dept. of Commerce, 518-523, 1976.

16. Hachey, D.L., Nakamura, K., Kreek, M.J. and Klein, P.D.: Analytical techniques for using multiple, simultaneous stable isotopic tracers. In: <u>Stable Isotopes</u>, H.L. Schmidt, H. Forstel and K. Heinzinger, eds., Amsterdam: Elsevier Scientific Publishing Company, 235-239, 1982.

17. Hahn, E.F., Lahita, R., Kreek, M.J., Duma, C., Inturrisi, C.E.: Naloxone radioimmunoassay: an improved antiserum. <u>J. Pharm. Pharmacol.</u>, <u>35</u>:,833-836, 1983.

18. Kaufmann, C.A., Kreek, M.J., Karoum, F. and Chuang, L.W.: Depression during methadone withdrawal: No role for beta-phenylethylamine. <u>Drug and Alcohol Dependence</u>, <u>13</u>:21-29, 1984.

19. Kaufmann, C.A., Kreek, M.J., Raghunath, J., Arns, P.: Methadone, monoamine oxidase and depression: Opioid dist-

ribution and acute effects on enzyme activity. Biol. Psychiatry, 18:1007-1021, 1983.

20. Kennedy, J.A., Hartman, N., Sbriglio, R., Khuri, E., Kreek, M.J.: Metyrapone-induced withdrawal symptoms. Brit J Addict 85:1133-1140, 1990.

21. Klein, P.D., Hachey, D.L., Kreek, M.J. and Schoeller, D.A.: Stable isotopes: Essential tools in biological and medical research. In: Stable Isotopes: Applications in Pharmacology, Toxicology and Clinical Research, T.A. Baillie, ed., Baltimore, MD: University Park Press, 3-14, 1978.

22. Kosten, T.R., Kreek, M.J., Raghunath, J., Kleber, H.D.: A preliminary study of beta-endorphin during chronic naltrexone maintenance treatment in ex-opiate addicts. Life Sciences 39: 55-59, 1986a.

23. Kosten, T.R., Kreek, M.J., Raghunath, J., Kleber, H.D.: Cortisol levels during chronic naltrexone maintenance treatment in ex-opiate addicts. Biological Psychiatry. 21:217-220, 1986b.

24. Kosten, T.R., Kreek, M.J., Swift, C., Carney M.K., Ferdinands, L.: Beta-endorphin levels in CSF during methadone maintenance. Life Sciences, 41:1071-1076, 1987.

25. Kreek, M.J.: Medical safety, side effects and toxicity of methadone. Proceedings of the Fourth National Conference on Methadone Treatment, NAPAN-NIMH, 171-174, 1972.

26. Kreek, M.J.: Medical safety and side effects of methadone in tolerant individuals. J. Amer. Med. Assn., 223:665-668, 1973a.

27. Kreek, M.J.: Physiological implications of methadone treatment. In: Methadone Treatment Manual, U.S. Dept. of Justice (USGPO) #2700-00227, Washington, D.C.: 85-91, 1973b.

28. Kreek, M.J.: Plasma and urine levels of methadone. N.Y. State J. Med., 73:2773-2777, 1973c.

29. Kreek, M.J.: Pharmacologic modalities of therapy: Methadone maintenance and the use of narcotic antagonists. In: Heroin dependency: Medical, economic and social aspects, B. Stimmel, ed., New York, NY: Stratton Intercontinental Medical Book Corp., 232-290, 1975.

30. Kreek, M.J.: The role of qualitative and quantitative analysis of drugs and their metabolites in maternal-neonatal studies. In: National Institute on Drug Abuse Symposium on Comprehensive Health Care for Addicted Families and Their Children, Services Research Report (USGPO), #017-024-00598-3, Washington, DC:67-73, 1977.

31. Kreek, M.J.: Medical complications in methadone patients. Ann. N.Y. Acad. Sci., 311:110-134, 1978a.

32. Kreek, M.J.: Effects of drugs and alcohol on opiate disposition and action. In: Factors Affecting the Action of Narcotics, M.W. Adler, L. Manara and R. Saminin, eds., New York, NY: Raven Press, 717-739, 1978b.

33. Kreek, M.J.: Methadone disposition during the perinatal period in humans. Pharmac. Biochem. Behav., 11, Suppl.:7-13, 1979a.

34. Kreek, M.J.: Methadone in treatment: Physiological and pharmacological issues. In: Handbook on Drug Abuse, R.L. Dupont, A. Goldstein and J. O'Connell, eds., NIDA-ADAMHA-DEW-ODAP-Executive Office of the President, 57-86, 1979b.

35. Kreek, M.J.: Metabolic interactions between opiates and alcohol. Ann. N.Y. Acad.Sci., 362:36-49, 1981.

36. Kreek, M.J.: Disposition of narcotics in the perinatal period. In : Publication of AMERSA and The Career Teacher Program in Alcohol and Drug Abuse, 3:7-10, 1981-82.

37. Kreek, M.J.: Opioid disposition and effects during chronic exposure in the perinatal period in man. In: <u>Journal of Addictive Diseases</u>, B. Stimmel, ed., New York, NY: The Haworth Press, Inc., <u>1</u>:21-53, 1982.

38. Kreek, M.J.: Factors modifying the pharmacological effectiveness of methadone. In: <u>Research in the Treatment of Narcotic Addiction: State of the Art</u>, J.R. Cooper, F. Altman, B.S. Brown, and D. Czechowicz, eds.,National Institutes of Drug Abuse Monograph, DHHS Pub. # (ADM) 83-1281, 95-114, 1983.

39. Kreek, M.J.: Opioid interactions with alcohol. <u>Journal of Addictive Diseases</u> New York, NY: The Haworth Press, <u>3</u>:35-46, 1984.

40. Kreek, M.J.: Drug interactions with methadone in humans. In: <u>Strategies for Research on the Interactions of Drugs of Abuse</u>, NIDA Research Monograph 68 Braude, M.C. and Ginzburg, H.M., eds., Rockville, MD., <u>68</u>:193-225, 1986a.

41. Kreek, M.J.: Exogenous Opioids: Drug-Disease Interactions, <u>Advances in Pain Research and Therapy</u>, eds. Foley, K.M., Inturrisi, C.E., New York, NY: Raven Press, <u>8</u>: 201-210, 1986b.

42. Kreek, M.J.: Multiple Drug Abuse Patterns and Medical Consequences. In: <u>Psychopharmacology: The Third Generation of Progress. Meltzer, H.Y., ed</u>. Raven Press, New York, NY 1597-1604, 1987a.

43. Kreek, M.J.: Tolerance and Dependence - Implications for the pharmacological treatment of addiction. In: <u>Problems of Drug Dependence, 1986: Proceedings of the 48th Annual Scientific Meeting of The Committee on Problems of Drug Dependence</u>. Harris, L.S., ed., <u>NIDA Research Monograph Series</u>, Rockville, MD, DHHS Publication No.(ADM) 87-1508 <u>76</u>:53-61, 1987b.

44. Kreek, M.J.: Opiate-ethanol interactions: Implications for the biological basis and treatment of combined addictive diseases.

In: Problems of Drug Dependence, 1987; Proceedings of the 49th Annual Scientific Meeting of the Committee on Problems of Drug Dependence. Harris, L.S., ed. NIDA Research Monograph Series Rockville, MD DHHS Publication No. (ADM)88-1564 81:428-439, 1988.

45. Kreek, M.J.: Immunological approaches to clinical issues in drug abuse. In: Problems of Drug Dependence, 1988; Proceedings of the 50th Annual Scientific Meeting of the Committee on Problems of Drug Dependence. Harris, L.S. ed., NIDA Research Monograph Series, Rockville, MD DHHS Publication No. (ADM)89-1605 90:77-86, 1989.

46. Kreek, M.J.: Drug interactions in humans related to drug abuse and its Treatment. Modern Methods in Pharmacology 6:265-282, 1990a.

47. Kreek, M.J.: Historical and medical aspects of methadone maintenance treatment: Effectiveness in treatment of heroin addiction and implications of such treatment in the setting of the AIDS epidemic. Evaluation of Different Programmes for Treatment of Drug Addicts Adamsson, C., Jansson, B., Rydberg, U., Westrin, C., (Eds.), Medicinska Forskningsradet, Stockholm, Sweden, 61-76, 1990b.

48. Kreek, M.J.: Methadone maintenance treatment for heroin addiction. The Effectiveness of Drug Abuse Treatment: Dutch and American Perspectives Platt, J.J., Kaplan, C.D., McKim, P.J., (Eds.), Malabar, Florida: Krieger Publishing Co. 275-293, 1990c.

49. Kreek, M.J.: HIV infection and parenteral drug abuse: ethical issues in diagnosis, treatment, research and the maintenance of confidentiality. In: Proceedings of the Third International Congress on Ethics in Medicine - Nobel Conference Series. P. Allebeck, B. Jansson, eds. Raven Press, New York, NY 181-187, 1990d.

50. Kreek, M.J.: Immune function in heroin addicts and former heroin addicts in treatment: pre/post AIDS epidemic. Current Chemical and Pharmacological Advances on Drugs of Abuse Which Alter Immune Function and Their Impact Upon HIV Infection: Pham, P.T.K., and Rice, K., eds. NIDA Research Monograph Series, Rockville, MD 96:192-219, 1990e.

51. Kreek, M.J.: Multiple Drug Abuse Patterns: Recent trends and associated medical consequences. Advances in Substance Abuse: Behavioral and Biological Research, Volume 4, Jessica Kingsley Publishers Ltd., London, England. In press 1990f.

52. Kreek, M.J.: Neuroendocrine (HPA) and Gastrointestinal Effects of Opiate Antagonists: Possible Therapeutic Application. In: Problems of Drug Dependence, 1990; Proceedings of the 52nd Annual Scientific Meeting of the Committee on Problems of Drug Dependence. Harris, L.S. ed., NIDA Research Monograph Series. Rockville, MD, in press 1991a.

53. Kreek, M.J.: Immunological Function in Active Heroin Addicts and Methadone Maintained Former Addicts: Observations and Possible Mechanisms. In: Problems of Drug Dependence, 1990; Proceedings of the 52nd Annual Scientific Meeting of the Committee on Problems of Drug Dependence. Harris, L.S. ed., NIDA Research Monograph Series. Rockville, MD, in press 1991b.

54. Kreek, M.J.: Using methadone effectively: achieving goals by application of laboratory, clinical, and evaluation research any by development of innovative programs. Improving Drug Abuse Treatment: Pickens, R., Leukefeld, C., Schuster, R. eds. NIDA Research Monograph Series Rockville, MD in press, 1991c.

55. Kreek, M.J., Bencsath, F.A., Fanizza, A. and Field, F.H.: Effects of liver disease on fecal excretion of methadone and its unconjugated metabolites in maintenance patients: Quantitation by direct probe chemical ionization mass spectrometry. Biomed Mass Spectrm., 10:544-549, 1983.

56. Kreek, M.J., Bencsath, F.A. and Field, F.H.: Effects of liver disease on urinary excretion of methadone and metabolites in maintenance patients: Quantitation by direct probe chemical ionization mass spectrometry. Biomedical Mass Spectrometry, 7:385-395, 1980.

57. Kreek, M.J., Brown, L.T., Bernstein, W.J. and Harte, E.H.: Estrogen treatment alters narcotic disposition in the rat. In: Proceedings of the 1979 International Narcotic Research Conference, E.L. Way, ed., New York: Pergamon Press, 405-407, 1980.

58. Kreek, M.J., Des Jarlais, D.C., Trepo, C.L., Novick, D.M., Abdul-Quader, A., Raghunath, J.: Contrasting prevalence of delta hepatitis markers in parenteral drug abusers with and without aids. J Infect Dis, 162:538-541, 1990.

59. Kreek, M.J., Dodes, L., Kane, S., Knobler, J. and Martin, R.: Long-term methadone maintenance therapy: Effects on liver function. Ann. Intern. Med., 77:598-602, 1972.

60. Kreek, M.J., Garfield, J.W., Gutjahr, C.L. and Giusti, L.M.: Rifampin-induced methadone withdrawal. New Engl. J. Med., 294:1104-1106, 1976.

61. Kreek, M.J., Gutjahr, C.L., Bowen, D.V. and Field, F.H.: Fecal excretion of methadone and its metabolites: A major pathway of elimination in man. In: Critical Concerns in the Field of Drug Abuse: Proceedings of the Third National Drug Abuse Conference, A. Schecter, H. Alksne and E. Kaufman, eds., New York, NY: Marcel Dekker, Inc., 1206-1210, 1978.

62. Kreek, M.J., Gutjahr, C.L., Garfield, J.W., Bowen, D.V. and Field, F.H.: Drug interactions with methadone. Ann. N.Y. Acad. Sci., 281:350-370, 1976.

63. Kreek, M.J., Hachey, D.L. and Klein, P.D.: Stereoselective disposition of methadone in man. Life Sci., 24:925-932, 1979.

64. Kreek, M.J. and Hartman, N.: Chronic use of opioids and antipsychotic drugs: Side effects, effects on endogenous opioids and toxicity. Ann. N.Y. Acad. Sci., 398:151-172, 1982.

65. Kreek, M.J., Kalisman, M., Irwin, M., Jaffery, N.F. and Scheflan, M.: Biliary secretion of methadone and methadone metabolites in man. Res. Comm. Chem. Path. Pharmacol., 29:67-78, 1980.

66. Kreek, M.J., Khuri, E., Fahey, L., Miescher, A., Arns, P., Spagnoli, D., Craig, J., Millman, R., Harte, E.: Long term follow-up studies of the medical status of adolescent former heroin addicts in chronic methadone maintenance treatment: Liver disease and immune status. In: Problems of Drug Dependence, 1985; Proceedings of the 47th Annual Scientific Meeting of The Committee on Problem of Drug Dependence. Harris, L.S., ed., NIDA Research Monograph Series Rockville, MD., DHHS Publication No.(ADM) 86-1448 67: 307-309, 1986.

67. Kreek, M.J., Khuri, E., Flomenberg, N., Albeck, H., Ochshorn, M.: Immune status of unselected methadone maintained former heroin addicts. International Narcotics Research Conference 1989 (INRC). Quirion, R., Jhamandas, K., Gianoulakis, C., eds., Alan R. Liss, Inc., New York, NY, 445-448, 1989.

68. Kreek, M.J., Khuri, E. and Joseph, H.: A new "heroin epidemic"? Ann. Intern. Med., 83:420-421, 1975.

69. Kreek, M.J., Oratz, M. and Rothschild, M.A.: Hepatic extraction of long- and short-acting narcotics in the isolated perfused rabbit liver. Gastroenterology, 75:88-94, 1978.

70. Kreek, M.J., Raghunath, J., Plevy, S., Hamer, D., Schneider, B., and Hartman, N.: ACTH, cortisol and beta-endorphin response to metyrapone testing during chronic methadone maintenance treatment in humans. Neuropeptides, 5:277-278, 1984.

71. Kreek, M.J., Rothschild, M.A., Oratz, M., Mongelli, J. and Handley, A.C.: Acute effects of ethanol on hepatic uptake and distribution of narcotics in the isolated perfused rabbit liver. Hepatology, 1:419-423, 1981.

72. Kreek, M.J., Schecter, A.J., Gutjahr, C.L. and Hecht, M.: Methadone use in patients with chronic renal disease. Drug and Alcohol Depend., 5:197-205, 1980.

73. Kreek, M.J., Wardlaw, S.L., Friedman, J., Schneider, B. and Frantz, A.G.: Effects of chronic exogenous opioid administration on levels of one endogenous opioid (beta-endorphin) in man. Advances in Endogenous and Exogenous Opioids, Simon E. and Takagi, H. eds., Tokyo, Japan: Kodansha Ltd. Publishers, 364-366, 1981.

74. Kreek, M.J., Wardlaw, S.L., Hartman, N., Raghunath, J., Friedman, J., Schneider, B. and Frantz, A.G.: Circadian rhythms and levels of beta-endorphin, ACTH, and cortisol during chronic methadone maintenance treatment in humans. Life Sciences, Sup. I, 33:409-411, 1983.

75. Nakamura, K., Hachey, D.L., Kreek, M.J., Irving, C.S. and Klein, P.D.: Quantitation of methadone enantiomers in humans using stable isotope-labeled $^2H_3$, $^2H_5$, $^2H_8$ methadone. J. Pharm. Sci., 71:39-43, 1982.

76. Nakamura, K., Kreek, M.J., Hachey, D.L., Irving, C.S. and Klein, P.D.: Studies on disposition of dl-methadone in former heroin addicts by the multiple deuterium labeling method. Proceedings of the Japanese Society for Medical Mass Spectrometry, 6:119-124, 1981.

77. Novick, D.M., Des Jarlais, D.C., Kreek, M.J., Spira, T.J., Friedman, S.R., Gelb, A.M., Stenger, R.J., Schable, C.A., Kalyanaraman, V.S.: The specificity of antibody tests for human immunodeficiency virus in alcohol and parenteral drug

abusers with chronic liver disease. Alcoholism: Clinical and Experimental Research 12, 687-690, 1988.

78. Novick, D.M., Farci, P. Croxson, S.T., Taylor, M.B., Schneebaum, C.W., Lai, E.M., Bach, N. Senie, R.T., Gelb, A.M., Kreek, M.J.: Hepatitis delta virus and human immunodeficiency virus antibodies in parenteral drug abusers who are hepatitis B surface antigen positive. J. Infect. Dis., 158: 795-803, 1988.

79. Novick, D.M., Khan, I., Kreek, M.J.: Acquired immunodeficiency syndrome and infection with hepatitis viruses in individuals abusing drugs by injection. United Nations Bulletin on Narcotics, 38:15-25, 1986.

80. Novick, D.M., Kreek, M.J., Arns, P.A. Lau, L.L., Yancovitz, S.R., and Gelb, A.M.: Effects of severe alcoholic liver disease on the disposition of methadone in maintenance patients. Alcoholism: Clin. Exp. Res., 9:349-354, 1985.

81. Novick, D., Kreek, M.J., Des Jarlais, D., Spira, T.J., Khuri, E.T., Raghunath, J., Kalyanaraman, V.S., Gelb, A.M., and Miescher, A.: Antibody to LAV, the putative agent of AIDS, in parenteral drug abusers and methadone-maintained patients: Abstract of clinical research findings: Therapeutic, historical, and ethical aspects. In: Problems of Drug Dependence, 1985: Proceedings of the 47th Annual Scientific Meeting of The Committee on Problems of Drug Dependence. Harris, L.S., ed.,NIDA Research Monograph Series., Rockville, MD., DHHS Publication No. (ADM)86-1448 67:318-320, 1986.

82. Novick, M., Kreek, M.J., Fanizza, A.M., Yancovitz, S.R., Gelb, A.M. and Stenger, R.J.: Methadone disposition in patients with chronic liver disease. Clin.Pharmacol. Ther., 30:353-362, 1981.

83. Novick, D.M., Ochshorn, M., Ghali, V., Croxson, T.S., Mercer, W.D., Chiorazzi, N., Kreek, M.J.: Natural Killer Cell Activity and Lymphocyte Subsets in Parenteral Heroin Abusers and Long-term Methadone Maintenance Patients. J. Pharm Exper Ther. 250:606-610, 1989.

84. Novick, D.M., Ochshorn, M., Kreek, M.J.: In vivo and in vitro studies of opiates and cellular immunity in narcotic addicts. In: Drugs of Abuse, Immunity and Immunodeficiency. Friedman, Herman, eds., Plenum Press, New York. In press 1991.

85. Novick, D.M., Trigg, H.L., Des Jarlais, D.C., Friedman, S.R., Vlahov, D., Kreek, M.J.: Cocaine injection and ethnicity in parenteral drug users during the early years of the human immunodeficiency virus (HIV) epidemic in New York City. J. Med. Virol. 29:181-185, 1989.

86. Ochshorn, M., Kreek, M.J., Hahn, E.F., Novick, D.M.: High Concentrations of naloxone lower natural killer (NK) activity. In: Problems of Drug Dependence, 1987: Proceedings of the 49th Annual Scientific Meeting of the Committee on Problems of Drug Dependence. Harris, L.S. ed., NIDA Research Monograph Series, Rockville, MD DHHS Publication No. (ADM)88-1564, 81:338, 1988.

87. Ochshorn, M., Kreek, M.J., Khuri, E., Fahey, L., Craig, J., Aldana, M.C., Albeck, H.: Normal and abnormal Natural Killer (NK) activity in methadone maintenance treatment patients. In: Problems of Drug Dependence, 1988: Proceedings of the 50th Annual Scientific Meeting of the Committee on Problems of Drug Dependence. Harris, L.S. ed., NIDA Research Monograph Series, Rockville, MD DHHS Publication No. (ADM) 89-1605, 90:369, 1989.

88. Ochshorn, M., Novick, D.M., Kreek, M.J.: In vitro studies of methadone effect on natural killer (NK) cell activity. Israel J of Med Sci 26:421-425, 1990.

89. Pond, S.M., Kreek, M.J., Tong, T.G., Raghunath, J., Benowitz, N.L.: Altered methadone pharmacokinetics in methadone-maintained pregnant women. J of Pharm. & Exper. Thera., 233:1-6, 1985.

90. Ragavan, V.V., Wardlaw, S.L., Kreek, M.J., Frantz, A.G.: Effect of chronic naltrexone and methadone administration on brain immunoreactive beta-endorphin in the rat. Neuroendocrinology, 37:266-268, 1983.

91. Rubenstein, R.B., Kreek, M.J., Mbawa, N., Wolff, W.I., Korn, R. and Gutjahr, C.L. and Wolff, W.I.: Human spinal fluid methadone levels. Drug and Alc. Dep., 3:103-106, 1978.

92. Stimmel, B. and Kreek, M.J.: Pharmacologic actions of heroin. In: Heroin dependency: Medical, economic and social aspects, B. Stimmel, ed., New York, NY: Stratton Intercontinental Medical Book Corp., 71-87, 1975a.

93. Stimmel, B. and Kreek, M.J.: Dependence, tolerance and withdrawal. In: Heroin dependency: Medical, economic and social aspects, B. Stimmel, ed., New York, NY: Stratton Intercontinental Medical Book Corp., 88-97, 1975b.

94. Tong, T.G., Benowitz, N.L. and Kreek, M.J.: Methadone-disulfiram interaction during methadone maintenance J. Clin. Pharmacol., 20:506-513, 1980.

95. Tong, T.G., Pond, S.M., Kreek, M.J., Jaffery, N.F. and Benowitz, N.L.: Phenytoin-induced methadone withdrawal. Ann. Intern. Med., 94:349-351, 1981.

96. Unterwald, E.M., Kreek, M.J.: Alterations in the expression of brain opioid receptors during senescence. In: New Leads in Opioid Research Eds: Van Ree, Mulder, Wiegant and Van Wimersma Greidanus, pgs. 200-201, 1990a.

97. Unterwald, E.M., and Kreek, M.J.: Age-related changes in the expression of brain opioid receptors. Society for Neuroscience Abstracts, 16:368, 1990b.

98. Unterwald, E.M., Nyberg, F., Terenius, L., Kreek, M.J.: Distribution of opioid peptides in brain and GI tract: Age and species-specific differences. In: Problems of Drug Dependence, 1990: Proceedings of the 52nd Annual Scientific Meeting of the Committee on Problems of Drug Dependence. Harris, L.S. ed., NIDA Research Monograph Series. Rockville, MD DHHS Publication No. (ADM) 91-1753 105:408-409, 1990.

99. Zhang, J.S., Plevy, S., Albeck, H., Culpepper-Morgan. J., Friedman, J., Kreek, M.J.: Effects of age on distribution of preproenkephalin-like mRNA in the gastrointestinal tract of the guinea pig. _Advances in the Biosciences_: Proceedings of 1988 INRC meeting _75_:349-350, 1989.

100. Ziring, B., Brown, L. and Kreek, M.J.: Effects of route of administration on methadone disposition in the rat. In: _Problems of Drug Dependence, 1980, Proceedings of the 42nd Annual Scientific Meeting of the Committee on Problems of Drug Dependence_, L.S. Harris, ed., _NIDA Research Monograph Series_, Rockville, MD DHHS Publication No. _34_:145-151, 1981.

101. Ziring, B.S., Kreek, M.J. and Brown, L.T.: Methadone disposition following oral versus parenteral dose administration in rats during chronic treatment. _Drug Alc. Depend._, _7_:311-318, 1981.

102. Ziring, B., Shepperd, S., and Kreek, M.J.: Reversed phase thin-layer chromatography for the separation of betaendorphin, beta-lipotropin and enkephalins. _Int. J. Peptide Protein Res._, _22_:32-38, 1983.

Methadone Maintenance: A Medical Approach to Heroin Addiction

A. Tagliamonte[1], I. Maremmani[2], and D. Meloni[1]

[1] Institute of Pharmacology and Biochemical Pathology, University of Cagliari,
Via Porcell 4, I-09124 Cagliari, Italy
[2] Institute of Psychiatry, University of Pisa, Via Roma 67, I-53100 Pisa, Italy

The issue of assistance to drug addicts in Italy still presents different elements of confusion. One of the main sources of confusion is the distinction between legal and illegal substances of abuse. Such distinction has two consequences: first, it leads to restrict the term "drug addict" to consumers of illecit drugs. Second, in the evaluation of the behavioral modifications produced by drug assumption, it brings a factor of uncertainty in distinguishing between pure psychiatric symptoms and crimes. Recently, the legislator has contributed to complicate even more the issue by punishing whoever carries illicit substancies, independently of the amount. The drug addict may be, thus, defined either as a patient criminalized for his disease or as a criminal who tries to take advantage from a disease.

Such a confusion heavily interferes with the evaluation of the different approaches used for treatment and rehabilitation of drug addicts. The emotional need for

a radical solution of the problem brings the social
community to prefer a therapeutic approach aimed to a
completely drug-free condition and to refuse the
pragmatism of the methadone maintenance program.On the
other hand, the concept that drug addiction is a chronic
disease with tendency to relapse has scientific grounds
that cannot be canceled by emotions.

The use of methadone in the therapy of heroin addiction
presents the same problems and has the same limits of any
other long term drug therapy.
Three main factors characterize a drug therapy: the
patient, the drug and the physician. The patient is a sick
person with peculiar personality traits that may or may
not be modified by the disease. The disease may or may not
be curable and its treatment may or may not result in
complete recovery.
However, in most cases long term therapy is finalized to
provide an exogenous support to an otherwise altered
functional equilibrium or to slow the progression of a
degenerative process. Drugs may be effective or not and
each of them is endowed with specific toxic effects, so
that long term use may produce peculiar medical problems.
Physicians have the duty to prescribe the right drug at
the correct dosage and to convince the patient to a valid
compliance.
It is the continuous interplay among these three factors
that characterizes a drug therapy.
We may consider in parallel three examples of disease that
needs chronic drug therapy:
- congestive heart failure
- bipolar depression
- heroin addiction
Congestive heart failure is treated with peripheral
vasodilators, diuretics and digitalis associated to strict
hygienic rules. The patient's personality is crucial for a
correct compliance, intended both as drug assumption and
obedience to the hygienic restrictions. For these
patients it is mandatory to stop smoking, follow an
appropriate diet, avoid emotions and excessive physical
efforts and maintain an adequate physical training.
The drugs used in heart failure are effective but, quite
often, may produce undesirable effects. Diuretics may
alter the electrolytic balance (Weiner, 1990), and
digitalis which has a very narrow therapeutic index, may
induce life threatening arrhythmias (Hoffman and Bigger,
1990).

Bipolar depression is treated with lithium (Bunney and Garland-Bunney, 1987; Dunner and Clayton, 1987), that should stabilize mood and prevent or reduce the intensity of both manic and depressive episodes. Lithium may be substituted with and/or associated to carbamazepine (Post, 1987) to which, if manic or depressive phases appear, the addition of neuroleptics, ECS and antidepressants, respectively, becomes mandatory. The patient compliance is strictly dependent on his mood. If it is equilibrated, he will be willing to take drugs, provided that he trusts the doctor. Any factor that will disconfirm the psychiatrist, may result in the abrupt interruption of therapy. If the patient becomes euphoric he may stop taking drugs and this fact may have dramatic consequences, since euphoria is the first symptom of an ensuing manic episode.

Thus, compliance in these patients is a serious problem and, no matter how professional the psychiatrist may be, many times it is not possible to prevent a relapse.

A point to be taken into consideration, is the low social acceptance that still exists towards lithium therapy and the misconceptions that label ECS as a kind of torture more than as a therapeutic tool. Any form of criticism addressed against a therapeutic approach may undermine the patient's confidence toward his doctor, and thus reduce compliance.

Heroin addiction may be treated in a closed institution where drugs are forbidden, and the interests of the patient are addressed toward those "values", that in the mind of the staff, will cancel haroin memory, and allow the soul finally free from negative influences, to express itself.

The impact of the therapeutic community (TC) on drug addiction is certainly positive (O'Brien and Biase, 1981), although controversial. In fact, only a low percentage of patients accept to spend years in a closed institution; furthermore no program guarantees from a possible relapse. The latter point is common to all known treatments of addiction and is crucial in raising criticisms against such treatments, in fact, drug addiction is a condition socially unaccepted so that its only possible solution has to be a radical one.

Unfortunately, a radical solution does not exist and the basic demand of such a solution rests upon a pure emotional basis.

Heroin addicts may be treated with long acting opiate agonists (methadone, LAAM) (Dole and Joseph, 1978; Blaine et al., 1981) or antagonists (O'Brien and Greenstein, 1981). Naltrexone is the most widely used antagonist. At therapeutic doses it blocks for more than 24 hours any possible effect of heroin. Thus, its long term administration should extinguish the desire of (i.e. the craving for) heroin. Given to a selected population of patients, this compound has produced positive outcomes (Jaffe, 1987). However, it does not guarantee from either precocious or delayed relapses.

Thus, both TC and opiate antagonists are valid indications for a selected population of patients which aim for a completely drug-free condition. The positive outcomes of both approaches are often used to criticize those patients who fail to obtain the expected advantages. They are considered responsible for the therapeutic failure, which is attributed to their insufficient endurance, low self-confidence and poor ego strenght.

In our culture, a relative who blamed a cardiopathic patient for health impairment would be considered a monster, while it is more frequent that friends and relatives blame a psychiatric patient because of his poor control of behaviour. In fact, although the concept of inadequate behaviour as a symptom of mental disease has been well clarified, sometimes it needs the authoritative opinion of the psychiatrist to be accepted.

On the other hand, drug addicts are regarded as personally responsible for their acts, symptoms and therapeutic failures as a rule.

The concept of patient fault arouses the projective attitudes of the therapist who, by blaming the patient, protects the deficiencies of both the approach used to cure him and the therapist's attitudes toward the patient itself.In other words, blaming the patient confers to the therapeutic approach a magic dimension of infallibility, which may be perceived by the staff as lack or absence of responsibility toward the patient. Such a condition is reassuring to the staff, but is persecutory to the patient and is detrimental to the development of a correct relationship between the two.

The magic dimension of an unfailing method that promises the complete recovery of drug addicts is easily accepted by the layman community, which is worried both emotionally and by the reality of the problems related to drug addiction.

This cultural context does not accept to classify the heroin addict as a psychiatric patient, as proposed by the DSM-III. In fact, if a patient is responsible for his own symptoms and he can avoid them by "just saying no", the conclusion is that he must be a simulator. If the symptoms are behavioural in nature, he may be defined as a criminal who is pretending to be insane in order to escape the due punishment.

In other words, the unacceptable point is the notion of drug addiction as a disease.

As a matter of fact, none of these prejudices will ever influence both the drawing and the outcome of the therapeutic protocol of a patient affected by heart failure. Indeed, also a cardiopathic patient is prone to relapse and such an accident is often due to his poor compliance to the hygienic prescriptions like, for instance, cigarette smoking.Tobacco produces a serious form of drug dependence and its use constitutes a serious hazard to cardiopathic patients.However, if they smoke and worsen, both the doctor and the relatives will strive to reassure them about their health and convince them to keep following the prescriptions. In other words, the patient is treated the way he should be.

Manic-depressive patients often relapse because they interrupt therapy. Again, nobody would blame a patient because he is having a florid manic episode, and both the psychiatrist and the relatives will feel committed to find the way to administer the neuroleptics.

The tactics used by the psychiatrist are different from those used by the cardiologist, but both have the same strategy aimed to cure the patient independently of his responsibilities towards himself or the community.

To a heroin addict, relapse may often cost the expulsion from the therapeutic program.

Drug addiction, by definition, is due to an extrinsic etiological factor and this point should be considered as a crucial one if any approach toward prevention has to be planned. On the other hand, it is difficult both to conceive and to accept the concept of a long term (if not a lifetime) therapy to prevent the relapse of a syndrome produced by a substance that can be administered only by purpose. However, both the axiom "once an alcoholic, always an alcoholic" and the definition of heroin addiction as "a chronic disease with the tendency to relapse" come from centuries of experience and from statistical data that cannot be denied. A patient who is suffering because of the consequences of his addiction to alcohol, heroin, or tobacco, is by definition incapable of controlling the use of the toxic substance, although he knows that his problems would vanish by "just saying no". If he could just say no, he would not be a drug addict. Such a chronically suffering patient needs a pragmatic response to his problems, not a moralistic one.

To the clinician, the only issue relevant to drug addiction must be the toxicity of the abused substance. Dependence per sè remains an unwanted drug effect, which becomes a medical problem only when it results in a compulsive behavior obsessively focalized on the drug consumption. In any case, a cigarette smoker sees the doctor and gets the prescription to stop smoking only if gastric, respiratory or cardiovascular symptoms are present. If medicine had an antidote to tobacco there would be no reason to stop smoking. In the era of diuretics, eccessive salt restrictions are a non-sense.

Similarly, a heroin addict will come to the attention of the psychiatrist only when he has lost the capacity to control heroin use, so that his behaviour becomes inadequate to the standards of a normal social life. The evaluation of a drug addict's behavioural symptoms presents several elements of confusion. For instance, the fact that the use of heroin or marijuana is illegal is not a medical problem, as it is not a medical problem the legal consequence of drinking champagne at dinner in Saudi Arabia, where alcohol is forbidden.

The main duty of a psychiatrist in front of a heroin addict asking for help is to reduce or eliminate the negative effects produced by the opiate. If the patient is determined to stop heroin use and is willing to enter a TC, he must be encouraged in this direction. If the patient does not accept the closed institution and lives in an environmental situation as requested by the protocol with opiate antagonists, he can be addressed to a naltrexone program. If these conditions are lacking or the patient already went through such experiences unsuccessfully, the prescription should be a methadone maintenance program.

Methadone maintenance is the most pragmatic and effective approach to heroin addiction in our hands. It is pragmatic since its main aim is the reduction, up to complete cessation, of heroin use, but it is not the eradication of opiate dependency up to the drug-free condition (Hargreaves, 1983). It is effective because, given orally once a day, it prevents or abolishes all withdrawal symptoms, eliminates craving, equilibrates mood and has little and well accepted side effects (Kreek, 1983).

Methadone is a full opiate agonist, with a selective affinity to the μ-receptor similar to that of morphine (Jaffe and Martin, 1990). Given chronically, it produces tolerance to most of its effects.

The use of illicit opioids decreases as a function of methadone dose: more than 90% of the patients treated at a daily dose ranging from 80 to 100 mg, stops using heroin (Dole, 1989). This means that an individual variability of response to methadone exists, so that the psychiatrist must tailor the correct dose on each single patient. Such a dose, should not produce by definition, sedation, nodding, euphoria nor any other acute, central opioid effect. The full dose is attained gradually, in order to favor the development of tolerance to the undesired effects.

In conclusion, methadone, given chronically at the optimal dose to heroin addicts: I) can prevent the compulsive use of heroin; II) normalizes the psycophysical function, thus allowing the process of social rehabilitation; III) may favor the attempt to reach a drug-free condition.

A comparative evaluation of the methadone trials is rather difficult, since there is no complete agreement either on the therapeutic protocols to be used or on the criteria to estimate the results (Hargreaves, 1983). These should be similar to the ones used to evaluate any other therapeutic protocol. For instance, the validity of a heart failure treatment is estimated in terms of measurable values of the hemodynamic parameters altered by the disease.

The validity of a bipolar depression treatment is evaluated in terms of manic-depressive episode frequency per year and of single episode intensity, evaluated by the use of approved rating scales.

On the other hand, the validity of a methadone maintenance program is evaluated in terms of:

- percentage versus time of retention in therapy;
- coincident use of heroin;
- employment rate;

- job keeping;
- family care;
- number of arrests.

The use of heroin is the cause, not a symptom, of addiction. Social parameters are usually altered as a consequence of heroinism, but constitute only an unspecific and indirect estimate of the disease.

The alterations of personality traits produced by chronic heroin use are only seldom taken into consideration. Thus, many questions related to the efficacy of chronic methadone remain officially unanswered. The staff members of a methadone clinic know, in fact, that many patients do very well although they keep using heroin episodically. I.e. methadone protects the patient from the dysphoric effects produced by heroin. However, such an effect is mentioned in the official literature only as a negative outcome. The reason for this, is that a positive conclusion could favor an excess of permissivism, certainly dangerous, since "heroin use, although episodic, is the gateway to relapse". We are forced to consider correct such a restrictive postulate since, until more data will disprove it, we may not conclude whether or not methadone permits a controlled use of heroin.

Thus, heroin use by methadone patients is considered evil even by the staff members of the clinic and remains a cause for blaming and punishing them.

More correctly, a urinalysis positive for morphine should be considered in the whole context of the therapeutic curriculum of a patient. A professional member of the staff, on whom the patient can rely being confident that he will never be punished by him, should have the responsibility to interpret and apply the clinic rules, not on a bureaucratic basis, but on a therapeutic one. I.e., rules, like methadone doses, should be tailored by the psychiatrist on each patient.

On the other hand, methadone clinics are often so overcrowded with patients that a really continuous and constructive relationship between them and a staff member becomes exceptional. In such a context, the imposition of rules on patients too often replaces a more personalized approach with them. Notwithstanding these problems, the therapeutic results obtained by methadone maintenance programs are unequivocally positive.

This fact does not mean that the pharmacologic approach to heroin addiction is universally accepted. Methadone maintenance remains the most criticized and less accepted therapeutic approach to heroin addiction, and the rationale of such opposition is certainly based on the fact that the drug-free condition is not the main target of the project.

To further improve the results obtained so far, a new professional figure should be created, the post-doc specialist in drug addiction. Such a specialist would guarantee a truly stable staff to the clinics and a professional assistance to the patients.

REFERENCE
Blaine JD, Thomas DB, Barnett G, Whysner JA, Renault PF (1981) Levo-alpha acetylmethadol (LAAM): clinical utility and pharmaceutical development. In: Lowinson JH and Ruiz P (eds) Substance abuse: Clinical problems and perspectives. Williams & Wilkins, Baltimore. pp 360-388.
of lithium in affective illness: Basic and clinical implications. In: Meltzer HY (ed) Psychopharmacology: The third generation of progress. Raven Press, New York, pp 553-566.
Dole VP, Joseph H (1978) Long term outcome of patients treated with methadone maintenance. Ann. N.Y. Acad. Sci. vol. 311, pp 181-189.
Dole PV (1989) Methadone treatment and acquired immunodeficiency syndrome epidemic. JAMA, september 22-29, vol. 262, pp 1601 1602.
Dunner DL, Clayton PJ (1987) Drug treatment of bipolar disorder. In: Meltzer HY (ed) Psychopharmacology: The third generation of progress. Raven Press, New York, pp 1077-1083.
Hargreaves WA (1983) Methadone dosage and duration for maintenance treatment. In: Cooper JR, Altman F, Brown BS, Czechowicz D (eds) Research on the treatment of narcotic addiction. State of the Art. Treatment Research Monograph Series. pp 19-79.
Hoffman BF, Bigger JT jr (1990) Digitalis and allied cardiac glycosides. In: Goodman and Gilman's (eds) The pharmacological basis of therapeutics. Pergamon Press, pp 814-839.
Jaffe JH (1987) Pharmacological agents in treatment of drug dependence. In: Meltzer HY (ed) Psychopharmacology: The third generation of progress. Raven Press, New York, pp 1605-1616.
Jaffe JH, Martin WR (1990) Opioid analgesics and antagonists. In: Goodman and Gilman's (eds) The pharmacological basis of therapeutics. Pergamon Press, pp 485-521.
Kreek MJ (1983) Health consequences associated with the use of methadone. In: Cooper JR, Altman F, Brown BS, Czechowicz D (eds) Research on the treatment of narcotic addiction. State of the Art. Treatment Research Monograph Series. pp 456-482.
O'Brien WB, Biase DV (1981) The therapeutic community: the family-milieu approach to recovery. In: Lowinson JH and Ruiz P (eds) Substance abuse: Clinical problems and perspectives. Williams & Wilkins, Baltimore. pp 303-316.
O'Brien CP, Greenstein RA (1981) treatment approaches: opiate antagonists. In: Lowinson JH and Ruiz P (eds) Substance abuse:Clinical problems and perspectives. Williams & Wilkins, Baltimore. pp 403-404.
Post RM (1987) Mechanisms of action of carbamazepine and related anticonvulsants in affective illness. In: Meltzer HY (ed) Psychopharmacology: The third generation of progress. Raven Press, New York, pp 567-576.

Weiner IM (1990) Diuretics and other agents employed in the mobilization of edema fluid. In: Goodman and Gilman's (eds) The pharmacological basis of therapeutics. Pergamon Press, pp 713-731.

Intravenous Methadone Maintenance: A British Response to Persistent Opiate Injectors

C. BREWER

Medical Director, The Stapleford Centre, 25a Eccleston, London SW1 9 NP,
United Kingdom

ABSTRACT

In drug abuse, the mode of administration of a drug and the
associated cues and rituals are often as important as its
pharmacology. Many tobacco smokers who found nicotine
chewing-gum an unacceptable alternative to cigarettes will
readily confirm this. Intravenous injection is evidently a
highly addictive behaviour and those who are strongly
addicted to it often find conventional oral methadone
maintenance and reduction programmes unhelpful, even if the
dosage is generous. Intravenous methadone maintenance appears
to make treatment acceptable to at least a proportion of
injectors who would not otherwise come forward. This paper
discusses some of the experiences and practices of one of the
largest injectable methadone programmes in Britain including
demographic data, assessment, dosage, safeguards, problems,
bureaucratic requirements and monitoring. It also touches on
certain historical and medico-political factors. Preliminary
results from a pilot study of hair-analysis for illicit drugs
indicate a surprisingly low incidence and level of continuing
heroin and cocaine use in our patients. Methadone doses up to
1100mg daily can be compatible with regular, skilled
employment. Both hair analysis and intravenous medication
assist the 'therapeutic bargaining' which is an intrinsic and
very useful feature (though often a neglected or undervalued
one) of methadone programmes.

INTRODUCTION

In the 19th Century, opiate dependence was common in Britain and other European countries, as well as in the US and much of the Orient. (Berridge and Edwards, 1987) As readers of Sherlock Holmes know, subcutaneous administration was an increasing feature of Victorian drug use, as intravenous injection has been in this century, and we cannot now disinvent the syringe, any more than we can disinvent nuclear bombs. Addiction (and its treatment) is not just a matter of pharmacology. Although many addicts use the intravenous route for the 'rush' or 'pharmacological orgasm', many are also clearly addicted to the process of injecting. The psychological factors involved are presumably similar to those which make cigarette smoking so notoriously difficult to give up, even when generous doses of nicotine are provided in other forms such as chewing gum or skin patches.

ORIGINS OF THE PRESENT BRITISH LEGISLATION

Following increasing pressure from the USA (Musto, 1973) opiate abuse was effectively criminalised in Britain during the First World War. Most other countries did not really share the American enthusiasm for prohibition but as on other occasions before and since, when America sniffed, the rest of the world caught cold. Nevertheless, in 1926, a committee headed by the distinguished physician Sir Humphrey Rolleston concluded that it was appropriate to prescribe maintenance opiates to the relatively small residue of addicts who continued to defy the new law. (Berridge, 1980) They numbered no more than a few hundred but their family doctors were free to prescribe oral or injectable opiates, or indeed cocaine, indefinitely. No official notification was required but they were all known to the Home Office (the British 'Interior Ministry') through officials who monitored the prescribing of all 'controlled' drugs.

RESPONSES TO THE ADDICTION EPIDEMIC

When the drug culture reached Britain from America in the 1960s, there was a rapid increase in the number of addicts but they were very different from the generally middle-class 'gentleman addicts' of the 1920s and 30s. The initial response was the setting up of prescribing clinics by the National Health Service (NHS) which were run by psychiatrists. Their philosophy sometimes seems to be have been: "Tell us how much you want and bring a wheelbarrow to take it home". Heroin, methadone, cocaine and mehthyl-amphetamine - oral and injectable - were freely prescribed. However, many addicts were helped by these clinics, in the sense that they were at least able to avoid crime and stay in work, and some have been on maintenance prescriptions from NHS clinics ever since the mid-1960s. Notification of addicts to the Home Office became mandatory around 1970.

The clinics soon faced two big problems. The first was that if they were 'user-friendly', they attracted many patients and were overwhelmed, since the initial funding and staffing of the clinics was generally static. Secondly, the initial enthusiasm of the staff tended to evaporate when they realised that few addicts were immediately interested in being steered towards lasting abstinence.

During the 1970s, disillusionment with methadone treatment, together with low morale, lack of funding (especially in London) and discontent in the NHS for a variety of reasons, led many clinics to terminate maintenance treatment, especially i/v maintenance. Some continued to dispense or prescribe 'courses' of standardised reducing doses of methadone but many dispensed little more than advice and exhortation. However, a few clinics continued to operate under the original system and prescribed injectable opiates indefinitely for those addicts who would not or could not detoxify. Although it is possible, with a special licence, to prescribe injectable heroin for addicts, this is now rare and is largely restricted to a few relatively old addicts. Private doctors cannot prescribe heroin for addicts, though there are no special restrictions on prescribing heroin for legitimate analgesic purposes.

As with abortion - another contentious medico-moral issue - methadone policy in a given area depends largely on the attitude of the local specialists. Cambridge and Liverpool, two very different cities, both continued traditional prescribing policies through the 1980s. In London, most clinics furtively maintain a few selected patients on injectables while refusing to take on new addicts for injectable maintenance. In contrast, Scotland was for many years almost a methadone-free zone and the first Scottish physician to prescribe methadone fairly freely in recent years was the doctor in change of infectious diseases when he was faced with the Edinburgh AIDS epidemic of the early 1980s. Even so, injectable prescribing is still almost unknown in Scotland.

THE STAPLEFORD CENTRE

The origins of the Stapleford Centre's methadone programme have been described elsewhere. (Brewer, 1988) The Centre began as a research-based organisation which provided private but relatively low-cost alcoholism treatment, rapid clonidine-naltrexone opiate withdrawal and naltrexone maintenance but prescribed no methadone. Following the disciplining of a private doctor who had a large i/v methadone maintenance practice and whose opiate licence was suspended, (Dally, 1990) her patients naturally sought alternative sources. Government departments and voluntary agencies supplied them with the names of a number of private and NHS doctors and units including ours. A senior civil servant told us that we would be doing a valuable public service if we could overcome our understandable reluctance to take them on, but indicated that we should not expect much official help if we got into trouble with other authorities. Three years later (as of February 1991) we now prescribe methadone for some 250 patients at the Stapleford Centre in London. 142 of these receive injectable methadone. We also continue to provide clonidine-naltrexone withdrawal under sedation during a 24 - 48 hour admission, three-day alcohol withdrawal and Antabuse and naltrexone programmes. Most patients come from the Greater London area but a significant proportion come from other towns within a 50 mile (80km) radius. A few come from as far away as Scotland (400 miles) and Tyneside (270 miles). We employ one full-time and three part-time doctors, one full-time and two part-time counsellors, who also write, but do not sign, prescriptions.

RUNNING AN INJECTABLE METHADONE PROGRAMME

SELECTION

Most patients are self-referred. About 15% are referred by various agencies. Few are referred by GPs, who are generally (and probably correctly) perceived as unsympathetic to opiate addicts. The fact that they have started to inject is commonly given by addicts as a reason for seeking detoxification or oral methadone treatment. About a third of the patients request only oral methadone. In some cases, the progressive disappearance of superficial veins is a powerful factor in discontinuing both injecting and unconventional drug use. However, others respond to this development by using femoral or jugular veins, or by injecting subcutaneously. Some are blessed (or cursed) with arm veins which do not collapse or thrombose despite repeated injection. Like smokers who cannot stop, these last two groups will continue to inject for many years whatever society, doctors or judges say. Many are in touch with needle exchanges but it seems inconsistent, in a harm-reduction model, to use clean syringes to inject dirty, illicit and impure drugs of unknown strength. If patients are ambiguous about injectable methadone, we suggest they try a generous oral programme first and in some cases they decide to stay on oral medication.

SCREENING AND DEMOGRAPHY

A comprehensive history is taken based on a self-completed questionnaire. Patients have to provide a urine specimen at the first interview but we do not usually wait for the results before beginning treatment. The average age is about 26 and about 20% are women. The patients are mainly white (black opiate abusers are still notably rare in Britain) but tattoos are common. They are mainly skilled or semi-skilled manual workers and their political views are often rather Thatcherite or, less commonly, 'green'. Many patients are initially unemployed, but their fees are paid by their families. However, we have several middle-class injecting patients. The Centre is located in a busy street in Belgravia, one of the smartest and most un-proletarian areas of London but despite the nature of our clientele, we have had no problems with our neighbours.

THE METHADONE DOSAGE

The initial methadone dose is based on the patient's estimate of heroin use. A few are primarily methadone addicts but most have some experience of methadone and of their tolerance to it. As a rough guide, we find 0.5G of street heroin is equivalent to 50mg - 70mg of methadone. To enable us to assess both their tolerance and their familiarity with injecting, injecting patients have to inject the test dose under supervision. If, as in most cases, they are prescribed a mixture of oral and injectable methadone, they must inject at least an hour after the agreed oral dose has been swallowed under supervision. For at least the next week, they must drink their methadone daily under supervision at their chosen pharmacy which is usually near their home or work. Some pharmacists will also let them inject daily in a back room at the start of treatment. A notable feature of i/v methadone test doses is the lack of obvious effect on mood, alertness or behaviour. In many cases, there is no more to see than if they had smoked an ordinary cigarette, even after as much as 150mg.

DOSAGE RANGE

The correct dose of most drugs is 'enough' - and not just barely enough. Another useful feature of the 'British system' is that there are no binding official regulations governing the maximum permitted dosage. Although the average daily dose for oral methadone, 79.2mg, is not particularly high, and the average total dose for injecting patients, 122mg, is not much greater, we have no upper limit. Anglin and McGlothlin (1984) have shown that generous methadone programmes give better results than stingy ones but apart from this general point,

some patients appear to need and to tolerate doses very much
higher than average.

Fig 1

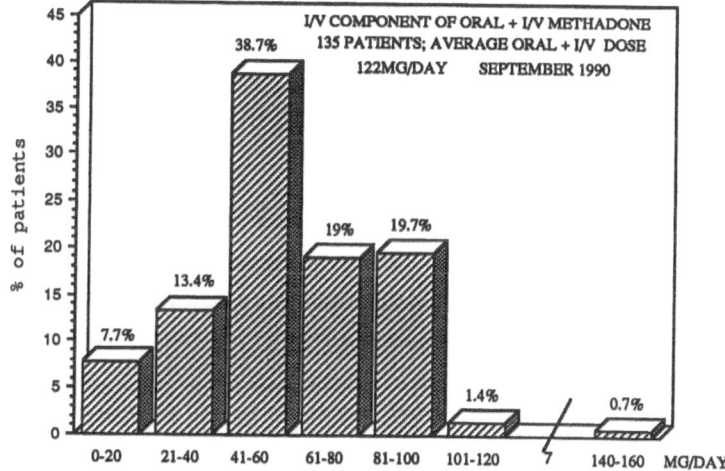

Daily Dosage Range

Fig 2

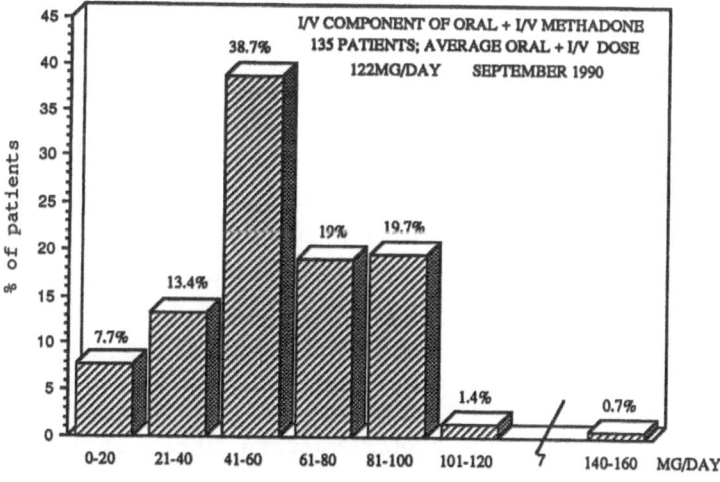

Daily Dosage Range

The most notable beneficiary of this policy has been an
opiate addict who used to abuse alcohol as well and had very
abnormal liver functions. He continued to drink without any
reaction despite large doses of supervised Antabuse but has

now managed to stop drinking completely for the first time as his methadone was progressively increased from its initial level of 150mg to the present dose of 1100mg daily.

MONITORING

HAIR ANALYSIS

One of the main aims of methadone treatment, whether oral or injectable, is to reduce or eliminate the use of illicit opiates, especially heroin. Urine testing is an inefficient and inaccurate method of assessing the pattern and extent of heroin use, especially in Britain where patients are not required to come to a clinic every day to take their methadone. Instead, they collect it from a convenient pharmacy at a frequency ranging from every day to every two weeks depending on their stability. They generally attend the clinic to renew their prescription and talk with a doctor or counsellor every two or three weeks. Irregular heroin use can easily be hidden under this system, although if the amount used is small, such occasional use may not be a serious problem.

Fortunately, quantitative radio-immunoassay (RIA) hair-analysis for opiates and other drugs has revolutionised our practice in this area. We can now detect even the occasional use of small amounts of heroin three months previously. More importantly, if heroin is being used regularly, we can tell fairly accurately what the average dose is. Hair-analysis is evasion-proof and avoids the humiliating aspects of urine testing. It is also repeatable if the results are disputed and it is not very expensive.

Equally importantly, hair testing makes it much easier for the courts to consider probation-linked treatment rather than imprisonment for serious or repeated heroin-related offences, since they know that the detection of any relapse can be virtually guaranteed. Two judgements of the Court of Appeal have specifically mentioned hair-testing (Brewer, 1989) and while this was in the context of treatment with naltrexone, there is no reason why the same principle should not apply to

methadone maintenance, since a common aim of both treatments
is to help patients avoid illicit drug use and the associated
criminal lifestyle.

<u>SAFEGUARDS</u>

A common criticism of injectable programmes is that some
addicts will sell their supplies. This applies to all
programmes involving unsupervised medication, oral or i/v,
but there are ways of minimising the problem. Firstly, hair-
testing ensures that if patients are selling methadone to
obtain and use heroin, the use of heroin will be discovered.
Secondly, we have introduced ampoules of 50mg in 5ml and 35mg
in 3.5ml in addition to the standard 10mg in 1ml size. This
not only reduces the cost of injectables considerably but
also means that the daily dose of most patients can be
contained in one or two ampoules which are large enough to be
individually labelled. Used ampoules have to be returned
either to us or to the pharmacy with their labels intact
before new ones are dispensed. This means that if someone is
arrested in possession of ampoules prescribed for another
person, the identity of his supplier will be quickly
revealed. Finally, the police drug squad know, from their
regular examinations of pharmacy records, who receives
regular methadone prescriptions. If they have doubts, they
can easily question or observe individual patients.
Dispensing methadone in the form of relatively high-dose
single ampoules encourages a pattern of injecting only once
daily.

<u>TREATMENT STRATEGIES</u>

Methadone has a number of uses which may have different
importance at different stages of an addict's career. The
aims of treatment may also change. Initially, simple
stabilisation is often the goal - a change from an irregular,
illegal, time-consuming and work-preventing pattern of drug
use to one which takes up much less time, effort and money
(the patient's money or other people's) and causes much less
variation in cerebral physiology. It may take months or years

196

on a regular dose for patients to settle into a more productive pattern of existence. Occasional or frequent crises, often unrelated to drug use, may occur as with more ordinary citizens.

At some stage, injecting patients will often want to try changing from partly or entirely injectable methadone to purely oral medication. This may be a prelude to complete withdrawal from opiates or merely to a further lengthy period of stabilisation without injecting. We encourage patients to make these experiments when the time is right (which means that we sometimes discourage them then we think the time is wrong) but we leave the timetable largely to them.

Some patients need injectables only for a few weeks, as a transition. Conversely, a few patients who have been satisfactorily maintained on oral medication for months may start regularly injecting heroin again, sometimes in response to a crisis, and may need to be given injectable methadone for a while. Weaning off injectables sometimes involves replacing the reduced i/v dose by a compensatory increase in oral methadone.

WITHDRAWAL

We offer patients the whole range of withdrawal techniques. These are:

1) Gradual reduction to zero as an out-patient. Clonidine and hypnotics are often helpful in the final stages.

2) Classic 2 - 3 week in-patient withdrawal with methadone and/or clonidine. This is expensive in private practice but is often available in NHS hospitals, so we generally refer patients to appropriate NHS centres if they wish. Patients with jobs may find it difficult to get enough time off work for this method.

3) Rapid withdrawal using clonidine, naltrexone and sedation. This involves only a 48 hour stay in hospital, sometimes less. It can be done, depending on the patient's

tastes and finances, under sedation with benzodiazepines and/or chlorpromazine (Brewer, Rezae and Bailey, 1988) or, as performed by Loimer et al (1988) in Vienna, under general anaesthesia. We have even detoxified one patient under anaesthesia and curare on a ventilator for 24 hours. After rapid detoxification, patients are fit to return home to family nursing within two days and can usually return to work within a week.

In all cases, we encourage detoxified patients to take naltrexone under family supervision for at least six months. Our observations indicate that for precipitated withdrawal, the severity of the withdrawal symptoms is largely unrelated to the usual daily opiate dosage and that recovery takes no longer for methadone than for heroin. We always make it clear that if abstinence fails, we will resume methadone – oral or i/v – if necessary. This makes it easier for patients to contemplate and attempt experiments with abstinence.

METHADONE AS AN AID TO PSYCHOTHERAPY

It has repeatedly been shown that methadone maintenance programmes have the highest retention rate of all the various treatments for opiate abuse. This point has been further emphasised in a paper presented at this conference by Kupfer-Gernun et al. If attendance is regular, some sort of relationship inevitably develops between the patient and the clinic and if the patient is usually seen by the same person, the relationship has much therapeutic potential. If psychotherapy can sometimes be seen as at least in part a bargaining process, methadone greatly increases the bargaining power of the therapist. The possibility of prescribing i/v methadone means that some patients can be drawn into the bargaining process who would not otherwise enter the therapeutic arena.

Inevitably there is a degree of paternalism about methadone programmes but benevolent paternalism is an old medical tradition and one which many patients appear to find quite comforting. The ability to be flexible about take-home privileges has an important corollary – that these privileges can be varied to modify the patient's behaviour. These modifications include improving timekeeping, reducing or avoiding the use of other illicit drugs and drinking less. Where necessary, troublesome coexisting alcohol abuse can be controlled in most cases by making continued methadone prescribing conditional on taking disulfiram under supervision. (Liebson, 1973) Withdrawing methadone before the patient is ready to do so is rarely helpful since the usual result is that the patient fails to attend the clinic and is thus no longer exposed to potential therapeutic influences.

The process of change often has to be measured in years rather than months, but few people familiar with psychotherapy would expect otherwise. Methadone is not a substitute for care, advice, support and concern, but not everyone needs intensive psychotherapy as opposed to consistent support from, and easy access to, someone who knows their history and cares about their welfare. Some addicts benefit more from pharmacological stability and control than from formal psychotherapeutic interventions. There is a significant rate of spontaneous remission in all addictions but an addict needs to stay alive to benefit from it.

REFERENCES

Anglin M D, McGlothlin W H, (1984) Outcome of Narcotic Addict Treatment in California, NIDA Research Monograph 51, DHHS Publication No. (ADM) 84-1349, Rockville, MD: NIDA

Berridge V, (1980) The making of the Rolleston report 1908-1926. Journal of Drug Issues, 10, 7-28

Berridge V, Edwards G, (1987) Opium And The People, Yale University Press, New Haven

Brewer C (1988) Dealing with Dr Dally's deluge. General Practitioner, 29th January, 55

Brewer C (1990) Hair-analysis for drugs of abuse. Lancet. 1:980

Brewer C, Rezae H, Bailey C (1988) Opioid withdrawal and naltrexone induction in 48-72 hours with minimal drop-out, using a modification of the naltrexone-clonidine technique. British Journal of Psychiatry, 153, 340-343

Dally A (1990,) A Doctor's Story. Macmillan. London

Kupfer-Gernun U, Busch H, Brunder ann H, et al (1991) Compliance of HIV infected IDVUs during methadone maintenance. Paper presented at First European Symposium on Drug Addiction and AIDS. Vienna. Feb 22-23

Liebson I (1973) Alcoholism among methadone patients: a specific treatment method. American Journal of Psychiatry, 130(4), 483-5

Loimer N, Schmid R, Presslich O, Lenz K (1988) Naloxone treatment for opiate withdrawal syndrome. British Journal of Psychiatry, 153, 851-52

Musto D (1973) The American Disease. Origins of Narcotic Control. Yale University Press. New Haven

The Impact of Methadone Maintenance Treatment on the Spread of HIV Among IV Heroin Addicts in Sweden

O. Blix and L. Grönbladh

University of Uppsala, Department of Psychiatry, Methadone Programme,
S-751 85 Uppsala, Sweden

Introduction

The epidemic spread of HIV among heroin addicts is well documented through reports from many countries (Des Jarlais et al 1989). Needle sharing is the main route of transmission. Effective HIV prevention must target this risk behaviour. Needle exchange programmes are showing promising results in various countries (Christensson, Ljungberg 1991, Stimson et al 1988). Carefully conducted Methadone Maintenance Treatment (MMT) has proven to be an efficient tool to prevent i.v. heroin addicts from contracting HIV (Novick et al 1988).

The situation in Sweden

Heroin was introduced on the Swedish drug scene in 1974. It has since then been the major opiate of abuse, replacing raw opium, morphine hydrochloride and morphine base from the late sixties and early seventies (Frykholm, Gunne 1980).

In 1981 the number of heroin abusers in Sweden was estimated to be 4000, of whom 2000 were daily users with a compulsive type of abuse. The heroin abusers comprise approximately 30% of the i.v. abusers. Amphetamine is still the most common street drug of injection (Olsson et al 1981). This situation is largely unchanged since that survey was performed.

HIV, as shown in retrospective studies of frozen sera, started to infect street addicts in Stockholm in 1983 (Pehrson et al 1988). Until December 31 1990 a total of 2655 HIV positive individuals were registered at the department of epidemiology at the National Bacteriological Laboratory in Stockholm. Of those, 575 were i.v. addicts and 367 had a history of opiate abuse. (M. Böttiger, 1991). The majority, 86 percent, of those were living in the Stockholm area. Most of the remaining 14 percent were former Stockholm addicts who have resettled elsewhere during and after treatment.

Methadone Treatment in Sweden

The Swedish MMT Programme was set up in 1966 in Uppsala by professor Gunne (Gunne 1966) and is based on the Dole-Nyswander programme (Dole, Nyswander 1965). Thus it is one of the oldest programmes still in operation in Europe. The admission to the programme was temporarily closed for political reasons 1979-1984. In 1981, the Swedish board of Health and Welfare formally accepted MMT as a treatment for opiate abuse, but only for a limited number of 150 persons at a time. As the regulations were somewhat hesitating, it took another 3 years until the programme was able to reopen. In 1988 the programme was allowed to expand to 300 patients. The regulations also allowed two new programmes to operate independently of the original National programme in Uppsala. There was an after-care unit set up in 1986 in Stockholm that has now developed a local independent programme, which is now the largest MMT programme in Sweden. Recently a new after care clinic opened in Lund for addicts from the southern parts of Sweden. The Uppsala programme has the rest of Sweden as catchment area.

The maximal number of patients allowed in treatment was again raised in October 1990 to 450. In January 1991 a total of 306 former opiate addicts received methadone treatment in Sweden. Of those 116 (38%) were HIV positive. The distribution between the 3 different programmes in Sweden is shown in table 1.

Table 1. MMT patients in Sweden by Jan.1 1991

	Total	HIV+	% HIV+
Stockholm	221	105	48
Uppsala	67	10	15
Lund	18	1	6
Total	306	116	38

Admission criteria

MMT has been reserved for opiate addicts with a documented history of at least 4 years of compulsive opiate abuse, a minimum age of 20 years, three previous inpatient detoxification attempts followed by relapses into opiate abuse, current i.v. opiate abuse, voluntary application and absence of dominating side abuse. These criteria were slightly changed in October 1990, excluding the need for earlier treatment. Current abuse is not necessary in case the patient is waiting for treatment in a drug free setting (compulsory drug free treatment, prison etc.) and has a well documented history of early relapses after similar treatment periods.

With regard to HIV infection there are no special inclusion criteria. There has been a tendency that the already infected addicts have been more frequently referred to MMT than the not yet infected.

MMT Organisation

The treatment programme in Uppsala is based upon in-patient initiation. Patients referred to the programme can also be started as out-patients, if local support in their home towns is possible and if they have proper housing situations. The local support can be a G.P. or a nurse. Departments of infectious diseases have also been a good support in some cases, as heroin addicts often are well known to these institutions due to repeated infections. Patients from southern Sweden are still referred to Uppsala for evaluation of admission criteria for formal acceptance. Some of them are then initiated as out patients at the new clinic in Lund while more complicated cases still are initiated as in-patients in Uppsala. The Stockholm programme has its own system. It has been based on out-patient treatment only but has recently opened a ward for in-patient treatment as well.

Evaluations

Evaluative studies of the Uppsala programme have shown that 74 percent of patients in treatment are free of abuse and hold down a work or full time studies (Gunne, Grönbladh 1981; Grönbladh, Gunne 1989). A study on mortality among MT patients and non treated heroin addicts reveals an increased death rate of 63 times the expected for that age group among the non treated cases while patients in treatment are approaching normal survival figures. (Gunne, Grönbladh, Öhlund 1990).

When the first HIV antibody tests were performed on i.v. drug abusers in 1984, 14 percent of the opiate abusers were found to be positive in Stockholm. In 1988 the prevalence of seropositive subjects among opiate addicts in custody in Stockholm was 45% (Olin, Käll 1988). The present study shows a rapid increase in seropositivity among patients referred to MMT while patients in treatment have remained negative.

Objective

The objective for this study is to verify differences in the prevalence of HIV among patients in MT treatment versus waiting list patients.

Methods and subjects

All patients admitted to the MMT programme before 1984 were tested and retested yearly for the presence of HIV antibodies 1985-1990. The blood tests were taken when patients came for regular counselling, but also - especially for those living far away - in local outpatient clinics or department for infectious diseases. Patients admitted 1984-1990 were tested upon admission to the treatment and retested yearly during treatment. The screening was performed with ELISA and positive tests were confirmed with the Western Blotting technique.

The MMT programme in Uppsala has an 8 bed ward with psychiatric trained nurses, social workers, psychologist and psychiatrist. An after-care treatment team is connected to the clinic and takes part in the resocialisation process already during the inpatient phase of the treatment (average 3 months). Patients were recruited from all parts of Sweden until 1988, when the local Stockholm programme took over also the initiating process. The last 33 patients from Stockholm treated by the Uppsala MMT programme were transferred back in 1990.

Results

When admission to the MMT reopened in September 1984 there were 67 patients still in treatment who were admitted before the temporary closedown in 1979. Two individuals (3%) were found to be HIV antibody positive. Both were females, living together with actively abusing men. Table 2 shows the prevalence of HIV antibodies among different cohorts. All patients who tested negative upon admission and all of the 65 who were negative in treatment in 1984 and still are in treatment have remained HIV antibody negative throughout the observation period 1985-1990.

Table 2. Attack rates of HIV infection among heroin addicts entering MMT in Sweden

Patients	N	HIV+	%
≤ 1983	67	2	3
1984 - 1986	32	5	16
1987	60	34	57
1988	83	49	59
1989	95	46	48
1990	97	40	41

(HIV started to infect addicts in Sweden in 1983)

Conclusions

Our findings - no seroconversion among MMT patients in treatment since 1984 and the rapid increase in HIV prevalence among patients entering treatment the following years - strongly suggest that Methadone Maintenance Treatment is effective in preventing opiate addicts from contracting HIV. This fact stresses the urgency to open up MMT programmes for opiate addicts who are still HIV negative and not reserve treatment for HIV positive patients alone. This has been a tendency in some countries, especially those with no earlier experience of MMT .

The levelling off of HIV seroprevalence during 1988-90 has similarly been observed in many countries (Des Jarlais 1989). It may reflect that the further spread of HIV has retarded, partly due to the many HIV positive patients in treatment who no longer spread the virus through needle sharing. This fact underlines the need for this treatment to a larger number of opiate addicts, regardless of HIV status. This does not exclude the need for continued information about risk behaviour with provision of clean needles and condoms to addicts.

MMT is still the treatment of choice for opiate addicts that have failed in drug free treatments. The problem today is that in different countries, and in different regions of some countries, there is a tendency to ignore the need for adequate treatment, or to provide this treatment too late.

Acknowledgements

We wish to thank Professor emeritus Lars Gunne for helpful comments on the manuscript and Professor Margaretha Böttiger for providing current data on HIV prevalence in Sweden.

Correspondance

Correspondence concerning this paper should be adressed to Dr. Olof Blix, Department of Psychiatry, Methadone Programme, Ulleråker, S-751 85 Uppsala.

References

Des Jarlais D C, Friedman S R, Novick D M et al(1989) HIV-1 infection among intravenous drug users in Manhattan, New York City, from 1977 through 1987. JAMA 1989, 261; 1008-1012

Dole WP, Nyswander M (1965) Medical Treatment for Diacetyl-morphine (Heroin) addiction. JAMA 193:646-650

Frykholm B, Gunne L (1980) A Swedish drug abuse warning network. Drug and Alcohol Depend 5(3) : 161-165

Grönbladh L, Gunne L (1989) Methadone-assisted rehabilitation of Swedish heroin addicts. Drug and Alcohol depend 24:31-37

Grönbladh L, Öhlund L S, Gunne L (1990) Mortality in heroin addiction: impact of methadone treatment Acta Psych Scand 82:223-227

Gunne L (1966) Behandling av narkomani med narkotikablockerande medicinering. Läkartidningen 63:4060-4065

Gunne L, Grönbladh L (1981) The Swedish Methadone Maintenance Program: A controlled study. Drug and Alcohol Depend 7:249-56

Ljungberg B, Christensson B, Tunving K et al (1991) HIV Prevention among injecting drug users: Three years of experience from a syringe exchange program in Sweden. J AIDS (in press).

Novick D M, Joseph H, Croxson T S et al (1990) Absence of antibody to human immunodeficiency virus in long-term, socially rehabilitated methadone maintenance patients. Arch Intern Med 150:97-99

Olin R, Käll K (1988) HIV status and risk behaviour among imprisoned iv drug abusers in Stockholm. Läkartidningen 85:334-5; 337-9

Olsson B, Carlsson G, Fant M, Johansson T, Olsson O, Roth C (1981) Heavy drug abuse in Sweden 1979 - A national case finding study in Sweden. Drug and Alcohol Depend 7:273-283

Pehrson P O, Gaines H, Gyllensten K et al (1988) HIV infection among iv drug abusers in Stockholm. IV´th international conference on AIDS, Stockholm 1988, abstract #4510.

Stimson G V, Donoghose M, Audritt L, Dolan K (1988) HIV transmission risk behaviour of clients attending syringe exchange schemes in England and Scotland. Br J Addict 83(12): 1449-55

Methadone Maintenance Treatment (MMT) in Stockholm, Sweden

G. BLENNOW

Karolinska Institute, Department of Psychiatry, S. t Gäran's Hospital, Box 12500, S-112 81 Stockholm, Sweden

INTRODUCTION AND BACKGROUND

Methadone is a synthetic opioid with effects on the opiate receptors of the brain. The craving for heroine is reduced, which enables the patient to concentrate all efforts to his or hers rehabilitation.

If methadon is given in a correct dosage, mixed in juice or a soft drink, and is taken once a day, it will neither give any "kicks" nor let the patient suffer from abstinence.

The goal for MMT in Sweden is that to certain intravenous heroin addicts - with social-psychiatric means and methadone-medication - give a possibility of education, work and a living of their own.

In other words to make it possible to break the destructive and life-threatening carrier as an addict.

Methadone maintenance treatment for opiate addicts was introduced by Vincent P Dole and Mary Nyswander in 1963. It was brought as a method to Sweden and our special circumstances in 1966 by L M Gunne in the Ulleråker hospital, Upsala. In 1981 the Swedish board of Health and Welfare decided to consider MMT as a regular treatment for certain opiate addiction.

In 1981 the method was considered as a regular treatment. Until October 1987 all Swedish patients were introduced to the program as inpatients for 3-6 months at the Ulleråker hospital. After this inpatient period they continued as outpatients.

By this time less than 100 patients were in treatment in Sweden, i.e. Stockholm and Ulleråker. Four of those were by then HIV positive. In the light of the risk of HIV spreading among intravenous addicts and of the liability to give already infected patients a better treatment we wanted to increase the capacity. In Stockholm we began to introduce patients, after only one week of detoxification, as outpatients from the first day.

Now three years later, in February 1991, we have about 240 patients in Stockholm of whom 50% are infected by HIV. About 20 patients suffer from HIV-related symptoms or AIDS. No patient have converted to HIV-positive while in treatment. But many of the patients we have received during the last three years were infected at admittance.

In March 1988 we received legal rights to admit patients in three regions in Sweden. Ulleråker became responsible for the northern region, Lund for the southern region and Stockholm for the region of the capital. The limit for patients to be treated in Sweden was by the same time raised to a maximum of 300. In October 1990 the limit was further raised to 450. But still the authorities preferred to keep a limit - to emphasize that the Swedish MMT is selective treatment program for certain opiate addicts. See Criteria (below).

ADMITTANCE OF PATIENTS

The Methadone Conference is a group dealing with applications for MMT. The group is constituted by delegates from social security, infection medicine, "drug-free" addict care, MMT Stockholm and Ulleråker. They meet every fortnight.

In order to keep the social goals, the patient´s psychiatrist has to refer the patient to our group, enclosing a statement from the patient´s social worker.

A secretary checks all data and reports to the methadone conference.

After discusing whether the patient fulfills the criteria, the conference comes to a decision. If accepted the patient is noted on a waiting list. This list now contains about 15 - 20 patients.

The criteria for entering the Swedish MMT are as follows:

- acceptable free-choice-situation
- 4 years of addiction, documented
- at least three earlier attempts of drug-free treatment

208

at least 20 years of age

absence of advanced mixing of drugs

ORGANIZATION

In our organization we have four teams for MMT outpatients, each team able to take care of 50 patients. We also have award for inpatient care. This ward is needed for detoxification when patients abuse drugs (mostly THC, bensodiazepines and alcohol) on the side. We also use the ward to take blood-samples for plasma-methadone. To help some patients with rehabilitation we have two treatment homes far away from Stockholm. The patients stay there for at least six months. We also have two consultant teams for the infection medicine, situated adjacent to two Stockholm infection clinics.

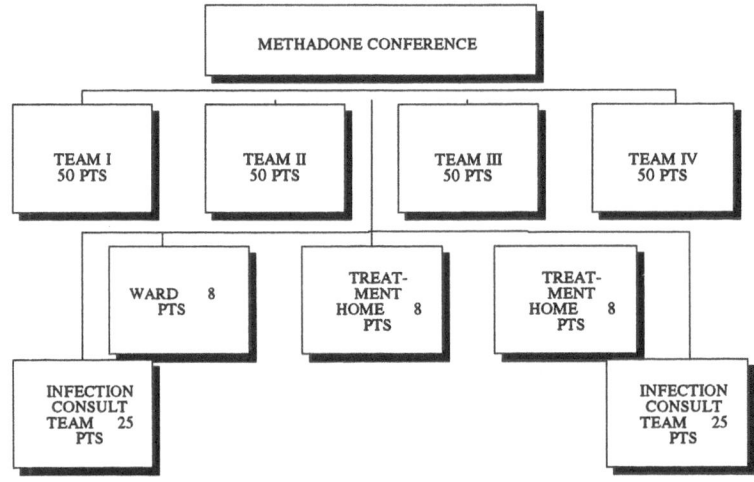

Figure 1. Organization table for the Stockholm MMT

CONCEPTS OF TREATMENT

The goal for MMT in Sweden is that to certain intravenous heroin addicts - with social-psychiatric means and methadone-medication - give a possibility of education, work and a living of their own.

In other words to make it possible to break the destructive and life-threatening carrier as an addict.

Entering the treatment the patients have to come daily to drink their methadone and to give carefully controlled urine samples. At least once a week they have a longer talk to their contact person. They also have opportunities to talk to a psychologist or a doctor. The urine samples are screened for:

- Methadone
- Opiates
- Central stimulants (CS)
- Benzodiazepines
- Cannabis (THC)
- Alcohol
- Urine-creatinine

If the samples shows that a patient is abusing drugs, we never let it be. But we don´t let the patient leave our program unwillingly unless we´ve tried all ways to keep him in treatment. We increase the frequency of visits, offer inpatient care, stay at a treatment home or whatever is considered necessary. If all our attempts to help the patient fail, the patient is excluded from our MMT. He might come back after 2 years or, if some circumstances, after 6 months.

The patients are encouraged to make efforts to achieve their own apartment and education or work. When the patients are in a stable social and psychiatric condition, they are encouraged to, under careful supervision, leave the MMT. A special program has been developed to assist patients with a long term tapping down procedure.

FUTURE

We have an upper limit of 450 patients in Sweden. Since Stockholm is considered to have about 80% of the opiate addicts, we should take care of about 340 patients. But at the moment we only have financial resources for 240 patients. But considering that few swedish addicts are pure opiate addicts and that MMT is of little or no help for addicts that mix different drugs, one really does not know if we need to treat any more patients than we already do. But this is a matter of debate - even in Sweden.

Methadone Treatment for Opiate-Addicted Patients. First Experiences of a Prospective Trial

M. Niederecker, D. Naber, C. Garwers, G. Völkl. M. Soyka, and H. Hippius

Department of Psychiatry, University of Munich, Nußbaumstraße 7, D-W-8000 München 2, Federal Republic of Germany

Methadone substitution in the treatment of opiate addiction was introduced by Dole and Nyswander (1965). 24 years later, 689 methadone treatment programs are conducted in the USA (Maany 1989). This therapy was and still is less popular in Europe, but particularly in Great Britain (Marx 1987), Sweden (Blix 1989), the Netherlands (Kooyman 1986), Austria (Pfersmann 1990), Switzerland (Uchtenhagen 1988) and Italy (Serraino and Franceschi 1989), numerous patients were treated. In Germany, the experience with methadone is rather limited and only a small number of publications exists (a.o. Elias 1990; Prütting 1990).

Due to the scarcity of methodologically well-conducted studies, differences in patient populations and their socio-cultural background and certainly also because of the political relevance benefits and risks of substitution treatment are still widely discussed (Dietzel 1990, Erlangen 1987, Krauthan 1989, Riedesser 1974, Soyka and Hippius 1990, Täschner 1990). Therefore, prospective studies which adhere to precisely defined proceedings, in- and exclusion criteria while reflecting the specific local situation, are still very much needed to replace political opinions by scientific facts when methadone is discussed.

At the Dept. of Psychiatry in the University of Munich, since 1988, HIV-positive drug addicts were first treated with methadone (Soyka et al. 1990). Two years later, in a German ur-

ban population, a prospective study was started, a) to evaluate wanted and unwanted effects of substitution therapy,
and b) to define the patient group which might benefit most
from this treatment. The preliminary experience with the
first 21 patients is hereby reported.

Inclusion and Exclusion Criteria

In order to be included, the patient has to fulfill the following criteria: He or she must be at least 21 years old and
must be i.v. opiate-addicted for at least three years. Moreover, the patient must have had two conventional long-term
abstinence treatments; at least one, if he is HIV-positive.
Further criteria are the refusal of any drug-free treatment
in spite of detailed consultation, and the willingness to re-
nounce any other illegal or recreational drugs aside from nicotine and coffein.

Exclusion criteria are continuation of polytoxicomania after
the beginning of methadone treatment, acute or chronic psychosis and inadequate social conditions (e.g. homelessness,
pending legal proceedings, illegal acts during methadone
treatment). The patient is excluded if he or she refuses to
participate in the weekly therapeutic group meetings.

Phases of Treatment

The course of the methadone treatment can be divided into
four phases: contact phase, in-patient phase, stabilization
phase, and, if possible, reduction phase.
During the contact phase, the patient has to participate subsequently three times in the once-weekly conducted "contact
group", where patients introduce themselves and are informed
about proceedings, in- and exclusion criteria. If criteria
for methadone treatment are fulfilled, the next step is the
consultation of the psychologist engaged in methadone treatment and finally the introduction to all the three psychiatrists involved . This contact phase usually takes 3-4 weeks.

After inclusion in the methadone treatment project, the patient enters the in-patient phase. During this time, which

usually lasts 1-2 weeks, the patient is admitted to the psychiatric ward where he later will be treated as an out-patient. In the in-patient phase, the individual dose is adjusted up to a maximum of 50 mg (=10 ml) of L-polamidone. Additionally, the patient is withdrawn from any other psychotropic drugs. A physical examination including a drug screening and a mandatory HIV-test is performed. After dismissal, the patient enters the phase of stabilization.

He or she is now treated as an out-patient. Under medical supervision, the constant daily dose of L-polamidone is administered after dilution in orange juice. The patient is not allowed to take the methadone home, the daily dose has to be consumed on the ward without any exception.

Alcohol consumption is tested daily by the use of an alcoholometer, urine is controlled about three times a month for intake of additional drugs. Patients have to attend weekly therapeutic meetings, further individual psychotherapy and other support is given by psychiatrists, psychologists, nurses and a social worker.

During this phase, the physical, psychological and social stabilization are the major goals. Most important are prevention and therapy of possible diseases (e.g. HIV-infection), the settlement of debts, improvement of living conditions, employment, improved relationships with family members and contact to non-addicts. Furthermore, patients are motivated to gradually reduce their daily methadone dose.

Principally, the stabilization phase is not limited, it may take 6 months to 2-3 years.

After the patient is succesfully stabilized and sufficiently motivated, his or her daily dose of L-polamidone is gradually reduced (e.g. 0.5 ml L-polamidone/week). Some patients prefer first a rather slow reduction as an out-patient and a final withdrawal as an in-patient, while others choose a more rapid reduction as an in-patient.

The reduction is scheduled according to the clinical impression and the subjective experience of the patient. If the dosage was reduced too fast, the former dose is re-administered for days or weeks. The phase of reduction usually takes about 1-6 months.

Until now, 21 patients participated, selected from about 120 patients who were originally interested in methadone treatment. From those patients who were rejected, about 25 % did not fulfill the inclusion criteria and 65 % wanted methadone treatment immedeately and refused to go through the contact phase.

Patients

Of the 21 patients, there are 10 females and 11 males. Their age (± SD) is 33 ± 10 (22-44) years. They have been addicted for 15 ± 11 (4-26) years and had about three (1-7) conventional drug therapies.

Until now, every patient gave permission to be tested for HIV-infection. 10 patients were HIV-negative, two had a positive test result, but were asymptomatic. Three patients suffered from LAS, two from ARC and four from AIDS.

The duration of methadone treatment is 9 ± 10 (1-38) months, the mean Levomethadone dose is 45 ± 10 (30-50) mg.

Results

Of the total group of 21 patients, nine are in the stabilization phase and five in the reduction phase. Two patients have finished the reduction, are drug-free and employed since three and 15 months, respectively.

The number of employed patients has increased from five before methadone treatment to nine under substitution therapy.

Before methadone treatment, seven patients had contact with their relatives, this number has increased to twelve.

Additional drug abuse or alcoholism was observed in eight patients. In three cases only once or twice, in five others at least three times with the consequence of exclusion from methadone treatment.

All the excluded patients continued to take methadone, administered by general practitioners, who usually do not adhere to the rather strict exclusion criteria used in this project. One patient who was excluded because of severe alcohol abuse, died four months afterwards because of an intoxication by ethanol, diazepam and methadone, prescribed by a general practitioner.

214

The most frequent side-effects of methadone were weight gain and sweating. Some patients showed symptoms of minor depression with nightmares and insomnia, which were mostly successfully treated with 25-50 mg of doxepine in the evening.

Conclusions

These preliminary data indicate the positive effects of methadone treatment in some, but certainly not all patients of a considerably selected subgroup of heroin addicts.

Efficacy seems to rely on the strict use of well-defined in- and exclusion criteria as well as on professional psycho-social support. The intake of methadone should be carefully supervised with regular urine screening.

Dosage of methadone, further definition of proceedings, particularly of in- and exclusion criteria, should be issues for further research which may lead to valid predictors for succesful methadone treatment.

References

Blix O (1989) Methadone maintenance programs in Sweden. JAMA 15: 2202

Dole VP, Nyswander M (1965) A medical treatment for diacetyl-morphine (heroin) addiction - a clinical trial with methadone hydrochloride J Amer. med. Ass 193: 646-650

Dietzel P (1990) Methadon als Drogenproblemlöser - eine Legende oder Hoffnungsschimmer? Deutsche Apothekerzeitung 5: 205

Elias H (1990) Ersatzstoffgestützte Behandlung Suchtkranker in der Praxis. Fortschr. Med. 13: 256-258

Erlangen A, Haas H, Baumann I (1987) Therapieerfolg von Methadonpatienten mit unterschiedlicher Indikation. Drogenalkohol 11: 3-15

Kooyman M (1986) Die Entwicklung der Behandlungsmaßnahmen für Drogenabhängige in den Niederlanden. Wiener Zeitschr. für Suchtforschung 9: 51-54

Krauthan G (1989) Einführung von Methadon-Erhaltungsprogramm in der Bundesrepublik Deutschland? Eine kritische Literaturübersicht. DHS Informationsdienst 3/4: 1-22

Maany I, Dhopesh V, Arnd JO (1989) Increase in desipramine serum levels associated with Methadone treatment. Am J Psychiatry 146: 1611-1613

Marx H (1987) Methadonpraxis in Europa. Deutscher Studien Verlag, Weinheim

Pfersmann D, Presslich O, Pakesch G, Hollerer E (1990) Gestaltung und Durchführung des österreichischen Methadonprogrammes und erste Ergebnisse. Nervenarzt 61: 438-443

Prütting D (1990) Das Methadonprogramm in Nordrhein-Westfalen. Deutsche Apotheker Zeitung 5: 217-222

Riedesser P (1974) Methadonprogramme in den USA. Med Klin 65: 671-680

Serraino D and Franceschi S (1989) Methadone maintenance programs and AIDS. Lancet I: 1522-1523

Soyka M and Hippius H (1990) Substitutionsbehandlung Drogenabhängiger mit Methadon. Münch Med Wschr 44: 689-690

Soyka M, Naber D, Niederecker M, Hippius M (1990) Methadonbehandlung HIV-infizierter Drogenabhängiger Münch. med. Wschr. 44: 691-694

Täschner KL (1990) Methadon-Stubstitution ist keine wirkungsvolle Alternative. Dtsch. Apothekerzeitung 5: 125

Uchtenhagen A (1988) Zur Behandlung Drogenabhängiger mit Methadon: Zürcherische Richtlinien und Auswertung der Therapieresultate. Schweiz. Med. Rundschau 13: 351-353

HIV and Methadone Treatment: The German Experience

F. M. Böcker

Psychiatric University Hospital, University of Erlangen-Nürnberg,
Schwabachanlage 6, D-W-8520 Erlangen, Federal Republic of Germany

Among physicians and politicians in Western Germany, attitudes towards opiate substitution and methadone maintenance treatment programs (MMTP's) have basically changed during the last four years. MMTP's are now perceived as indispensable tools of modern health policy. Beginning in 1987, different types of maintenance treatment for narcotic addicts with or without HIV infections have been established in 7 out of 11 Western German Federal States. This reversal of opinion cannot be explained without the HIV- epidemic and the widely shared belief that MMTP's can prevent the spread of HIV- infections among active intravenous drug users and reduce the AIDS risk for the society (an expectation, however, which is lacking empirical support from epidemiological studies [Böcker 1991]).

HISTORICAL REMARKS

Beginning in 1972, a controversial debate on MMTP's has been going on in Western Germany for more than two decades. Official authorities have previously taken the view that MMTP's do not represent an appropriate treatment method for narcotic addiction. Some physicians have always engaged in uncontrolled prescriptions of codeine, dihydrocodeine (Remedacen[R]) or even levomethadone (Polamidon[R]) and had in some cases to defend their action against criminal prosecution (suspected violation of the German Law on Narcotics). A clinical investigation was started in Hanover in 1973 with 20 patients (9 of whom left prematurely) and terminated in 1975 because of poor results. The long-time-effects, evaluated by following-up the remaining 11 clients in 1987, have been discussed controversially. With this one exception, however, no MMTP's have been established. The Federal Government has in 1986 and 1987 repeatedly confirmed to disapprove of further experiments. The administrations of some Federal States with different political majorities, however, refused to accept this "drug free treatment only"- philosophy.

The present situation, as described below, reflects political power and public opinion rather than scientific knowledge. The major objections against MMTP's, which previously have been regarded as decisive, have not yet been ruled out. Critics are concerned, for example, about weakening of abstinence motivation among addicts, continued illegal and polyvalent drug use [e.g. cocaine], problems of levomethadone toxicity [e.g. combined with other drugs], side effects [e.g. depression?] and withdrawal [e.g. if clients have to be excluded from further participation].

A Joint Working Group on "Narcotic Substitution" of the Federal Medical Council has commented on exceptional indications for opiates in special individual cases (February 1988): Temporary substitution is considered as appropriate in narcotic addicts with life-threatening withdrawal symptoms, opiate withdrawal with severe physical illness or uncontrollable organic pain syndromes, and late stages of pregnancy. Long- term maintenance may be advisable in opiate addicts with advanced stages of AIDS (Gerchow et al 1988). According to a second statement (March 1990), intake of drugs of abuse (including alcohol) should be terminated within three months of maintenance treatment, and patients with continued abuse of habit-forming drugs should be excluded (Gerchow et al 1990). This suggestion, however, is not observed by the majority of programs.

NORTH-RHINE-WESTFALIA

The State Government of North- Rhine- Westfalia (Dusseldorf), acting on request of the Minister of Labour, Health and Social Affairs, decided in July 1987 to conduct a "SCIENTIFIC TRIAL OF DRUG-SUPPORTED REHABILITATION OF INTRAVENOUS OPIATE ADDICTS" planned for five years. After the consent of the State's two Medical Councils had been obtained, levomethadone maintenance treatment of a limited number of narcotic addicts has been started in Dusseldorf, Essen and Bochum in March 1988, and in Cologne and Bielefeld in September 1989. Applicants have to be at least 22 years old and opiate-addicted for several years (patients with politoxicomania or untreated alcohol dependence shall be excluded), must have taken part in drug-free treatment programs at least twice for several months without success, and have to sign a written contract, committing themselves to participate in a counseling center's program of psychosocial care. HIV- infected patients have to be at least 18 years old and must have attempted several detoxifications. Enrolment decisions are made by a state commission. Non- injectable levomethadone (dissolved in fruit juice) is taken daily (including weekends) under medical supervision. Neither narcotics nor prescriptions are handed out to patients or relatives. Continued use of street drugs is supervised by regular urinary screening.

According to the annual report published in 1990, 93 clients had been admitted up to December 1989 (of whom 1 left on his own, 6 were expelled for disciplinary reasons, two died, 84 were in treatment [Nowak et al 1990]). 19 % of the sample had HIV-antibodies. Polyvalent abuse of psychotropic substances was common (Table 1). 68 % had previously used methadone (54 % daily, 15 % intravenously). Data of a one-year-follow-up available for 29 patients admitted in 1988 revealed modest results, as regards social adjustment (some previously unemployed patients found a regular occupation [N= 3] or occasional jobs [N= 4], but the majority [N= 20] remained unemployed) and illegal drug use (Table 2). The authors of the study have classified the outcome as

TABLE 1   MMTP OF NORTH-RHINE-WESTFALIA

PARTICIPANTS DRUG EXPERIENCE	(N= 91)
Hypnotics, Analgesics:	74 %
Minor Tranquilizers (Benzodiazepines):	70 %
Marihuana:	87 %
Lysergic acid diethylamide:	63 %
Amphetamines:	60 %
Cocaine:	87 %
Opiates:	100 %
Methadone:	68 %

TABLE 2   MMTP OF NORTH-RHINE-WESTFALIA
FOLLOW-UP: SECOND HALF-YEAR OF TREATMENT

URINARY SCREENING FINDINGS:	(N= 28)
Alcohol	not determined
Amphetamines	not determined
Cannabinol	not determined
Opiates:	75 %
Benzodiazepines:	68 %
Barbiturates:	54 %
Cocaine:	32 %

DRUG USE PATTERNS:	(N= 28)
Drug- free:	4
Opiate- free*:	3
Decrease of heroin use**:	12
Delayed decrease of heroin use**:	3
Continued heavy polyvalent drug use:	6

*: psychoactive drug use,
**: heroin use   related to stressful life events

"at least some success" in 19 cases. According to the 1990's suggestions of the Federal Medical Council, however, 24 out of 28 patients would have been excluded from further participation.

The scientific value of this open, uncontrolled study (no blind ratings, no control group) will be limited. The main reason to label the program as a clinical trial was of a legal nature, since a review of the legal position revealed that the use of narcotics in scientific investigations, approved for by the state's medical council, represents no violation of the Law on Narcotics (Hellebrand 1988).

In December 1987, the said Minister released a decree concerning the prescription of narcotics to opiate addicts suffering from AIDS and stated that intravenous drug users with symptomatic HIV infections (CDC IV, WR III) can receive levomethadone maintenance treatment from general practitioners. Cooperation with the local narcotic counseling center is recommended as well as a notification of the local health authority. As a consequence, extensive "FAMILY DOCTOR SUBSTITUTION" has developed in many cities. Very favourable results, compared to the program presented above, have been obtained in a follow-up-study of 50 patients (AIDS outpatient clinic, Münster; open uncontrolled study; maintenance treatment for a minimum of 3 and an average of 12 months; LAS: N= 34; ARC: N= 13; AIDS: N= 3): Improved physical health and social adjustment, a complete stop of prostitution and delinquency, and a nearly complete cessation of intravenous heroin use have been reported (Walger et al 1989).

BERLIN

Individual levomethadone treatment in private practice, with knowledge and approval of the Medical Council of Berlin (West), has begun in 1987 (Jacobowski 1989). The Medical Council has provided recommendations and offers counseling to physicians and hospitals. All treatment decisions, however, are left entirely to the discretion of the physician in charge. A maximum case load of 3 patients is suggested for a private practice. In June 1990, the Medical Council knew of 130 patients in maintenance treatment.

HAMBURG

Health Authority, Social Authority and Medical Council agreed in June 1988 to allow substitution of narcotics (daily supervised oral intake) in individual cases, provided the practitioner is in agreement with a social worker of a narcotics counseling centre and applies for approval of a special commission.

BREMEN

A "Joint Recommendation" of the Senator of Health and the Medical Council of Bremen, brought into line with the Federal Public Health Office and released in January 1990 states that individual levomethadone treatment in private practice may be offered to opiate addicts (including patients with severe psychiatric disorders, e.g. psychoses, as well as patients with physical diseases who need hospital treatment and are not willing to undergo detoxification [temporary substitution]). Practitioners planning long-term-prescription of narcotics should have special experience and skill and are expected to contact a counseling commission. In spring 1990, 41 addicts, 21 of whom were HIV- infected, received maintenance treatment.

SCHLESWIG-HOLSTEIN

Sick fund organisations, Medical Council, Pharmacist's Council, several other committees and the Government (Minister of Social Affairs, Health and Energy) agreed on a contract, valid from April 1990, to March 1993, "to investigate whether treatment with levomethadone is a suitable way to accomplish long-lasting rehabilitation of narcotic addicts". Clients shall be accepted only if there is a realistic chance to achieve opiate abstinence and if maintenance treatment is the only promising medical measure. The decision is left to a special commission. A written agreement has to be signed by the responsible physician and the patient. Until June 1990, 6 patients had been admitted. In comparison, a general practitioner from Kiel has been providing long-term-codeine-treatment to 323 patients in 1988 (Grimm et al 1989).

LOWER SAXONY: MMTP in preparation (10/1990).

HESSEN

A pilot trial for HIV- infected long-term-drug-dependent prostitutes has been established in Frankfurt, maintaining 35 clients on levomethadone in June 1990. A practitioner from Frankfurt's Central Station quarter has offered dihydrocodeine- prescriptions to 319 patients (100 in treatment in December 1989 [Elias 1990]). Dr. Walter Wallmann, CDU, then Minister President of Hessen, gave notice of a new "Hesse Narcotics Initiative" in June 1990 and announced to establish MMTP's as a regular part of narcotic addiction treatment programs, but failed to win the State's parliament elections in January 1991. The new government, however, is expected to pursue even more extensive plans.

SAARLAND

A scientific trial of "drug-supported rehabilitation of intravenous opiate addicts", similar to North-Rhine-Westfalia, located at the State's Public Health
Office in Saarbrücken, limited to 20 clients and planned for a time of 3-5
years, has been initiated by the Minister of Health and Social Affairs without
participation of the Medical Council.

RHINELAND-PALATINATE, BADEN-WÜRTTEMBERG, BAVARIA

With the exception of an open, uncontrolled study conducted at the Psychiatric University Hospital of Munich (Naber et al 1991), no MMTP's have been
set up. An unknown number of physicians and hospitals provide prescriptions
of narcotics to an unknown number of drug users, sometimes after consulting
the local health authority or obtaining psychiatric expert opinion. In Stuttgart, for example, dihydrocodeine has been offered to 39 patients attending a
private practice between January and October 1989. In November 1989, 21
patients (10 HIV+) received an average daily dose of 600 mg (Ulmer 1990).

REFERENCES

BÖCKER FM (1991) Methadone and AIDS: Are methadone maintenance treatment
   programs (MMTP's) apt to prevent HIV infections among intravenous drug
   users? First European Symposium on Drug Addiction and AIDS, Vienna,
   Austria, February 22-23, 1991.

ELIAS H (1990) Ersatzstoffgestützte Behandlung Suchtkranker in der Praxis.
   Fortschr Med 108:256-258.

GERCHOW J, HEINRICH K, JANSSEN PL, KIMBEL KH, POSER W, RETZLAFF I,
   TÄSCHNER KL, WALDMANN H, WANKE K (1988) Ersatzdrogen: Stellungnahme
   des gemeinsamen Arbeitskreises des Wissenschaftlichen Beirates und des
   Ausschusses "Psychiatrie, Psychotherapie und Psychohygiene" der Bundesärztekammer. Deutsches Ärzteblatt 85:192-193.

GERCHOW J, HEINRICH K, JANSSEN PL, KIMBEL KH, POSER W, RETZLAFF I,
   TÄSCHNER KL, WALDMANN H, WANKE K (1990) Beschluß des Vorstandes der
   Bundesärztekammer vom 9. Februar 1990. Ergänzende Stellungnahme des
   Arbeitskreises "Ersatzdrogen". Deutsches Ärzteblatt 87:575-577.

GRIMM G, WOLF B, BORNEMANN R, BSCHOR F (1989) Prevention of HIV-Infection
   in Parenteral Drug Abusers (PDA's): About Evaluation and Efficiacy of
   Opiate-Substitution Treatment. Poster No. TAP 28 (p 103): V. International
   Conference on AIDS, Montreal, June 4-9, 1989.

HELLEBRAND J (1988) Methadon: Chance oder Illusion? Der Einsatz von Methadon in der Drogen- und AIDS- Hilfe am Beispiel Nordrhein-Westfalens.
   Forum-Verlag Godesberg, Bonn.

JACOBOWSKI C (1989) Drogensucht und Methadon: Zum Stand der Diskussion
   über Methadon in der Behandlung Drogensüchtiger. Mitteilungsblatt der Berliner Ärztekammer 26:623-635.

NABER D, NIEDERECKER M, GARWERD C, SOYKA M (1991) Methadone Treatment for Opiate-Addicted Patients: First Experiences in a Prospective Clinical Trial. First European Symposium on Drug Addiction and AIDS, Vienna, Austria, February 22-23, 1991.

NOWAK M, SCHLEIFER L, SCHMIDT EH, GASTPAR M, RÖSINGER C, LODEMANN E, MAY B (1990) Wissenschaftliches Erprobungsvorhaben medikamentengestützte Rehabilitation bei i.v. Opiatabhängigen: Jahresbericht 1989 vom 12.3.1990. Prognos AG, Köln.

ULMER A (1990) Dihydrocodein bei Drogenabhängigen: Ein Zwischenbericht. Fortschr Med 108:261.

WALGER P, BAUMGART P, WILKE G, KUPFER U, EIFF M v, DORST KG (1989) Medizinische und psychosoziale Effekte der Methadon-Substitution HIV-infizierter Drogenabhängiger. Psychother Psychosom med Psychol 39:381-389.

Drug Addiction Treatment in Italy in the 80s Fear of Treatment

I. MAREMMANI[1, 4], O. ZOLESI[1, 4], M. CIRILLO[2, 4], R. NARDINI[4],
P. CASTROGIOVANNI[1], and A. TAGLIAMONTE[3, 4]

[1] Psychiatric Institute, University of Pisa, I-56100 Pisa
[2] Psychiatric Unit USL 4, Regione Toscana
[3] Pharmacology Institute, University of Siena, I-53100 Siena
[4] Social Diseases Study and Intervention Association, Italy

It is a widespread opinion that the treatment and recovery of drug addicts must necessarily and absolutely be the result of psychotherapy or therapeutic community. Medical intervention, on the contrary, is considered one of the least important and necessary methods of dealing with the addict and his problem.

The causes of drug addiction are surely not only medical. However, when a physical dependence on an opioid substance develops, this dependency has the peculiar features of a long term illness, characterized by a tendency toward relapse, even after an apparent recovery (Maremmani e Castrogiovanni, 1990).

This hypothesis was first expressed in the U.S.A. in the early 1960's, confirmed successively in international clinical experiences (Deglon, 1982; Cooper, 1983), and definitively assumed as the most credible idea in the mid 70's. In those years, Hughes in England, Terenius in Sweden and Goldstein in the U.S.A., almost simultaneously discovered the existence of a system of biochemical functions regulated by natural endogenous opioid substances produced by the brain. Since then, scientific research on drug addiction has been particularly concerned with the intake of opioids and the probable imbalance resulting within the complex neurotransmitter system, which regulates the most important of human functions (Verebey, 1982). The results suggest the biochemical nature of drug addiction, and strengthen the hypothesis of a possible long term chemical treatment and cure for this disease (Cooper, 1983).

Such being the case, in order to recuperate a patient we:

- circumscribe the primary damage
- repair the secondary damage, namely the global functional imbalance, both organic and psychologic, caused by the primary damage
- prevent, correct, or, at least, contain the tertiary damage, that is, the functional consequences or the psychic sequences deriving from the organic pathology and from the inadequate environmental stimulus.

The primary damage can be confronted by psychopharmacological means in order to stabilize the endorphinergic system.

To control the secondary damage it is necessary to resolve the pathologies which, as a result of addict's behaviour, directly affected the various organs and apparatuses.

The tertiary stage of the illness can be considered separately. If, once the first two stages are resolved, some physical or psychic disability persists, then a psychological and social support program can surely be beneficial. On the other hand, in cases where the individual's abilities are no longer impeded by addict's practices, the medical intervention alone will have been sufficient.

Detoxification programs that followed rigourous scientific methodology and included medical intervention according an integrated biopsychosocial approach, and not solely extemporized intervention, as has been the case in Italy, have thus far shown the best results. On the contrary, notwithstanding the considerable amount of resources employed, every attempt to approach drug addiction as a matter of re-education has furnished very little reliable information.

In light of this evidence, it is unreasonable to suppose that social aggregation, psychological support, work programs or isolation can do other than effect a clamorous failure in the majority of cases.

A drug addict demonstrates specific pathologies in his major functioning systems, and this is reflected in his behaviour. Moreover, he suffers from all the pathologies caused by this behaviour. Given this situation, he must be treated with a specific medical cure for drug addiction, along with all the other medical interventions required by his concomitant diseases. Only a public, highly specialized structure can provide such treatment. At present, this approach is absent in non-medical institutions.

When a patient, is properly cared for, he soon rediscovers the inner resources, that were obscured by his illness, and, at least, he returns to the conditions exact before his substance abuse. We can also intervene in cases of need, which persist apart from the drug addiction, and so create the favourable condition for a complete rehabilitation. As a result of these strategies, patients come in off the street, and their familial and social nods tend once again toward normalcy.

Those accustomed to working with agonist opiate drugs knows that a biological therapeutic program, far from being a pure and simple medical intervention has a well defined strategy, that involves a myriad of professional resources, and also includes the patient's family.

Rigours scientific controls notwithstanding, such programs have been severely hindered in Italy for the last decade by public opinion, and by those civil servants responsible for public health services in general. The prevailing 'conventional wisdom' is most often supported by a prejudices and inexact beliefs.

For example, it is widely believed that the medical aspect of drug addiction is limited to the so-called 'detoxification' stage. In this approach, once the doctor has overseen the elimination of the abused drug, or its substitute, he should then consign the patient to the care of the psychologist or re-educator who will in turn, once having entered into the dynamics of the subject's behaviour, prevent his return to drug addiction Some of these 'psychosocial workers' claim they want "to remove the profound causes", that brought the subject to addiction and even ask us to believe in a real 'reconstruction process' for the individual. Very seldom, however, is an addict treated by the most capable psycho-analysts, partly because he is not able to withstand the rigid structure of the interviews. Unfortunately, statements of intent to 'remove the profound causes", or to effect a 'reconstruction process' are most often intended to elicit an emotional response.

Also, within the Italian social service structures, often times an addict cannot be placed into a physician's care, if he has not first seen a psychologist, and so much the better if the visit included parents, girlfriends or boyfriends. In other words, the psychologist stands between the addict and the available,.if ineffective cure. As it is now, we are able to obtain doses of substitute drugs only for those addicts considered 'incurable', and the priority of psychological intervention over the medical intervention continues to be almost universally recognized. This seems a peculiar belief, if we consider that, within the current state of therapeutic analysis, there is no school of psychology, or a psychologist able produce evidences for the cure of having consistently cured a significant number of addicts

Generally, psychologists report on an individual's case history and the mechanisms within it which they retain responsible for the addiction . But 'Peter's story', or 'Mark's histories', told within a framework which evokes fragile, broken shells and cracked mirrors, rarely conclude in results. Should some results be achieved, it is never repeated in a significant number of subjects. Most of the time, the best a psychologist can do is to extract a promise from the addict to enter a therapeutic community. This is, in fact, delegating total responsibility to an institution which will administer a "psychotherapy" all the more undefined and disputable.

At certain levels of conditioning, it can sometimes happen that a candidate patient, if he is desperate enough, will resign himself to attempting the proposed 'therapeutic community life'. On the other hand, he is made to believe that there are no alternatives. Nonetheless, the majority of the addicts channelled in this way abandon the program in the initial phases. Those who drop out are almost always those most in need of care, that is the long term addicts, for which preventative detoxification only temporarily masked many of the major, and minor, symptoms of a disease which had persisted for years. When the real symptom reappears, that is the addict's recidivist behaviour, his departure from the community is inevitable.

The most serious problem for closed residential programs is their inability to detain patients for sufficient periods. This 'drawback' is circumvented at San Patrignano by the use of chains. The chains used in other communities are not quite so visible. If a youth abandons the community, because he cannot manage within it, then, outside, he must find "scorched earth", that is the family is instructed to leave him on the street without any help whatever, and often public services will not accept him. That they must "touch the bottom" is the order of the day! Some returns to the community, run away again, then return. Others, the majority, completely ruin themselves by causing irreversible damage. Still others, in the early stages of their 'escape', completely deprived of their opiate tolerance but still prey to the typical compulsive 'craving', end up 'shooting up' the one that kills them.

In many therapeutic communities, the re-education practice there are more or less debatable. They are practices improvised by operatives, who are themselves improvised, programs created on the spot, based on immediate experience in the field, with no scientific supervision 'upstream,' and no control of the results 'downstream'. 'Frustrating' punishment are often in use, such as making the subject face a wall for period of time, or hanging an offensive sign around his neck, or the practice of spying within the group, and reciprocal aggression. Often, one's "sense of guilt" must be confessed publicly, and the questioning periods can be cruel and irreverent, or filled with complacency and affectations. This is truly a Medieval approach, re-proposed with 'drugs' as an excuse, imposed on desperate people, who would accept anything, including exorcism.

But, what about the results? Neither in the United States, where the therapeutic community first came into being, nor in Europe, where they have been spreading for years, is there any credible data available. Very often the 'patients' are in a continual rotation, and for every one that abandons the program there is a ready replacement at the top of a long waiting list. So that this 'revolving' mechanism can function, it is necessary that certain public services do not function, or, are at least limited to furnishing detoxified subjects to place within the community. And such is the current political attitude in Italy, even after the passage into law of Bill 162/1990. The therapeutic community, which is the most selective and costly therapy known, offers itself as the only viable solution, since most public services have been seriously disabled by the diffusion of distorted images and all too conventional wisdom.

The true is, in Italy, that the typical social services available to the drug addict do not dedicate themselves to a patient's cure, but rather, to the repression of the use of methadone as a means of therapeutic care. The average operative in Italy in the 1980's reached his 'goal' when he was able to reduce the dosage of substitute drugs as quickly as possible. The addict could go back to the street, he could be ill, he could even die and his physician would be none the less satisfied. As long as the doctor kept the dosages below the ceiling imposed or suggested here and there by norms more rhetorical than substantive, he would have no problems. In fact, the prerogatives available of all other doctors have been canceled for the physician treating drug addicts in Italy. No one would dream of limiting the medicinal doses proscribed by a psychiatrist, or a gynaecologist or a dentist. Every doctor must draw his information from educational institutions, from scientific literature and from clinical practice. He must prescribe pharmaceuticals in the quantities and for the duration he retains to be opportune "in science and conscience". But not so for the doctor working with drug addicts! For these physicians there exists a subtle but repressive program, which has already established well defined limits within which therapeutic action must take place. Within these confines, failure is certain.

Current scientific understanding tells us that medical programs for heroin addicts should be protracted in time and that doses of substitute drugs must be 'tailored' to suit the individual patient. The regimen must continue until the patient discontinues to use street heroin, and until he demonstrates the behaviour modifications which are the foundations of success in this type of program..

Even though, at present, some 85% of the heroin addicts in the United States are in long term methadone programs, and even though these programs have constituted the primary and most efficient structure for fighting addiction over the last 25 years, Italians are certain, because they have been so informed, that these programs have failed. The problem is not so much that the prevailing ideas are incorrect and that they contrast sharply with the scientific data available on the subject. Rather, the problem resides in our inability to understand what is behind the development of such a distorted image in Italy, for the most part diffused through channels with capillary roots throughout the country.

Ideology? Some other interests? Convincement or emotivity? Unrefined information, or a clear design to influence opinion? Or something else? It is not easy to say.

Perhaps, this is one of the knots that sociologists or psychologists could undo, if they turned their attention not so much toward the addict, but toward society's confused and frightened attitudes when dealing with this new kind of illness. In general we are dealing with a genuine escape into confusion and fear, which is resolved by denying, against all evidence to the contrary, that a 'drug disease' even exists.

And so, a medical doctor is denied to the drug addict, because it would be minimizing the issue to say that the core of "mans'" problem, within himself and society, is a medical one. And above all he is denied a specialist able to work within the range of a body of scientific literature and clinical experiences. We define this approach as truly fraudulent, a no-win situation which will fall upon the entire community.

In fact, in this age we can no longer ignore the need for disciplined application of scientific method in the analysis of social phenomenon. Each of us is bound, also as regard drug addiction, to effect a rigourous analysis and formulate consequent proposals, so that it cannot be said, to paraphrase Einstein, that 'we are living in a period in which is it is easier to smash an atom than a prejudice'.

REFERENCES

Cooper J.R. (Ed.) (1983): Research on the treatment of narcotic addiction. State of the art. Treatment research monograph series. U.S. Department of Health and Human Services. N.I.D.A., Rockville, Maryland

Deglon J.J. (1982): Le treatement a long terme des hèroinomanes par la mèthadone. Editions Mèdicine et Hygiéne, Genéve

Maremmani I., Castrogiovanni P.: (1990): Tossicodipendenza da eroina fra progresso scientifico e pregiudizio culturale. Grasso Editori. Bologna

Verebey K. (Ed) (1982) : Opioids in mental Illness: Theories, Clinical Observations, and Treatment Possibilities. Ann. N.Y. Acad. V. 398. The New York Academy of Sciences, N.Y.

Psycho-Social and Psychopathological Features as Predictors of Response to Long Term and High Dosages Methadone Treatment

I. Maremmani[1, 2], O. Zolesi[1], and P. Castrogiovanni[1]

[1] Psychiatric Institute, University of Pisa
[2] Social Diseases Study and Intervention Association, Italy

Pharmacological treatment of heroin addiction with opiate agonists, if carried out according to a correct methodology, produces the most consistent results nowadays. Though United States government authorities and the Italian Health Ministry (Circular 87, 1984) advise it, in the public services it is very difficult to carry out this kind of intervention, because some regional governments, by means of special laws, prevent the realization of long term and "so-called" high dosage treatments.

One of the problems most strongly felt by the workers in this field is therefore the identification of clear diagnostical standards for the inclusion of heroin addicts in opiate agonist programs. The need for carrying out a further screening between low or high dosages is even more strongly felt. The "need" for establishing a maximum methadone dosage and the treatment length would not exist, if long term methadone detoxification was considered a usual medical-psychiatric treatment.

Unfortunately, although this medical intervention is effective in the behavioural control of the drug addicts, cultural prejudices provoke opposition from the political arena and from the literary academy against this kind of treatment (Weppner, 1979; Smith & Kronick, 1979).

In the original "discussion" about methadone maintenance, Dole and Nyswander (1965; 1966) used about 100 mg or more in daily dosages. At the beginning of the 70's, research, published in the United States, even proposed that about 30 mg dosages were therapeutic. Nevertheless, the twenty years experience of the New York State Methadone Clinics and a series of controlled studies, reported by Hargreaves (1983) with a very critical attitude, enable one to assert that doses higher than 60 mg prove to be more effective in the control of drug addiction behaviour and very often represent the minimum effective dose to prevent relapse.

This dose's extreme variability seems to depend on the presence of various methadone idiosyncratic metabolizes, such as pharmacological interactions or certain medical conditions, which can modify this drug bio-availability (Walton et al., 1978; Kreek, 1983); it also can depend on associated psychopathological components. Schizoid patients, schizotypical, and paranoid personalities respond to higher dosages than subjects with histrionic, narcissistic, antisocial personalities and "borderline" subjects. Dependent, coercive and passive-aggressive individuals need a lower average dose (Treece & Nicholson, 1980).

Aim

The aim of this research is to show, by means of the comparison of subjects in long term detoxification programs at high or low doses, the psychological, behavioural and illness course components, which are able to direct patient's screening towards one therapeutic modality or the other.

Material and Methods

Patients, treated by two public services of Central Italy, were considered. Subjects were evaluated for their socio-anagraphic variables, and also by means of a special questionnaire, which surveyed drug addiction state at the start of the treatment, and in particular:

- the presence or less of illness which often superimposed drug addiction practice, such as hepatitis, vascular pathologies, lymphoadenopathologies, gastroenteritis, genital sphere and odontalgic disorders,

- psychiatric problems concerning anxiety disorders, mood anomalies, sleep disturbances, ideation and sense-perception disorders, and aggressive behaviour,
- legal situation and family relations,
- other substances abuse, such as cannabinoids, stimulants, psychotomimetic substances, alcohol and psychotropic drugs, so that we could select homogeneous subjects as far as these variables were concerned.

Thus, 17 subjects, 13 males, 4 females, mean age 25 (sd 5,5), were included in this study; all of them followed a long term methadone treatment, in the metabolic stabilization phase. By means of the urinary opiate metabolizes control, it was possible to document that they had not been using heroin. 9 of them took a higher than 50 mg/die dosage (High dosages Group, H-Group). The doses of the remaining 8 persons were limited under 30 mg/die (Low dosages Group, L-Group). The two groups were strictly homogeneous as for sex, age, education (mean-low), socio-environmental condition (poor), drug addiction length (more than two years).

Subjective symptomatology was evaluated by means of the Self-Report Symptom Inventory (SCL-90) by Derogatis et al. (1973), composed of 90 items, according to ten dimensions: Somatization, Obsessive, Compulsive, Interpersonal Sensitivity, Depression, Anxiety, Hostility, Phobic Anxiety, Paranoid Ideation, Psychoticism.

Social Adjustment was studied by means of S.A.S. "Social Adjustment Scale", by Schooler et al. (1979). It is a semi-structured interview composed of 52 items investigating various social adjustment fields, subdivided in five areas: Work, Family, External Family, Socialization-Leisure Time, Personal Well-Being.

Aggressive behaviour was evaluated by means of the italian version of B.D.I (Buss and Durkee Inventory for Assessing Different Kinds of Hostility) (Castrogiovanni et al., 1982), which as well as providing a global aggressiveness index (BDI Total score), gives the assessment of an aggressive behaviour profile, composed of seven factors (Assault, Indirect Aggression, Irritability, Negativism, Resentment, Suspiciousness, Verbal Aggression).

The Rosenzweig Picture Frustration Test, in its Italian version by Nencini and Belcecchi (1956), was used for the evaluation of the kinds of *reaction to frustration* : through a projective procedure, it can reveal the kind and the direction of aggressiveness. Obstacle Dominance responses show the frustrated subject blocked on considerations concerning the damage suffered; he stresses its severity (in case of extrapunitive responses), ascribing to himself the responsibility for not having been able to face the situation (in case of intrapunitive response), or minimizing and denying damage, so that he even finds the situation advantageous (in case of impunitive responses). Ego Defense responses tend to protect the subject's Ego, ascribing the guilt to somebody else (Extrapunitivity), to himself (Intrapunitivity) or not ascribing the blame to anyone (Impunitivity). Finally, in Need Persistence responses, the subject worries about the positive solution of the frustrating situation; for this purpose, he asks for external environment help (sometimes to the same frustrating subject) (Extrapunitivity), tries to find the solution by himself (Intrapunitivity), or places his trust in time or circumstance by waiting passively (Impunitivity). Subjects filled in their forms and self-evaluation questionnaires in a single session. Social adjustment was recorder by a researcher, who did not know each patient's kind of treatment and who also collected the special drug addiction form, referring to the present situation.

Results and Comment

The toxicological state of the two groups does not differ significantly during the stabilization phase as far as physical conditions and other substances concomitant abuse are concerned.

The subject's psychopathology and social adjustment, which were briefly evaluated for an anamnestic assessment, show the same trend. Nevertheless, the longitudinal evaluation of the single parameters reveals more positive variations in the H-Group (Table 1).

With regard to the observations during the metabolic stabilization period, the low mean SCL-90 values in the two groups (Table 2) testify a good recovery of psychophysical balance independently of the dosages. Yet, psychiatric symptoms are greater in high dosage subjects, especially with respect to psychoticism and hostility. Low dosage subjects reveal a greater sensitivity.

234

Table 1.
Toxicomanic Characteristics of two samples at beginning and in
Methadone Maintenance Program (Low dosages L-GR or
High dosages H-GR)

	Beginning		MMTP		Diff. Beg./MMTP	
	L-GR	H-GR	L-GR	H-GR	L-GR	H-GR
Liver diseases	75%	55%	50%	33%	33%	40%
LAS	75%	22%	50%	11%	33%	50%
Digestive tract dis.	62%	33%	50%	22%	19%	33%
Genital diseases	12%	33%	12%	0%	0%	100%
Dental diseases	50%	55%	25%	55%	50%	0%
Anxiety	62%	50%	77%	33%	19%	57%
Mood	75%	62%	77%	55%	17%	29%
Sleep disturbances	75%	62%	66%	33%	17%	50%
Hostility-out	12%	25%	66%	33%	-52%	50%
Hostility-in	62%	25%	55%	33%	60%	40%
Thought disturb.	50%	37%	33%	33%	26%	0%
Hallucinations	25%	12%	11%	33%	52%	-66%
Abuse of Cannabinoids	87%	66%	37%	33%	24%	11%
Abuse of Stimulants	62%	33%	12%	0%	47%	100%
Abuse of Psychedelics	50%	55%	12%	0%	-9%	100%
Abuse of Alcohol	37%	55%	0%	22%	-33%	-100%
Abuse of BDZ	75%	55%	37%	0%	27%	100%

Table 2.
SCL-90 and SAS Student's T-Test between Low (L-GROUP) and
High (H-GROUP) Dosages Methadone Maintenance Programs

	L-GROUP		H-GROUP			
	M	s	M	s	T	p
SCL-90						
1. Somatization	0,86	0,5	0,96	0,8	-0,32	ns
2. Obsessive-Compulsive	0,87	0,6	1,03	0,8	-0,47	ns
3. Interpersonal Sensitivity	0,70	0,4	0,69	0,9	0,05	ns
4. Depression	0,86	0,6	1,05	0,7	-0,59	ns
5. Anxiety	0,72	0,6	0,94	0,8	-0,65	ns
6. Anger-Hostility	0,73	0,7	1,11	1,2	-0,84	ns
7. Phobic Anxiety	0,72	0,6	0,64	0,8	-0,65	ns
8. Paranoid Ideation	0,81	0,5	0,96	0,8	-0,45	ns
9. Psychoticism	0,38	0,4	0,73	0,5	-1,63	ns
10. SCL-90 Total Score	0,72	0,4	0,89	0,6	-0,67	ns
SAS						
1. WORK	2,23	0,6	2,09	1,3	0,30	ns
2.1 PFM Relation*	2,25	0,8	1,42	0,9	2,02	ns
2,2 Sex Impairment	1,12	1,0	1,01	0,9	1,22	ns
2.3 Parental Role	1,40	0,7	1,25	0,5	0,49	ns
2.4 Concerns with relatives	2,29	0,4	2,14	0,9	0,40	ns
3. EXTERNAL FAMILY	1,87	1,2	1,01	0,9	1,97	ns
4.1 Leisure activity	3,37	1,4	2,88	1,7	0,65	ns
4.2 Social contacts	2,83	1,1	1,59	0,9	2,58	<,05
4.3 Interpersonal contacts	2,40	1,0	1,41	0,7	2,16	<,05
5. PERSONAL WELL-BEING	2,25	0,8	1,97	0,8	0,71	ns

* PFM = Principal Family Member

There are no significant differences between the two groups (Table 2) with regards to Social Adjustment quality and degree. The L-Group trend however show the maintaining a certain discomfort, testified by the higher mean values. Social contacts and leisure time utilization is especially problematic. High dosage subjects seem to be able to recover social and interpersonal contacts in a very good way.

Within the Family Area, there is a trend towards a better relation with the principle family member in the H-Group, with less sexual problems.

Aggressive behaviour (Table 3) is in the norm for the two groups, even if a certain elevation of the dyed resentment-suspiciousness remains. The L-Group is characterized by resentment, direct and indirect aggressiveness, while the H-Group proves more irritable, negative and suspicious.

Table 3.
Buss-Durkee Inventory (BDI) and Picture Frustration Study
(PFS by Rosenzweig) Student's T-Test between
Low (L-GROUP) and High (H-GROUP)
Dosages Methadone Maintenance Programs

	L-GROUP		H-GROUP			
	M	s	M	s	T	p
BDI						
Assault	57	11	54	11	0,50	ns
Indirect	57	11	56	10	0,21	ns
Irritability	52	11	56	9	-0,74	ns
Negativism	53	10	54	10	-0,24	ns
Resentment	62	13	59	9	0,62	ns
Suspiciousness	58	15	60	12	-0,29	ns
Verbal	58	13	58	11	-0,04	ns
Guilt	55	13	56	7	-0,05	ns
BDI Total score	55	11	55	9	-0,01	ns
PFS						
1.1. EOD	47	10	46	9	0,23	ns
1.2. IOD	51	6	45	7	1,86	ns
1.3. MOD	53	9	44	6	2,44	<,05
2.1. EED	49	8	52	18	-0,47	ns
2.2. IED	51	9	51	14	-0,12	ns
2.3. MED	53	16	53	9	0,05	ns
3.1. ENP	53	14	59	15	-0,82	ns
3.2. INP	47	9	43	9	0,83	ns
3.3. MNP	50	7	53	18	-0,48	ns

At an inner level, through PFS (Table 3), two significant different kinds of reaction to frustration can be pointed out. The L-Group tends to give more Obstacle Dominance responses, blocking itself on considerations about the suffered damage and minimizing its severity, while the H-Group, even if it does not have a manifest aggressive behaviour, shows the tendency to direct its aggressiveness, with various modalities and intensity degrees, towards objects and individuals of the external environment.

Conclusions

The low incidence of psychopathological manifestations and the good social adjustment of long term methadone treatment subjects demonstrate its effectiveness either at high or low dosages. Nevertheless, the ideal drug dose, able to stop heroin use, seems to imply the metabolic factors supposed by Kreek (1983), Walton et al. (1978), as well as the subject's psychopathological and aggressive aspects, according to Treece and Nicholson (1980) observations.

Subjects with a psychiatric symptomatology, included in high dosage treatments, show a significant recovery of social relations, of sexual activity, of leisure time utilization; these are signs of hedonist function recovery. Moreover, aggressivity-out, which can be noticed at the projective level, are behaviourally more limited than in the low dosage group subjects, in whom a certain hostility remains.

A correct psychopathological diagnosis of the drug addict, with particular regard to his aggressive experiences and social adjustment, is therefore necessary in the screening of patients, who must be included in a long term opiate agonists program.

"High" dosage methadone proves itself a better mood stabilizer especially for those subjects who show, beside the usual inclusion criteria, psychopathological and aggressive problems, with loss of hedonist functions. It confirms indirectly Dole and Nyswander's (1968) initial data.

REFERENCES

Castrogiovanni P., Andreani M.F., Maremmani I., Nannini-Innocenti M.A.(1982): Per una valutazione dell'aggressività nell'uomo: contributo alla validazione di un questionario per la tipizzazione del comportamento aggressivo. Rivista di Psichiatria, 17, 276-295

Derogatis L.R., Lipman R.S., Rickels K., (1973): The Hopkins Symptoms Checklist (HSCL): A measure of Primary Symptom Dimensions. In P. Pichot (Ed) "Modern Problems in Pharmacopsychiatry. Karger, Basle, 189-204

Dole V.P., Nyswander M.E. (1965): A medical treatment for diacetylmorphine (heroin) addiction. J.A.M.A. 193: 646-650

Dole V.P., Nyswander M.E. (1966) : Heroin Addiction: a metabolic disease. Arch. Intern. Med. 120: 19-24.

Dole V.P., Nyswander M.E., Warner A. (1968): Successful treatment of 750 criminal addicts. J.A.M.A. 206: 2708-2712.

Hargreaves W.A.(1983): Methadone dose and duration for maintenance. In J.R. Cooper (Ed) "Research on the treatment of narcotic addiction. State of the art. N.I.D.A. Rockville, Maryland, 19-82

Kreek M.J. (1983): Health consequences associated with the use of Methadone. In: J.R. Cooper (Ed) "Research on the treatment of narcotic addiction. State of the art. N.I.D.A. Rockville, Maryland, 456-491

Nencini R, Belcecchi M.V (1956). Guida alla forma per adulti del P.F.S. di Rosenzweig O.S. Firenze

Schooler N.R., Hogarty G.E., Weissman M.M. (1979): Social Adjustment Scale II.In "Resource material for community mental health program evaluation" (Hargreaves W.A. et al. Editors), A.D.M. 79, 328, 291 (Printing Authors, Washington, D.C.,)

Smith T.A., Kronick R.F. (1979): The policy culture of drug: ritalin, methadone, and the control of deviant behaviour. Int. J. Addict 12: 993-946

Treece C., Nicholson B (1980).: DSM III personality type and dose levels in methadone maintenance patients. J. Nerv. Men. Dis. 168: 621-628

Walton R.G., Thornton T.L., Wahl G.F.(1978) : Serum methadone as an aid in managing methadone maintenance patients. Int J. Addicts 13: 689-694

Weppner R.S.(1979): Conflicting world views and the delivery of treatment to narcotics addicts: some socio-cultural observations. Soc. SCI. Med. 13: 257-262

Methadone Maintenance and Delinquency Rates of Opioid Drug Users

D. Pfersmann[1], W. Prosche[1], W. Werdenich[2], G. Pakesch[1],
V. Pfersmann[1], O. Presslich[1], N. Loimer[1], and M. Neider[3]

[1] Department of Psychiatry, University of Vienna, Wien
[2] Sonderanstalt Favoriten, Ministery of Justice, Wien
[3] Ministery of Justice, Wien, Austria

INTRODUCTION

The methadone maintenance therapy still stays controversal, pro- and contra aspects are discussed as well. Besides scientific - medical, social - psychological aspects also economical ("economy of drug use") are pointed out and become more and more of interest. According to the latter costs have been listed for the consumption of drugs, the court, long time arrest and the costs for rehabilitation and prevention of crime. An alternative which makes sense is the long time therapy in an outpatient department with a dosage, which is adapted gently to the patient. In accordance with Haas (1) especially the methadone maintenance therapy in this group of patients is working palliative for an unlimited period of time.

In this study we are presenting preliminary results, organized by the Department of Psychiatry of the University of Vienna together with the Ministery of Justice. Besides the group of patients suffering on AIDS there is the group of criminal drug addicts, which is a very sensitive group you are not really able to handle with the established methods (drugfree longtime therapy, short time therapy requiring admission to hospital). Many of these patients cannot deny that they can't live without the drug, esp. if the drug history is 10 to 15 years of duration. Only after a long time of methadone maintenance in this sensible phase the patient is able to create a sufficient private and social life. Out of this feeling there often results the intrinsic wish of the patient himself to start the methadone reduction therapy with detoxification at the end.

The long time prognosis for opioid addicts show a trend to heal the addiction and elimination of social deficiency after adolescence. If one can help the young to cope with this very dangerous interval and to protect them from greater misery, which leads to a criminal career, the prognosis consecutively increases.

EXECUTION OF THE METHADONE PROGRAM

In 1987 and 1991 the supplementary law of the narcotic drug law made it possible, that patients with confirmed opioid addict for years and two or more unseccessful detoxifications are allowed to receive methadone as methadone maintenance or methadone detoxification therapy. Furthermore methadone is legal for patients who are HIV seropositive.

The criterias for admission to methadone maintenance program are as follows (2):
- the application mode is obligatory,
- the patient has to undergo the control of his doctor, esp. the urine samples (positive for drugs or not),
- the patient is not allowed to refuse additional treatment (e.g. psychotherapy)
- the patient has to avoid any use of narcotic drugs,
- the onset of treatment has to be reported to the authorities (in Austria this department is called "Suchtgiftüberwachungsstelle des Bundeskanzleramtes, Sektion 6, Volksgesundheit").

Only a medical doctor, who is familiar with the special problems of drug addicts and who is experienced in drug therapy is allowed to decide, if this very patient is responsible for methadone maintenance or not and it is his decision to admit this patient to the methadone maintenance program. In general a district officer of health or a consultant of psychiatry and neurology is regarded as such a specialist. To find the right dose the patient should be admitted to hospital; only in special case and for good reason an experienced medical doctor could start the therapy in an outpatient department or in his surgery. After prescribing a permanent prescription for methadone for the patient the prescription has to be validated by the district officer of health in that district where the drug addict is living. Undergoing this procedure and not earlier the patient is allowed to get methadone at any pharmacy of his choice and to drink methadone there under visible control of the pharmacist. This threefold controlmechanism (first the medical doctor, than the district officer of health and last but not least the chemist) is to ensure that there is no misuse and to emphasze that you treat the patient efficiently. The permanent prescription usually is prescribed for 31 days and has to be left at the pharmacy. So the daily dosage is no subject to discuss as long as the next time the patient will come to see his doctor. A therapy-planner for the dosage will be ruled out for the following 31 days (to reduce the dosage for 5 mg a week - or to start with an initial dosage, e.g. 60 mg, and to stay with this initial dosage till the patient is used to the oral application mode and than you reduce the dosage weekly very gently. The initial dosage depends on the kind of drug (heroin, paracodeinum or poppy-head-tea) on which the patient has been addicted. The rate of weekly reduction of methadone has to be adjusted by the intimate situation of the patient - this is the only way for a resonable compliance what assumes a very good relationship between the doctor and the drug addict. There is coercion to go to the pharmacy daily and to undergo urine samples regularely. If the patient uses drugs he will be withdrawn from the Methadone Maintenance Program. Of course there is exception for drugs which are prescribed by his doctor, e.g. to treat anxiety.

The benefits of methadone maintenance is not only HIV prevention - caused by it's oral application mode - it is crime prevention as well (2,3,4,5). The reason why is, thatmethadone is given daily - resulting in no stress and fear of getting no drug today; it is legal to receive this "drug" - so the addict is not in conflict with the authorities getting, holding and consuming this "drug". So the physical and psychical stress how to get the drug, very often leading to property offenses and other offenses, vanished.

METHODS

The goals of this study still is to investigate the influence of methadone maintenance therapy on prevention of crime, the progression of HIV infection to full blown AIDS and psychiatric sensations. With the purpose of these we created an enhanced questionaire, where we summarized social conditions, drug history, pychiatric history and datas from criminal records (Table 1, 2). To begin with the patients have been asked once - the observation period was 2.5 years (01.10.1987 - 01.03.1990) - nevertheless we are planning to repeat questioning the patient once a year for three years to be able to observe the progression.

264 patients on methadone maintenance have been investigated, 175 out of it with previous convictions (140 men and 35 women) and 89 drug addicts without previous convictions. The mean age was 29.6 years, the mean duration of drug history 8.5 years. 35 % have been classified as polytoxicomaniac (opioids plus tabletts; key according to ICD-9: 304.7), 65 % have only been opioid drug users (ICD-9: 304.0). The patients stayed in the methadone maintenace program by means 11 months (from 6 months to 29 months). The mean initial dosage was 60 mg a day. 80 % of the patients hold on with methadone, 6 % had a successful detoxification therapy and are drug free at the moment, 6 % have been admitted to hospital for detoxification and 8 % have withdrawn therapy for unknown reason.

46 % of the patients needed additional medication (major- and minor tranquillizer) because of depression, anxiety psychosis and disturbed sleep (somnipathies). The relapse rate on illegal drugs decreased significantely under therapy but the relapse rate on alcohol increased.

In detail we have been evaluating:

- the total number of convictions

- the number of fines

- the number of suspended sentences of imprisonment

- the number of unsuspended sentences of imprisonment

- duration of imprisonment (months)

Table 1

- categories of offences:

       - property offences

       (forgery and fraud as subgroups)

       - narcotic drug law violation

       - violent crimes, assault

       - rape and sexual offences

       - illegal possession of firearms

       - negligence against minors

Table 2

The point is: every item has been considered before and during methadone maintenance therapy. In order to evaluate the total and relative reduction of crime as success of treating the drug abuser we compared all items before and during therapy.

RESULTS

The crime rate at entering the methadone maintenance program was very similar to other studies: 66.3 % ; 85 % out of these patients showed narcotic drug law violation , 85 % (n = 175) property offences, 51 % violent crimes, 41 % illegal possession of firearms and other offenses, 0.05 % negligence against minors and 0.04 % sexual offenses (the latter reduced to a zero level during therapy!).

38 % of the patients had 1 - 5 previous convictions (31 % of the male and 65 % of the female), 40 % had 6 - 9 previous convictions (42 % of the male and 31 % of the female) and 22 % had 10 or more previous convictions (26 % of the male and 3 % of the female).

27 % of the criminal drug addicts (n = 175) stayed less than 6 months in prison (17 % of the male and 7 % of the female). 16 % stayed 6 months to one year in prison (11 % of the male and 5 % of the female). 19 % stayed one to two years in prison (17 % of the male and 2 % of the female). 38 % of the criminal drug addicts stayed more than two years in jail (35 % of the male and 1 % of the female).

The duration of unsuspended sentenses of imprisonment before onset of therapy have been by means 30.55 months in male and 19.7 months in female drug addicts.

One patient showed by means 6.13 convictions before onset of therapy, 2.68 fines, 2.14 suspended sentences of crime and 3.99 unsuspended sentences of crime. Narcotic drug law violation has been found 2.89 times in one patient by means before onset of therapy, property offences 3.73 times, violent crimes 2.19 times, sexual offences 1.75 times, possession of firearms and others 1.67 times and negligence against minors 1.44 times in one patient.

Crime Rates in Methadone Patients						
n = 264 number of previous convictions	total		male		female	
	n	%	n	%	n	%
1 - 5	67	25.38	44	16.67	23	8.71
6 - 9	70	26.52	59	22.35	11	4.17
> 10	38	14.39	37	14.02	1	0.38
total	175	66.29	140	53.03	35	13.26

Number of Methadone Patients in arrest						
duration of imprisonment (male = 140; female = 35)	total (n = 175)		male		female	
	n	%	n	%	n	%
< 6 months	46	27	30	17	16	9
6 - 12 months	27	16	19	11	8	5
13 - 24 months	32	19	29	17	3	2
> 24 months	64	38	62	35	2	1

Table 3

Narcotic Drug Law Violation						
Number of sentences	total n = 175	%	male	%	female	%
1 - 5	23	13	16	9	7	4
6 - 9	135	77	108	45	27	15
> 10	18	10	16	9	2	1

Property Offences						
Number of sentences	total n = 175	%	male	%	female	%
1 - 5	22	13	16	9	6	3
6 - 9	109	62	85	49	24	14
> 10	46	25	39	21	7	4

Violent Crimes						
Number of sentences	total n = 175	%	male	%	female	%
1 - 5	80	46	49	26	31	13
6 - 9	91	52	87	50	4	2
> 10	4	2	4	2	0	0

Table 4

Considering all patients on methadone (n = 264) 25 % had 1 - 5 previous convictions (16 % of all male and 8 % of all female, both criminal and non-sentenced for crime), 26 % had 4 - 9 previous convictions (22 % of all male and 4 % of all female) and 14 % had 10 or more previous convictions (14 % of all male and 0.3 % of the female).

17 % of the criminal plus non criminal drug addicts (n = 264) stayed less than 6 months in prison (11 % male and 6 % female). 10 % overall stayed 6 months to one year in prison (7 % male and 3 % female). 12 % stayed one to two years in prison

(11 % male 1 % female with respect to n = 264). 24 % of the drug addicts stayed more than two years in jail (23 % male 1 % female).

Evaluating the categories of crime we have found that 13 % of the criminal drug addicts showed narcotic drug law violation (in the group 1 - 5 previous convictions); 9 % of the male and 4 % of the female. For the group with 6 - 9 previous convictions the big amount of 77 % (n = 175) were sentenced for drug law violation (45 % male and 15 % female) and for 10 and more previous convictions the rate was 10 % (9 % male and 1 % female). With property offences we recorded for the group with 1 - 6 previous convictions: 13 % sentenced for property offences (9 % male and 3 % female); 6 - 9 previous convictions: 62 % (43 % male and 14 % female); 10 or more previous convistions: 25 % (21 % male and 4 % female). For violent crime the values are: 1 - 6 previous convictions: 46 % (26 % male and 18 % female); 6 - 9 previous convictions: 52 % (50 % male and 2 % female) and 10 or more previous convictions - that's interesting: a markedly decline of only 2 % involved in violent crimes, all male.

DISCUSSION

Our results show a relatively high rate of delinquency in our population examined (66.29 % previous convictions, 64.01 % previous imprisonments. The crime rate of males in our population was significantly higher than of the females. This result is consistent with the distribution of crime in the austrian population in general. Most of the offences originate from the stress to get the drug ("Beschaffungskriminalität").

We assume there is a trend that methadone maintenance has a reducing effect on the absolute number of property offences, violent crimes and on the outstanding number of narcotic drug law violation.

American investigators found a negative correlation between the absolute number of patients in the methadone maintenance program and the monthly report of crime rates of property offences (3). That means the more patients you treat with methadone, the less the crime rate is. Robbery, burglary and larceny decreased significantely. Total crime rates needs to be considered carefully, because there are crime acts of great extend which stay uninvestigated (3). More information you get to know using a questionaire asking the patient about his income modalities (anonymous) for the time prior to therapy and under therapy. The american group found a reduction in self-reported, partly uninvestigated illegal income of drug abusers from 6.937 US$ per year before methadone maintenance therapy down to 2.546 US$ during therapy.

A marked reduction in crime accurs after patients are integrated into methadone maintenance treatment (4). This reduction in criminality is evident with respect to all types of crime. Indeed, the general uniformity of the rate of reduction of criminality for 14 types of crime is striking. In 10 out of the 14 types of crime investigated declined by 80 percent or even more.

```
┌─────────────────────────────────────────────────────────────────┐
│                   Mean Crime Days Per Year                         │
│                                                                    │
│  Pre-treatment:    When addicted,                                  │
│                    "on the street"    n = 600    306.6  crime days │
│  In-treatment:     0.5 - 2.5 years    n = 345     24.0  crime days │
│  In-treatment:     2.5 - 4.5 years    n = 145     18.0  crime days │
│                                                                    │
└─────────────────────────────────────────────────────────────────┘
```

By the time patients had been in treatment over 4.5 years, both heroin use and crime had almost ceased ! Thus, 83 percent of the long-stay group were complete successes; 13 percent reported either some heroin use or crime - but only 4 percent reported both. The frequency of heroin use or crime was - 0.9 days per month for those who addicted heroin and 1.5 days per month for those still involved in crime. It was found that length of stay in treatment was significantly related to this reduction in drug abuse and crime; heroin use and crime continued to decrease after one or more years in treatment. These findings support the efficacy of long-term methadone maintenance treatment (4, 10).

Concomitantly there is a decrease of danger to be the victim of a crime offended by drug addicts in order to spoil their habbit.

While values based on criminal act counts often only reflect modest reduction in costs between pretreatment and posttreatment, the self-reported values of illegal income indicate major reductions as therapy success (5).

1. The most efficacy you achieve is combining methadone maintenance therapy with psychiatric and social help. The sense of methadone is that the patient gets time to recover physically, psychically and socially. This takes time and nobody should push anything. Very important is a sufficient dosage during a sufficient time interval (6).

2. Methadone maintenance is not only effective in the time of being under arrest, the positive effect also stays permanent thereafter.

3. Relapses have been found, but remarkably reduced, depending on to the time staying in treatment (4).

4. A therapy success is breaking off the circulus vitiosus (7):
The patients are feeling physically down - in order to try to escape from troubles in partnership, having no money because of being mentally and physically not able to work, being on the street again and facing the drug offered on the street which pretends that you could overcome misery, surrended to prostitution with all the risks (AIDS and sexually transmitted diseases) and crime. Relapses of drug addict will

follow, the need of drugs and money - crime - arrest - increased social misery - outlaws . . .

Breaking off the circulus vitiosus

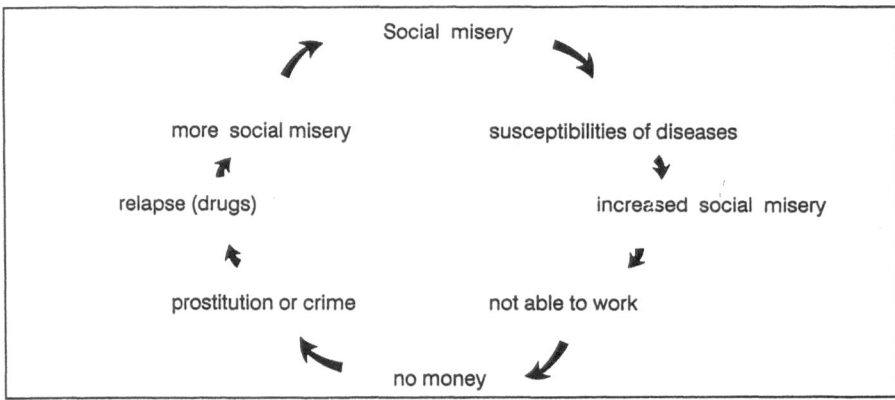

Kreek (11) concludes that methadone is a safe therapy, even when used in high doses (120 mg per day) for long term treatment of opioid addiction. Careful evaluation of each individual client to assess readiness for detoxification is the best approach.

Stimmel et al. (12) found that, of persons detoxified from methadone maintenance and followed up 5-6 years later, 35 % were doing well in terms of freedom of criminal activity and drug abuse. Methadone maintenance seems to have an impact on reducing the period being unemployed and a reduction of illegal income in those patient who originally started to live from welfare (9).

Guiding the patient becomes difficult because of the hypesthetic emotional weakness following an acute detoxification on opioids. The patients are suffering an heavy variation in the mood and heavy vegetative complaints, which are definitely reinforced by the extreme burden of arrest. If the patient doesn't voluntarily agree to detoxification you should abstain from trying to achieve detoxification under the conditions of arrest!

We conclude that methadone maintenance is a great help to stabilize the social and physical situation of the drug addict: sixtyseven percent achieved an inprovement of social productivity: employment, education (returned to school), household -- to give him enough time to calm down and to be prepared for detoxification at the right time. In summary, it has been shown that, for many opioid abusers, methadone maintenance is a viable method (8) of treatment, allowing an individual to satisfy a narcotic craving and at the same time seek to accomplish changes or funding of employment, family life and significant reduction of criminal activity in some kind with values about 80 %.

REFERENCES

1. Haas H, Fuchs WJ, Olgiati M, Uchtenhagen A (1990) Methadonabgabe in der Apotheke. Deutsche Apotheker Zeitung 130: 210 - 216

2. Pfersmann D, Presslich 0, Pakesch G, Hollerer E, Pfersmann V (1990) Gestaltung und Durchführung des Österreichischen Methadonprogrammes und erste Ergebnisse. Nervenarzt 61: 438 - 443

3. Maddux JF, Desmond D (1979)   Crime and Treatment of Heroin Users. The Int J of the Addiction 14: 891 - 904

4. Ball J, Corty H, Bond C, Myers C, Tommasello A (1988) The Reduction of Intravenous Heroin Use, Non-Opiate Abuse and Crime During Methadone Maintenance Treatment: Further Findings. Natl Inst Drug Abuse Res Monogr Ser 81: 224 - 230

5. Harwood HJ, Hubbard RL, Collins JJ, Rachal JV (1988) The Costs of Crime and the Benefits of Drug Abuse Treatment: A Cost - Benefit Analysis Using TOPS (Treatment Outcome Prospective Study) Data. NIDA Res Monogr 86: 209 - 235

6. Presslich O (1990) Patienten sind keine Objekte für ideologische Spielchen. Spectrum AIDS 1: 83 - 84

7. Pfersmann D (1990) HIV - positiv und Drogen, ein auswegsloser Teufels-kreis. Spektrum AIDS 1: 91 - 93

8. Doyle KM, Quinones MA, Louria DB (1982) Treating the Drug Abuser. Public Health Rev 10: 77 - 98

9. Kosten TR, Rounsville BJ (1987) Source of income as a predictor in opioid addicts. J of the Addiction 76: 196 - 199

10. Dole VP, Nyswander ME, Warner A (1968) Successful treatment of 750 criminal addicts. Am J Med Assoc 206: 2708 - 2711

11. Kreek MJ (1979) Methadone in treatment: Physiological and pharmacological issues. In: Dupont, Goldstein and O'Donell, Handbook on Drug Abuse. Natl. Institute of Drug Abuse, Washington, D.C. 19079

12. Stimmel B, Goldberg J, Rotkopf E, Cohen M (1977) Ability to remain abstinent after methadone detoxification: A six-year study. Am J Med Assoc 237: 1216 - 1220

Course and Outcome of HIV-Positive Drug Addicts in a Methadone Treatment Program

H. Rittmannsberger[1], Ch. Bayer[2], M. Ruschak[2], Ch. Silberbauer[2],
M. Geit[3], R. Simma[3], L. Binder[4], and H. Mittermayer[4]

[1] Outpatient Centre for Drug Addicts "Point", Wagner Jauregg Krankenhaus,
A-4020 Linz
[2] Coordination Bureau for the MTP, Public Health Authority of Upper Austria
[3] General Hospital Linz
[4] Hospital "Elisabethinen", Linz, Austria

Introduction

In 1987 a methadone treatment program (MTP) was created in Austria following a decree from the federal ministry of health. Target groups are long time drug addicts with HIV infection or those who underwent unsuccessful prior treatments. One of the aims of the MTP was to reduce the spreading of HIV infection.

In Austria a prevalence for HIV infection from 12% to 44% was found among drug addicts in several studies (Blecha et al. 1985, Erlacher 1990, Loimer&Hollerer 1990).

We will introduce the results of the first three years of the MTP in the region of Linz, Upper Austria. The organization of the MTP in Upper Austria provides that several institutions are resposible for the treatment of the participants: the psychiatric state hospital "Wagner-Jauregg-Krankenhaus", the outpatient centre for drug addicts "Point" and the coordination bureau for the MTP of the public health authority of Upper Austria. Specialized treatment for AIDS is supplied in the General Hospital Linz and the hospital "Elisabethinen".

The aim of our study was to examine the social and medical situation of the participants in the MTP three years after its start and to compare the HIV positive group with the HIV negative group regarding their social reintegration (work situation, drug use). For this reason we tried to examine all patients who were in the MTP in November and December 1990, provided that they had participated for at least half a year. We also looked at their reasons for ending the MTP. We also examined the progression of HIV infection among the HIV· group since being in the MTP.

Results

Population studied

In the three years from December 1987 to December 1990, 120 persons were treated with methadone, 31 of them had left the program as of November 1990. Of the 89 patients still in treatment 71 could be interviewed; 18 had been in MTP for less than half a year or did not want to answer our questions. The average time of treatment in the MTP was 21 months.

Among the 71 patients, 39 (24 male, 15 female) were HIV positive and 19 (13 male, 6 female) were negative. In 13 patients the HIV status could not be properly assessed. Regarding the social situation at the beginning of treatment, there were no differences between the HIV positive and negative group: the average age was 29 years, the average duration of addiction 11 years. 85% had been at least once in prison.

Dropouts. Among the 31 dropouts from the program 19 persons were HIV positve, 12 HIV negative. In the HIV positive group 8 patients died (3 died of AIDS, the others by suicide or accidents), 5 patients stopped on their own request and 6 persons were suspended from the program. Among the HIV negative group 2 died, 4 stopped on their own request and 6 were suspended.

Medical treatment and progression of HIV infection

72% of the HIV positive participants of the MTP came to an outpatient examination or treatment 4 or more times a year. A similarly high percent were in hospital at least once a year, 35% more than 5 times a year. Most of these stays were only for 2 or 3 days since these patients were mostly stationary due to examination rather than from being very sick.

During methadone treatment 16% of patients showed progression (measured by the stage of illness) and 58% remained stable; in 26% no assessment could be done.

asymptomatic infection (II)	5%
PGL (III)	65%
Constitutional disease (IVA)	16%
AIDS (IV B-E)	14%

Table 1: Stages of HIV infection of patients in the MTP (December 1990, CDC-classification (CDC 1986))

Employment situation

Generally speaking a marked improvement in the employment situation could be assessed, with an increase of persons working and a decrease of persons being on welfare (Table 2). Comparing the rate of employed persons at the beginning and at the follow up, statistical significance reaches p=0,08 (chi-square test).

	start	follow up
Employed	20%	35%
Registered unemployed (worked previously)	37%	29%
Disability pension	1%	17%
Others (welfare, illegal, ...)	41%	19%

Table 2: Employment and subsistence (N=71)

The employment situation at follow up was much better in the HIV negative group than in the HIV positive group (Table 3). Comparing the rate of persons in the two groups who either worked at follow up or had worked previously a highly significant difference could be shown (p=0,01, chi-square test)

	HIV neg	HIV pos
Employed	46%	33%
Registered unemployed (worked previously)	46%	21%
Diability pension	---	28%
Others (welfare, illegal, ...)	7%	18%

Table 3: Employment and subsistence at follow up: HIV negative vs HIV positive patients (N=58)

Drug use

At least once a month an urine sample was taken and examined for different drug metabolites. Table 4 shows the percentage of patients, who during the examination period, tested positive at least once for one of the investigated substances.

Drug metabolite	HIV neg	HIV pos
Cannabis	61%	67%
Opiates	58%	68%
Benzodiazepines	29%	45%
Barbiturates	26%	37%
Amphetamines	19%	22%
Cocaine	16%	16%
All drugs	71%	84%

Table 4: Positive testing for drug metabolites in HIV positive and negative patients

The consumption of alcohol was assessed by interview: 43% of the HIV negative and 56% of the HIV positive patients drank alcohol occasionaly or more often.

Subjective feeling

Patients and counsellors of the outpatient center were asked to rate the patients' physical and psychological condition and the overall· satisfaction and usefulness of the MTP (table 5).

	Patients		Counsellors	
HIV	neg	pos	neg	pos
psychological state	60%	58%	68%	46%
physical state	73%	58%	73%	31%
overall satisfaction	79%	77%	67%	75%

Table 5: Ratings of the patients' physical and psychological state by themselves and by the counsellors: percents of ratings "good" or "very good" in HIV negative and positve patients

Discussion

The WHO has recommended the installation of MTPs to stop the spreading of HIV infection (WHO 1989). Drug addicts have become the risk group of most concern, since common strategies for the prevention of spreading of HIV infection like "safer sex" showed little success among drug addicts: "safe addiction" is an illusion (Dole 1989). There are some positive results (Cooper 1989, Serriano 1989), but it must wait to be seen if the expectations for stopping the spreading of HIV infection by MTPs will be fullfilled.

In our view a second impact point of the MTP is the support for treatment of patients, who are already HIV positive. As our data showed, about 75% of our patients are in close contact with AIDS treatment centers, though more than two-thirds were asymptomatic or merely in the stage of PGL. In 16% of the patients we found a progession towards a higher stage of illness; this seems to be no high figure, but whether it is a good result cannot be judged, since there is no control group. Yet there is some evidence that treatment in a MTP significantly reduces the risk of progession of HIV infection compared with those still living in the scene (Weber et al. 1990). This improvement seems to be attributable to the changing of general living conditions and cessation of i.v. injecting rather than drug consumption by itself, since other studies had found no influence of alcohol and psychoactive drugs on the course of HIV infection (Kaslow et al. 1989). In our experience compliance with medical treatment of HIV infection is linked closely to participation in the MTP; on the other hand, those patients who comply poorly in the MTP (little contact to the outpatient center, frequent positive testing for other drugs), do likewise in the medical treatment.

Improvement in the social sphere is documented best by the employment situation, with a marked increase in working persons. Yet there is a striking difference between HIV positive and negative persons. Almost all HIV negative participants are working now or have previously worked. This can be said about only 50% of the HIV positives. Among 30% of the HIV positives the financial situation was stabilized through receiving an invalid pension.

Less encouraging are the results of urine samples. Only 29% of HIV negative and 19% of HIV positive patients never used other drugs than methadone (as registerd by the urine tests). Yet it has to be considered that polytoxicomanic drug use was a common pattern prior to MTP in almost all participants. Also here, though statistically not significant, the HIV positive group fares worse with a higher rate of consumption of additional drugs. This might be attributed to a worseened physical and psychological state with more urge for relief through psychotropic drugs on the one hand and to a lesser fear of being expelled from the program on the other hand. At any rate our experience shows that polytoxicomanic drug use decreases with time due to frequent consultations, but the decrease in this behaviour is less among the HIV positive group.

The majority of participants generally judge their physical and psychological state to be good; but from the counsellor's point of view especially the state of those with HIV infection is especially viewed less optimistically. Yet the overall satisfaction with the MTP is high in all groups, despite several conditions complicating life like the daily visit to the pharmacy, frequent contacts to the outpatient center, numerous urin samples and a limited freedom of movement.

In conclusion the HIV positive patients in MTP are faring less well than the HIV negative in almost all outcome variables; on the other hand the possible benefits from this treatment are to be estimated especially high for these persons, since the MTP often offers the only chance to reduce the speed of the infection's progression.

References

Blecha HG, Deinhart F, Dierich MP et al (1985) Drogenabhängige in Österreich – eine Risikogruppe für AIDS. Neuropsychiatrie 1:24-28

Centers for Disease Control (1986) Classification System for Human T-lymphotropic virus type III/lymphadenopathy-associated virus infections. JAMA 256:20-24

Cooper RC (1989) Methadone treatment and acquiried immunodeficiency syndrome. JAMA 262:1664-68

Dole VP (1989) Methadone treatment and the acquired immunodeficiency syndrome epidemic. JAMA 262:1681-82

Kaslow RA, Blackwelder WC, Ostrow DG et al (1989) No evidence for a role of alcohol or other psychoactive drugs in accelerating immunodeficiency in HIV-1-positive individuals. JAMA 261:3424-3429

Loimer N, Hollerer EM (1990) Harte Drogen und AIDS. Wiener Z f Suchtforschung 13:27-32

Serraino D, Franceschi S (1989) Methadone maintenance programmes and AIDS. Lancet 334:1522-23

Weber R, Ledergerber B, Opravil M et al (1990) Progression of HIV infection in misusers of injected drugs who stop injecting or follow a programme of maintenance treatment with methadone. BMJ 301:1362-1365

World Health Organisation (1989) Options for the use of methadone in the treatment of drug dependence. WHO, Division of Mental Health; Geneva

Managing AIDS: The European Centre/WHO Collaborative Study and Database Project

K. Guzei and P. Kenis

European Centre for Social Welfare Policy and Research, Berggasse 17,
A-1090 Wien, Austria

In the following, two major databases will be presented which directly result from the research project "MANAGING AIDS — The Role of Private Nonprofit Institutions and Nongovernmental Organizations in Public Health and Welfare Policy". MANAGING AIDS is a collaborative study of the Regional Programme on AIDS of the World Health Organization (WHO) and the European Centre for Social Welfare Policy and Research in Vienna.[*]

A. The Study of Organizations When Dealing with AIDS

The starting points of the MANAGING AIDS project are as follows:
- that a medical solution to the AIDS problem is not to be expected in the near future;
- that people in general do not change their behaviour, or do so only under very specific circumstances; and
- that in most countries, the state reacted to the social dimensions of the AIDS problem only hesitantly and often contradictorily, and that one can expect that the state will continue to do so in the future.

In contrast, there are clear empirical indications that *organizations* constitute a possibility of coping with the HIV/AIDS problem in a encouraging, adequate, and positive way. It appears that in most countries and in a short period of time, a variety of HIV/AIDS organizations have developed — e.g., counselling and prevention centres, interest organizations, self-help groups, etc. Without the activity of these HIV/AIDS organizations, AIDS management in most countries would be non-existent or, at least, inadequate.

---

[*] For the elaborated research design with theoretical background, see Marin and Kenis (1989).

It can be stated that there is consensus regarding the fact that these organizations play a crucial role in overall AIDS management and in health and welfare policy. Nevertheless, there does not exist any systematic and comparative study on these associations. This is particularly striking when compared with the overwhelming number of (a) studies which produce epidemiological data respectively studies which map and investigate behavioral changes (or better, non-changes in behaviour) and (b) studies which discuss models of how one should deal with the problem on a political level or from a public policy point of view. There seems to exist a *micro-macro bias*: the *micro-level* being the level of behaviour and the *macro-level* being the level of political discourse and planning. Not only from a theoretical point of view but also in practical terms, we think that the concrete and significant accomplishments, changes, reactions, and innovations in the field of HIV/AIDS are to be located at the *meso-level* — or, in other words, at the level of concrete HIV/AIDS organizations.

Given this deficit in research as well as the significance of these organizations in daily practice, we think it most important to study in detail the following points: how in different countries these organizational structures developed; which groups with which interests and which means could establish themselves in the HIV/AIDS policy field; how these different groups compete or cooperate; and for which groups in society services are provided with which intensity, which spread and quality, etc. At the same time, studying the existing organizational responses allows us to observe those groups which are not at all organized or are organized only to a limited extent. In a next step, the study might define the circumstances which are needed for groups to get organized in such a way that they can cope effectively with the HIV/AIDS problem. This last aspect might be especially relevant to the case of drugs, since we know that drug users are among the most difficult groups to either help or to persuade to help themselves through organizational modes.

B. The Research Project MANAGING AIDS: A Brief Summary

The MANAGING AIDS project is considered to be an organizational study with policy implications. That means that we primarily focus on the analysis of organizations — their functional capacities, their organizational and managerial properties, their interorganizational linkages, their cooperation, division of labor, competition, etc. Secondly, we are interested how these associations cope with the HIV/AIDS epidemic in the different national health and welfare systems.

At the time being there have been ten countries involved in this international comparative study: Austria, Belgium, Britain, France, Hungary, Italy, the Netherlands, Portugal, Sweden and Switzerland. Every country is represented by its own research team composed of two or three persons.

In general, the field research is divided into two phases: in a first phase, a Directory will be produced containing all existing AIDS service organizations in the different countries. This we do by gathering information based on a standardized Inventory Sheet (for more detailed information, see point "C"). This research will result in a database called AIDSINST. The database can be used for empirical research, but it will also be available to the public as a Directory telling where to find what kind of services in a specific area.

In a second phase, a representative sample of fifty AIDS service organizations will be taken from each National Directory. These selected organizations will be studied in detail through a standardized questionnaire (for more detailed information, see point "D"). This research will lead to a database called MANAGAIDS and will be used exclusively for research. It will help to answer questions about the functioning of different kinds of AIDS service organizations in relation to the services provided, their clients, managerial aspects, decision processes, etc.

In both databases, the unit is the AIDS service organization (ASO). In general terms and within the scope of this project, ASOs are defined as those organizations engaged in at least one HIV/AIDS-related activity in the field of (a) prevention, education, information, (b) health care and social services, (c) control, intelligence, surveillance, monitoring, (d) policy advocacy, interest organization, civil and human rights, or (e) fund-raising for AIDS programmes.

C. AIDSINST / AIDS Institutions Directory

Goal, Purpose, and Usage for Different Groups

AIDSINST will provide a complete list of all private, nonprofit, and public AIDS prevention/service/policy institutions in the aforementioned countries. Dependent on the specific group concerned, the AIDSINST database offers the following possibilities for its usage:

(a)   Persons Concerned: Persons who are HIV positive can, for instance, easily find out where to get specific professional help. Persons who are part of risk groups can be provided with information: e.g., what kind of services are offered by specific organizations in a specific area. Persons who are in a kinship relation with HIV/AIDS persons or live together with them can, for example, find out if there exists — and if yes, where — a self-help group for relatives and friends.

(b)   Streetworkers, Social Workers, Teachers, Social Administrators, Medical Professionals, etc.: Firstly, these groups of people — many of whom are confronted on a daily basis with HIV-positive persons or people with AIDS — can get information on where which services are offered in order to refer concerned persons to specific institutions. Secondly, they can be provided with information about programme activities which are set up in other places so as to learn from these programmes.

(c)   Persons Working in ASOs: The AIDSINST database can be useful also for ASOs in terms of contributing to the implementation of international ASO networks and to the exchange of information.

(d)   Policy-makers: Policy-makers on different levels (local, regional, national, international) — as well as policy-makers from different organizations (governmental, private, or nonprofit voluntary) — might, on the one hand, be informed about individual experiences, innovations, etc. and, on the other, might have the possibility to avoid duplications, deficiencies, etc.

(e)   Researchers: The AIDSINST database can also be useful for researchers dealing with the HIV/AIDS problem in order to learn about the complexity of the organizational pattern of ASOs, the organizational mix, the organizational structure, etc.

Procedure for Gathering Data

A standardized, two-page Directory Sheet is sent to all AIDS service organizations in a given country. These sheets have to be filled in by the organizations themselves. A cover letter is included which, on the one hand, describes the general goal of the study, and, on the other, tries to offer an incentive so that the organizations take part in the study. If there is no response within a limited period, we remind the respective organizations by phoning them or writing them so as to raise the return rate. The quality of the ASO Directory is in great part dependent on its being complete.

Identification of Organizations

The procedure of identifying the relevant ASOs takes place in different steps. Firstly, all generally "known" organizations in the field are requested to answer. Secondly, we ask all organizations of a specific type who theoretically could provide the kind of services the project is interested in — e.g., hospitals, prisons, counselling centres, etc. Thirdly, we ask experts in the field — such as care providers, doctors, experts of other ASOs, etc. — to name potential ASOs. Fourthly, we use the so-called "reputational method". This means that we ask organizations which have been already identified, whether they know of any other organizations in their geographical area which provide HIV/AIDS-related services.

Variables

(1)   Name, Acronym and Address of the Organization

(2)   Legal Status of the Organization: The Directory compiles (a) governmental, public agencies; (b) private firms or companies; and (c) nonprofit, voluntary organizations. In the initial stage of the research, it became clear that this dimension has to be considered as crucial. As far as research interests are concerned, this differentiation helps to adequately judge the role of state agencies as well as of the civil society in coping with HIV/AIDS. We are aware of the fact that many, as private classified organizations, depend on state subsidies.

Nevertheless, we think that the legal status of an ASO is a rough indicator for the specific AIDS policy in a given country. For clients, it might be helpful to know whether the initiative to set up a specific ASO came from the state or from "below".

(3)   Founding Date of the Organization, Year in which HIV/AIDS Programmes were started, and Founding Date as an AIDS Service Organization/Unit: These questions are important for researchers as well as for clients. From a theoretical point of view, we are interested in analyzing developmental cycles of organizations. Moreover, first indications seem to show that there exists no clear correlation between the founding of ASOs and the epidemiological situation in a given country. For clients, it might be useful to know about the age of a specific organization and how long specific activities have been carried out by this institution, since some clients might be in favour of an "old, well-established" organization — whereas other clients might prefer a "young, non-establishment" organization.

(4)   Whether the organization is specialized in HIV/AIDS only or whether it is a general organization including HIV/AIDS programmes among other activities: Crucial within the theoretical framework of our study, is the present differentiation in organizations dealing exclusively with HIV/AIDS-related issues, as opposed to organizations dealing with HIV/AIDS among other activities. Examples of "specialized, exclusive organizations" are National AIDS committees, AIDS hotlines, self-help groups for people with HIV/AIDS, etc. Examples of "encompassing, inclusive organizations" are hospitals with HIV/AIDS units, drug treatment/counselling centres, civil and human rights organizations, etc. Several hypotheses regarding this key concept were set up. Specialized, exclusive organizations might have the advantages of clear, even monopolistic mandates, political and financial support, regulatory authority, task specialization, etc. However, they might simultaneously lack the embedded nature, high reputation, professional recognition, organic linkages, and resource access of an old, non-specialized institution performing AIDS programmes among others. Encompassing, inclusive organizations might incorporate AIDS programmes within a generally advantageous institutional texture, thereby having the ability to cross-subsidize and professionally support them in an optimal way. However, they might also prove to be unable or unwilling to occupy themselves with a disease which is new, scientifically ill-understood, institutionally difficult to handle, risky, medically unhealable, and culturally often stigmatized.

(5)   Kind of Organization in General, and Kind of Organization in Particular (regarding HIV/AIDS): Some of the different possibilities given here are, for instance, AIDS-specialized foundations; inpatient health care centres; policy advocacy, civil and human rights organizations; social work agencies; AIDS policy coordination and implementation bodies; homes for persons with HIV/AIDS; drug treatment counselling centres, etc. Given the fact that clients are interested in a specific kind of services, it might be helpful to know the general type of organization. There are clear indications that organizations of a total different kind might carry out the same services or activities — e.g., home care services can be provided by

home care service organizations, by local health initiatives/mutual aid networks, by community care centres, and by social work agencies as well as by PWA case management organizations and so on.

(6)   Main HIV/AIDS-related activities: This question is in some way the core of the Directory, since we are not interested in just introducing various organizations but rather in presenting the service mix offered by the respective organization. One main purpose is to inform clients where they can obtain which kinds of services or activities. Moreover, it might be useful for clients to know where they can find an organization which offers several services which the client needs — e.g., a person, who wants to be HIV-tested might be in favour of an organization, which provides HIV tests as well as face-to-face counselling, instead of being tested without therapeutical advice.

(7)   Geographical Scope of the Organization: We ask whether it is local, regional, national or multinational and also in which concrete geographical area the organization is active. This is not only important for clients but also for policy-makers, so as to find out in which areas there are duplicates or deficiencies. This question helps to clarify how a certain area is covered by AIDS programmes or services. Moreover, we are especially interested if epidemiology and organizational density correlate — or in other words, if the epidemiological situation influences the organizational density or *vice versa*.

(8)   Organizational Resources in General, and Organizational Resources for HIV/AIDS in Particular: These questions help to describe to which extend the national field is equipped with HIV/AIDS-related resources. Based on the results of these questions, we are also enabled to analyze the variation or spread of HIV/AIDS programmes or activities within a given national context. Moreover, these data indicate, e.g., both how many resources are provided for a certain HIV/AIDS programme and which role volunteers play with regard to specific services.

Presentation and publication

One *European Directory* in English and single *National Directories* for each country in its respective language(s), are expected to be published during the course of 1991.

Updating

A continuously updating is foreseen if there is response to it — i.e., if clients, policy-makers, or the organizations themselves are interested in updating the AIDS Institutions Directory.

D. MANAGAIDS

Goal, Purpose, and Usage for Different Groups

MANAGAIDS is an integrated AIDS Policy Management Information System which provides a comprehensive description of the up to 50 most significant ASOs in each of the ten countries studied. The aim of the database is to empirically and cross-nationally investigate questions regarding the internal functioning and external relations of ASOs. This is done in order to ultimately address the following questions: what the contribution of ASOs is to the social dimension of AIDS; what forms such ASOs take in different social, economic and political environments; and what tasks such ASOs perform. For example, is the "Buddy" system available in a certain area? What explains the absence or presence of the Buddy system: is it demand, organizational resources, legal regulations, a tradition of volunteering, the kind of organization providing it (private, nonprofit, public), the kind of groups affected, etc.?

The crude data within the MANAGAIDS database will be only accessible to the country teams of the MANAGING AIDS project and will be treated in a fully confidential manner. However, on the basis of the database, aggregate data analysis will be carried out for academic purposes — as well as to advice policy-makers and ASOs on the specificities and logics of institutional devices and developments in the field of AIDS.

Procedure for Gathering Data

The entries to the database is information collected primarily through a structured questionnaire. Interviews on the average last between 4 and 5 hours and are conducted exclusively by the research groups in the different countries themselves.

Identification of Organizations

Using Cluster Analysis, a sampling procedure has been developed which allows for two things: on the one hand, it pictures the AIDS policy field in a specific country; and on the other hand, it allows for organizational analysis of ASOs on the basis of a data set comprising 500 (= 10 x 50) organizations.

Variables for Analysis

The database will not contain any information on individual persons but will only represent organizational characteristics. Any individual organization is described by approximately 600 to 800 variables which reflect the following 11 main areas of interest:

(1)   Status, Organizational History, Development: This group of variables describes basic characteristics of the ASO. For example, is it a private, public or nonprofit organization? Is it an old or new organization? Is it a social work agency, nursing home, fund-raising organization, biomedical research centre, self-help group etc.? Is it a political or secular organization? Is it an organization which deals exclusively with HIV/AIDS, or do they also other things than HIV/AIDS activities? Firstly, this set of variables is crucial in describing the policy field of AIDS Management, both in a specific country and in general. For example, is it predominantly private nonprofit organizations or public organizations which are active in the field of AIDS? Did new organizations especially develop to deal with the problem or was

it rather the old established organizations which took on the problem? Secondly, on an organizational level, we expect these variables to have explanatory value regarding the kind of services and programmes performed.

(2) Formal Organization: Here a group of variables is given which describes the degree of formalization of the organization. For example, are there written statutes? Is there an organogram? Are there outlets or branches? Are there committees and working groups? From an organizational point of view, these variables would allow to test hypotheses. For example, does the degree of formalization depend on environmental structures (e.g., the country), the kind of organization (private vs nonprofit, new vs old, etc.), or the kind of resources on which the organization is dependent? Or is it rather the other way around, being the kind of output (service/programmes) the organization performs?

(3) Decision-making and Managerial Processes: Some questions are asked here to get a rough idea of how the organization is internally structured. For example, is it a highly differentiated or integrated organization? Are there conflicts over specific issues? Who formally and actually participates in the organizational decision-making process?

(4) Volunteering, Professionalism, Leadership: Questions in this category relate to characteristics regarding the persons working and/or volunteering in the organization. From a policy-level point of view, these variables allow to describe the kind of personal resources of which the sector consists: is it mainly, professionals, laypeople, volunteers, part-time workers, males, females, persons personally involved or not, etc.? Generally speaking, do HIV/AIDS services programmes imply a specific personal input? Moreover, does the kind of personal input vary according the type of organization (private, public, nonprofit)? For example, are women more represented in the nonprofit sector as compared to the other type of organizations, and as compared to other sectors of society in general? From an organizational point of view, the main questions raised with these variables will address the relationship between programmes and activities performed and the kind of personal resources of the organization.

(5) Activities: Task Profiles: Here the main question is on the domain the organization is active regarding HIV/AIDS programmes and activities. The MANAGING AIDS project is unique since it is simultaneously interested in activities regarding prevention, care and social services, control/intelligence/ surveillance/monitoring, policy advocacy/interest organization/civil and human rights and support activities. From a policy-field point of view, we believe that it is very difficult to understand how a national context reacted to the problem of HIV/AIDS when concentrating on any singular type of activity. All of them are equally important in a comprehensive policy towards HIV/AIDS. On the organizational level, such a "mix" of activities seems equally to play an important role. First findings clearly indicate that most ASOs provide several types of activities at the same time. What this means is not clear yet, but it is a clear proof for the importance of combining an analysis of the different types of activities in one single study.

(6) Activities: Work Organization and Processes: Variables in this group try to picture how organizations internally organize their task performances and under which conditions they perform their tasks. For example, do people carrying out programmes and activities work in team or individually? Are there specific professional "techniques" used in the organization? How is time organized: is there overtime, night work, what are the operating and opening hours, etc.?

(7) Activities Output/Service Statistics and Performance Indicators: In this section, the organization is asked to indicate — from a list of 100 programme and service activities — which of these they perform. This is a central question, since most of the project is organized around HIV/AIDS activities. From a policy-field point of view, the question on activities will picture a specific country according to types of services performed and not performed, existing duplications, divisions of labour between types of organization and *regio*, etc. From an organizational point of view, the type of activities performed will be treated as a dependent variable in order to understand why and when specific tasks are performed or not performed.

(8) Membership Structures: Questions in this section apply only to membership organizations. The single questions address number of members, coverage, assessment of dues, exclusivity of membership, etc. The main reason for investigating these question is to find out the potential a membership organization inherits for organizing HIV/AIDS activities when compared to other forms of organization.

(9) Input and Allocation of Resources: Questions in this section apply to the availability and source of non-personal resources within the organization. From a policy-field point of view, it is interesting to learn what the constraints and possibilities are to mobilize financial and extra-financial resources for organizations (in this case, primarily nonprofit organizations) in different social, political and economic environments. Is it really the source and availability of resources which defines the activities of an organization, or are other factors important as well?

(10) Interorganizational/Intersectoral/International Cooperation and Competition: From an organizational point of view, it is nowadays stressed that interorganizational linkages seem to become more and more important for organizations to fulfil their tasks and to deal with their environment. At the same time, however, it is not yet well understood exactly what the function of such linkages is. On the other hand, it is equally stressed nowadays that — on a policy-field level — there exist many unnecessary duplications and overlaps in activities as well as counter-productive sectoral configurations. Both phenomena, as well as the relationship between them, will be analyzed on the basis of interorganizational variables.

(11) Institutionalization: Variables in this category only apply to private organizations, since they measure the degree to which organizations perform state-like functions: e.g., administration of state grants, representation for the public or semi-public areas, etc. Interesting here is how countries differ in the extent to which tasks are transferred to private actors and how this capacity relates the programmes and activities performed.

MANAGAIDS is the result of rather time-consuming field research and will only be carried out once. Arriving at structural insights in how organizations deal with the social aspects of HIV/AIDS, is the primary goal here — in contrast to AIDSINST, where the main goal is to provide up-to-date information on existing activities and programmes.

We hope that both AIDSINST and MANAGAIDS will contribute by giving insight and direction in how to prevent HIV transmissions, how to reduce the personal and social impact of HIV/AIDS and how to unify efforts against AIDS.

References

Marin, B. and Kenis, P. (1989) 'Managing AIDS: The Role of Private Nonprofit Institutions in Public Health and Welfare Policy. A Research Proposal for an International Comparative Study'. Vienna: European Centre for Social Welfare Policy and Research.

AIDS Fear and Risk Behavior in Intravenous Drug Users

K. O. Karamustafalioğlu, M. Y. Ağargün, N. Karamustasfalloğlu,
L. Alpkan, N. Eradamlar, and M. Beyazyürek

Bakirköy Ruh ve Sinir Hastaliklari, Hastanesi,
34747 Istanbul, Turkey

Although the association between the use of needles and syringes by drug users and transmission of virus infection was noted as far back as 1958, suggestions for prevention of this mode of transmission have only recently been widely published. Until recently, official schemes to distribute clean equipment or advice about sterilizing existing equipment have not been established. This intervention strategy is clearly an attempt to divert widespread dissemination of HIV infection among parenteral drug users and more specifically to attempt to prevent epidemics similar to those recorded in Edinburgh, Milan and New York (Robertson 1988)

There are other dimensions of attempts to reduce AIDS infection in drug users. Attempts to reduce the impact of HIV infection on society currently depend largely on public health measures, in particular health education. The effects of health education comprise cognitive and behavioral aspects, education seeks to increase knowledge and change beliefs about health risks and then exhorts people to modify their behavior accordingly so as to reduce the incidence of disease in a community (Coleman 1988a).

Intravenous drug users are one of the important risk groups for HIV infection. They are an important group when to predict the likely future incidence of infection in the community (Moss 1987). In order to make such predictions it is essential to know what are the levels of sexual and equipment sharing behavior through which infection can be transmitted. It may be also important to know something about the ways in which risk behavior is distributed and organized among drug users (Coleman 1988b).

Even though HIV transmission and AIDS are sporadic in Turkey, they still have a potential of risk. It was reported that there were 4 HIV positives' among 183 intravenous drug users (Beyazyürek 1988).

Intravenous drug users may change their injecting, sharing of injecting equipment and sexual behavior because of various reasons and AIDS fear is one of them. In this study, we aimed to find out the risk behavior for AIDS, perception of AIDS and change of behavior related to their perception of AIDS in intravenous drug users.

Method

4 female and 40 male, totally 44 patients who were admitted to Bakırköy Neuro-Psychiatric Hospital Drug Abuse Treatment Center were taken into our study. They were interviewed by clinic doctors using a standard questionnaire aiming to assess their AIDS perception and risk behaviors.

Results

The mean age of 40 male, 4 female totally 44 patients were 32.93 and the mean duration of IV drug use were 4.89 years. All of the patients supplied their injecting equipment from the drugstore. 64 %(N=28) of the patients shared their injecting equipment. The leading reasons for sharing were not finding an open drugstore, withdrawal symptoms and being prisoned. Table 1 illustrates sexual behavior and being abroad characteristics of IV users.

TABLE 1

Sexual behavior and being abroad characteristics of IV users

	YES	NO	TOTAL
Sharing injecting equipment	28	16	44
Being abroad	16	28	44
Abusing drugs abroad	9	7	16
Sexual intercourse with multiple partners	28	16	44
IV drug abuse of sexual partners	12	32	44
Sharing injecting equipment with sexual partners	12	--	12
Sexual partner sharing with someoneelse	12	--	12

All of our patients knew that they were under the risk of AIDS.
Table 2 illustrates the perception of AIDS

TABLE 2

AIDS PERCEPTION

	YES	NO	TOTAL
Thinks exposed to AIDS	27	17	44
Screening tests done upon request of			
patient before admission	18	26	44
Don't want to be screened	10	16	26

Table 3 illustrates the change of behavior in order to prevent AIDS
infection. The methods patients prefered in prevention of AIDS were
washing, boiling, using alcohol or using lemon juice to sterilize the
injecting equipment.

TABLE 3

Change of behavior for prevention of AIDS

	YES	NO	TOTAL
No cleaning	9	35	44
Using injecting equipment only once	4	40	44
Cleaning	21	9	30
Change to nasal use	8	36	44

39 %(N=17) of the patients believe that prohibition of the sale of
injecting equipment will end up with effective prevention. 7 of the 17
thought this prohibition will cause the nasal use of heroin.

Discussion

Drug abusers are not hereditary uninteligable behaving people. They
have a potential towards reducing their high risk behavior. All of our
patients knew that they were under the risk of AIDS, half of them thought

that they were exposed to AIDS, half of this group had screening tests for AIDS before their admission to our hospital and changed some of their behavior.

In reality, some of the abusers will continue their injecting behavior. Hence 32 %(N=14) of patients don't think of changing the pattern of abuse or quit abusing drugs. In this case, the most important thing is to prevent the sharing behavior of injecting equipment (Power 1988). The problems faced in supply of sterile injecting equipment is a cause of sharing behavior. Our patients were facing problems in supply of sterile injecting equipment. 48 %(N=21) of our patients were not sterilizing their injecting equipment adequately in their successive use even if they supply it from the drugstore. The education of this group will abolish an important risk group.

Only to inform the drug abusers about the risk of AIDS and risk behavior does not solve the problem. With the suppression of immune system various illnesses could be seen in HIV(+) patients (Guegen 1988). Because of this, there is a need for multidiciplinary and specialized consultatory approach in the clinics involved in drug abuse treatment (Oddou 1987).

AIDS have changed the perpectives to drug addiction in which amazing problems have been faced in intervention strategies. This new perspective may bring new dimensions even though it is associated with AIDS. It is noteworthy that even if AIDS or HIV transmission is very sporadic, this is the case in Turkey.

R E F E R E N C E S

Beyazyürek M, Tuncer C, Ersül Ç, Samancı AY, Karamustafalıoğlu KO, Möröy A(1988) Uyuşturucu madde bağımlılığı ve AIDS. XXIV. Ulusal Psikiyatri ve Nörolojik Bilimler Kongre Kitabı. Saypa, Ankara.

Coleman RM, Curtis D, Feinmann C(1988a) Perception of Risk of HIV Infection by Injecting Drug Users and Effects on Medical Clinic Attandance. Brit J Addiction 83: 1325 - 1329.

Coleman RM, Curtis MA(1988b) Distribution of Risk Behavior for HIV
Infection Amongst Intravenous Drug Users. Brit J Addiction 83: 1331 - 1334.

Guegen JP(1988) SIDA: et si les Intervenants en Toxicomanie n'étaietent pas
vraiment concernés? Intervention 17: 29 - 31.

Moss AR(1987) AIDS and intravenous drug use-the real heterosexual epidemic.
Brit Med. Journal 294: 389 - 390.

Oddou A(1987) Le Toximanie Malade du SIDA? Intervention Hors Serie,53-56.

Power R, Hartnoll R, Daviand E(1988) Drug Injecting, AIDS and Risk
Behavior: Potential for change and intervention strategies. Brit J
Addiction 83: 649 - 654.

Robertson JR, Skidmore CA, Roberts JJK (1988) HIV Infection in Intravenous
Drug Users: a follow-up study indicating changes in risk behavior. Brit J
Addiction 83: 387 - 391.

HIV-Risk and Social Integration in Groups of Drug-Addicts

A. Dobler-Michola, D. Zimmer Höfler, R. Korbel, and
A. Uchtenhagen

Sozialpsychiatrischer Dienst, Forschung und Dokumentation, Militärstraße 8,
CH-8021 Zürich, Switzerland

Looking for the association between HIV-risk and social integration, we were
interested in whether HIV-positive drug-addicts disclose more characteristics of social
desintegration and less social resources - currently and in their social background -
than their HIV-negative counterparts. The basis of the empirical analysis was made
from two samples consisting of clients of methadone maintenance (n=73) and
therapeutic communities (n=177) respectively.

In both samples, HIV-positive and HIV-negative clients were compared according to
their familiy situations in childhood and youth, social and psychological deviance,
vocational integration and social contacts.

No difference was seen in their social background-status. They are less integrated in
their job and demonstrate a higher rate of deviant behaviour. They report more suicide
attempts and either have repeatedly been to prison or/and judged by court. They are
also less integrated in social networks. In case of problems, emotional parental support
is practically non-existent and they have less friends.

Summarizing, we can hypothesize that HIV-positive drug-addicts are especially
socially isolated and display many characteristics of social marginality, even more than
drug-addicts in average.

1. INTRODUCTION

During the eighties, HIV-infection was continuously increasing among IV-drug addicts.
The resulting dangers became a main issue within the discussion of HIV-prevention.
(Friedland GH, Harris C, Butkus-Small C, Shine D, Moll B, Darrow W, Klein R, 1985;
Des Jarlais DC & Friedman SR, 1988; Robertson JR, Skidmore C, Roberts M, 1988). For
IV-drug-addicts, transmission and prevention have special aspects and a conceptual basis
for undestanding behaviour change among intravenous drug users is needed for
generating cumulative knowledge and rational design of prevention programmes (Des
Jarlais DC & Friedman SR, 1988). It is necessary to develop prevention programmes,
which fit the real situation of drug-addicts and which are efficient to produce behavioral

changes and expecially diminish risktaking-behaviour. For that, however, more knowledge has to be gained about addicts' every-day life and factors which are associated with increasing seroprevalence rates in drug-addicts.

A first step is observation of the real situation at a time for the epidemiology of HIV in a country. For Switzerland, IV-drug addicts were found to be a risk population with high infection-rates, (Uchtenhagen A, 1988a; Uchtenhagen A & Fuchs W, 1989; Bauer G, Heusser R, Kerker M, 1990) at least as high as reported in other countries (e.g. Des Jarlais DC, 1989; Schoenbaum EE, Hartel D, Selwyn P, Klein RS, Davenny K, Rogers M, Feiner C, Friedland G, 1989). The probability to get infected, however, varies in groups of addicts.

That is why studies about risk taking behaviour are a second step (e.g. Des Jarlais DC & Friedman SR, 1988; McKeganey N, Barnard M, Watson H, 1989), showing, that especially non-clinic addicts still disclose a high risk of needle sharing "...there is a continuous tendency for individuals to be asked and to make their equipment available for others to use and to accomodate such requestes" and, additionally sexual transmission is a high risk, since "an overwhelming majority of the drug injectors who provided information on their sexual partners were involved with individuals who were not injecting drugs". Especially "males stated that they would never choose a drug injecting female partner". This is of concern since "there appears to be such a low level of condom use between the drug injectors interviewed in this study" (McKeganey N, Barnard M, Watson H, 1989, p 1486-1488). It seems, however, that behavioural change occurs and risk reduction among intravenious drug users has been reported since 1985 (Des Jarlais DC & Friedman SR, 1988). For an international comparison of risk-taking behavior or active prevention, interesting results can be expected from a multinational study, which is being performed.

It is a third step and a major interest, to find out, what the triggers of behavioural change are, how they happen and how they can be settled and established. As an overview and a research agenda - given by Kaplan HB, Johnson RJ, Bailey CA, Simon W (1987) - for HIV-infections show there are until now only few studies focusing on this sociological issue. We see our project localized at this very point of the third step and tried to fit our investigation concept accordingly (Zimmer Höfler D & Dobler-Mikola A, Uchtenhagen A, in work). The presented results in this paper focus on the background conditions and current social integration or desintegration on entering a therapeutic programme. The

---

[1]Project supported by grant 4026-026872 from the Swiss National Science Foundation

corresponding impact on attitudes toward HIV shall be evaluated by the ongoing project. The main questions here are, whether there are statistically significant differences between the HIV-seropositive and HIV-seronegative drug-addicts, especially, do HIV-seropositive and HIV-seronegative drug addicts differ in terms of :

(1) their structural and psychosocial ressources in childhood and youth?

(2) their current living conditions and their social network?

(3) parameters of deviant behavior and delinquency?

The results are, due to the complexity of the sample and the comprehensive data-basis, volumious. It would go far beyond our presentation to show them all. Therefore we have decided to highlight just some results here, indicating the mainline of our analysis.

2. SAMPLE UND METHODS

The presented results are based on preliminary analysis of basic-data from the first investigation of a prospective follow-up study performed by the researchgroup of the Socialpsychiatric Service of the Psychiatric University Hospital, Burghölzli, in Zürich, Switzerland. The project includes a second investigation and a special evaluation of the impact of HIV on individuals.

The basis is given in two roots: the first one is a follow-up study, concerning social integration of heroin-addicts in Switzerland which started in 1978. This study has been followed for three times since. A comparison with a normal Swiss cohort of the same age and other results are published or are still in print or in work (e.g. Zimmer-Höfler D, Uchtenhagen A, Christen St, 1984; Uchtenhagen A & Zimmer-Höfler D, 1985a; Uchtenhagen, A & Zimmer-Höfler D, 1985b; Zimmer-Höfler D, Dobler-Mikola A, Harte B, 1987; Dobler-Mikola A & Zimmer-Höfler D, 1989).

Secondly, an "Evaluative Research Association" of several therapeutic institutions (therapeutic communities and methadonprogrammes) and our research group have been conducting interviews with all indivuduals entering these institutions since 1985 (Zimmer Höfler & Uchtenhagen, 1990). Out of the pool of the interviewed individuals between 1985 and 1989 a sub-sample for the abovementioned project was selected. In the sampling, however, we have to take into consideration that we have to start off with a bigger sample and thus enable us to replace dead or lost individuals in our cohort for interviewing in order to have 200 final second interviews which would be a sufficient number of objects for complex statistical analysis.

In the first phase of our project we selected a sample of 250 subjects. The first interviews of this selected sample are databasis of the results presented here. Selection criteria for the sample were defined as follows:

- 125 HIV-seropositive clients at the time of first interview at intake in the therapeutic community or methadone programme.
- 125 HIV-seronegative clients at this time.
- There should be at least one third women in the whole cohort, also consisting of two comparable subgroups of HIV-seropositive and seronegative subjects.

3.RESULTS

3.1. Structural and Psychological Integration in Childhood and Youth

Occupational status of father, nationality of parents and educational level of the addicts themselves, are indicators of structural ressources. Comparing those indicators in these two described groups, we could not find significant differences.

Early pycho-social distress was defined by parameters such as: "divorce of parents", "addiction" or "psychological disorder of close relatives". In a first pilot-analysis of the differences between the seropositive and the seronegative subgroup we had results, indicating more difference than we could reproduce, when analyzing a larger sample in a broader time-span of intake in the institutions. The only thing that stayed was a slight tendency of mothers who were proned to have depressions and/or nervous breakdowns in the subgroup of HIV-seropositve individuals. The question is still open to discussion whether this finding out of individuals reports reflects the real situation or the perception of the indviduals, because biographic data are diffcult to validate. For our interpretation, thus, we stay on the conservative point of view and conclude, that there is no relevant association between the described and investigated early family-ressources and the later HIV-risk.

3.2. Current Integration

Our earlier studies, comparing drug addicts with non addicted controls (Uchtenhagen A & Zimmer-Höfler D, 1985a) show, that drug addicts are considerably less integrated in most aspects. We wonder, whether a similar difference could be found between HIV-seropositive heroin addicts and the HIV-seronegative group.

Looking at their housing accomodation (Fig. 1) we see, that the HIV-seropositve group is characterized by poorer housing. They are more often homeless or stay in rented single rooms. Their HIV-seronegative counterparts, on the contrary, more often live in their own appartements or with their parents.

276

Figure 1: Housing situation

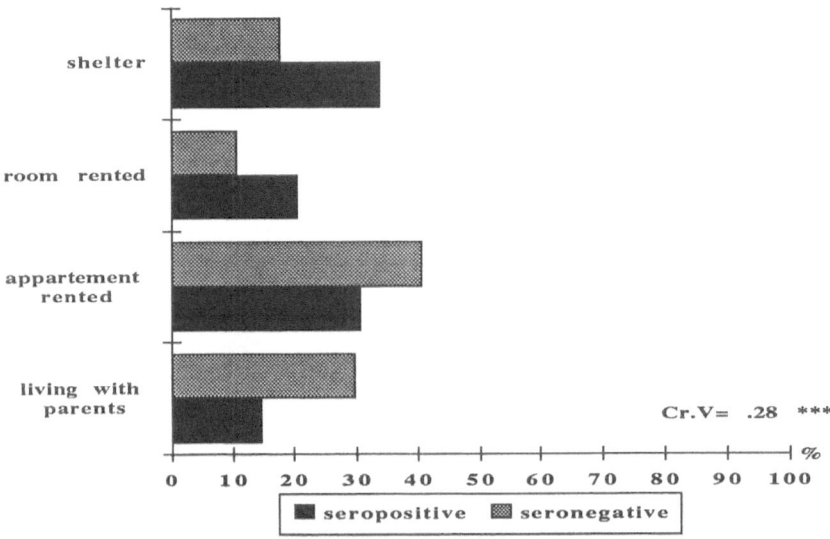

Regarding their job-performance, the HIV-seropositive group indicates again a lower degree of social integration. 44% in this group have not worked during the past twelve months and only 23% were working during more than half of that period (Fig. 2).

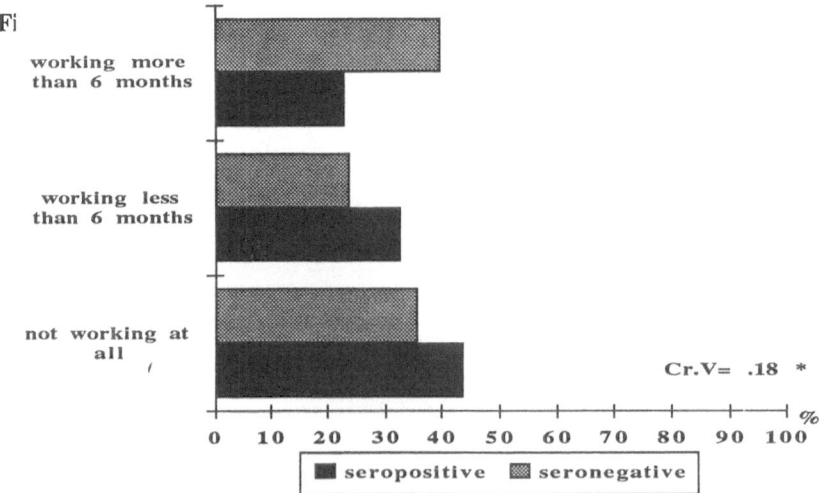

Accordingly the HIV-seronegative subjects supported themselves to a higher extend by their own income from a main job or were supported privately by their parents, whereas the seropositve group more often depended on social welfare (Fig. 3). Still it is interesting, to remark, that dealing with drugs occur as often in both groups.

Figure 3: Sources of income

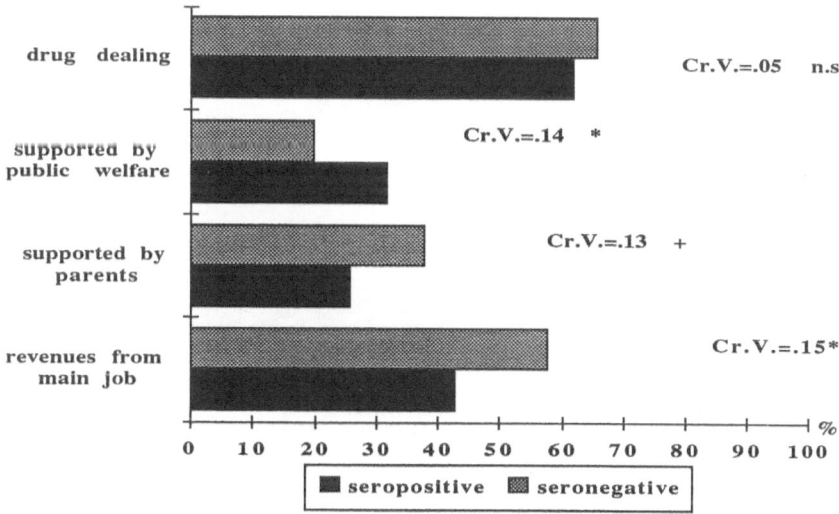

3.3. Integration in social networks

Regarding social integration within social networks we were interested to look at possible differences between the groups, concerning their possibilities to receive emotional support from their parents or friends. Figure 4 shows on the left the existence (if any) of parental contact and on the right the emotional quality of the contact respectively.

278

Figure 4: Parents: contact and emotional support

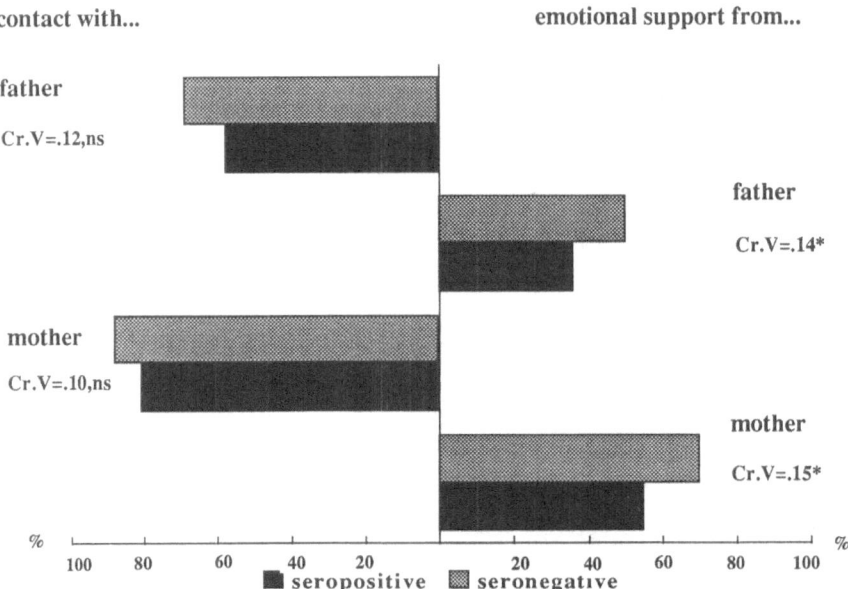

Contact with parents is equally common in both groups, and in both cases, slightly more with mothers. Significant differences, however, are found concerning the question if they also can speak about their problems with their parents. HIV-seropositive subjects have less emotional support from their parents in terms of having a possibility to speak with them about personal difficulties.

Concerning social support we were additionally interested, whether the compared groups differ in the number of reported friends or confidents they have outside of their families. Figure 5 shows the distribution of this issue in both groups.

Figure 5: Having close friends

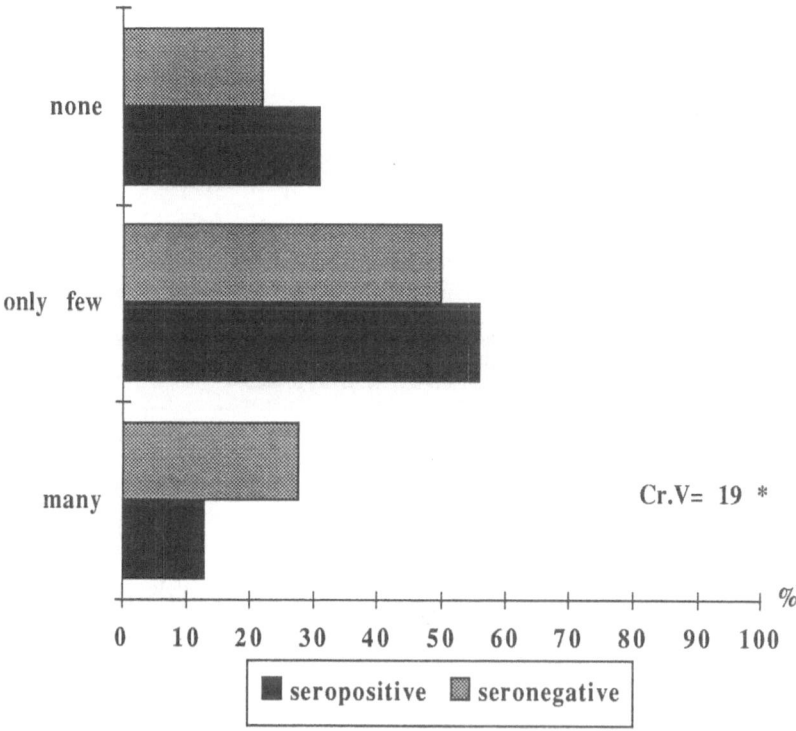

Again, the HIV-positive group is less supported also outside of their families, which means that they have less often close friends, or in other words they more often report having no close friends at all.

3.4. Delinquency and drug consumption

Additionally to the parameters of social integration and available social support, we looked at the social desintegration. Delinquency and drug consumption are the classical parameters for this.

Delinquency was measured for both groups by experiences with court, by experience with prison and, third, by the kind of delinquent behaviour, if committed. As we see in figure 6, significant differences can be identified: the HIV-positive group has been more often sentenced by court and also more often in prison.

Figure 6: Experiencies with court and prison

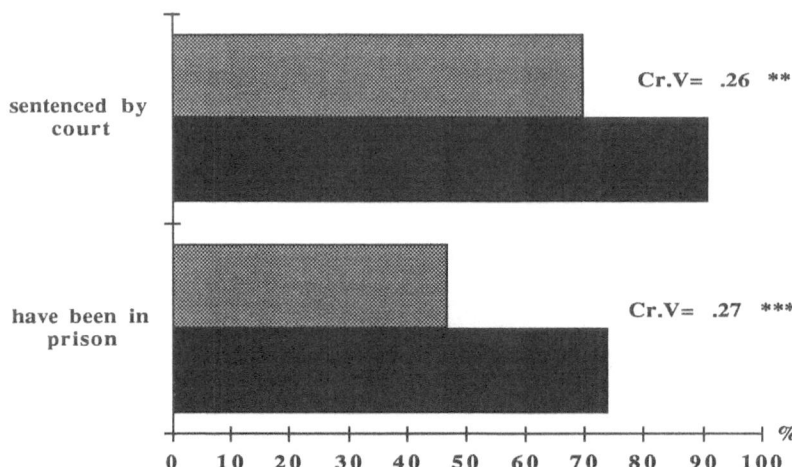

Regarding the kind of delinquent behaviour, we see, that all kinds of delinquent behaviour are more often committed by the seropositive group (Fig. 7). This means, the main difference is in quantity of all aspects of reported delinquency, not in their quality.

Figure 7: Kind of delinquent behavior

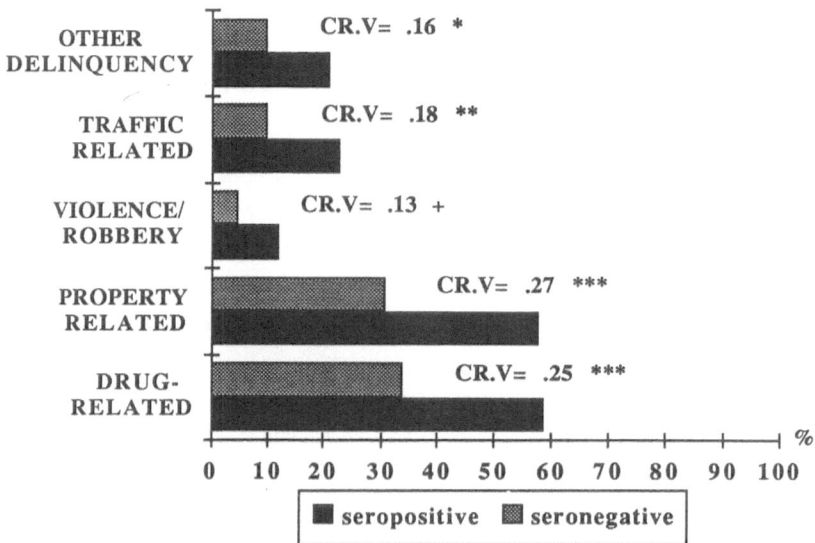

Finally we wanted to know, whether the two groups show different patterns of drug use. We looked especially at the self reported consumption of cannabis and heroin being the most popular drugs in the sample. Seropositive subjects disclose daily heroin-use within the last 12 months more than the seronegative group. Those, however, took more often cannabis within the same period (Fig. 8).

Figure 8: Consumption of cannabis and opiates

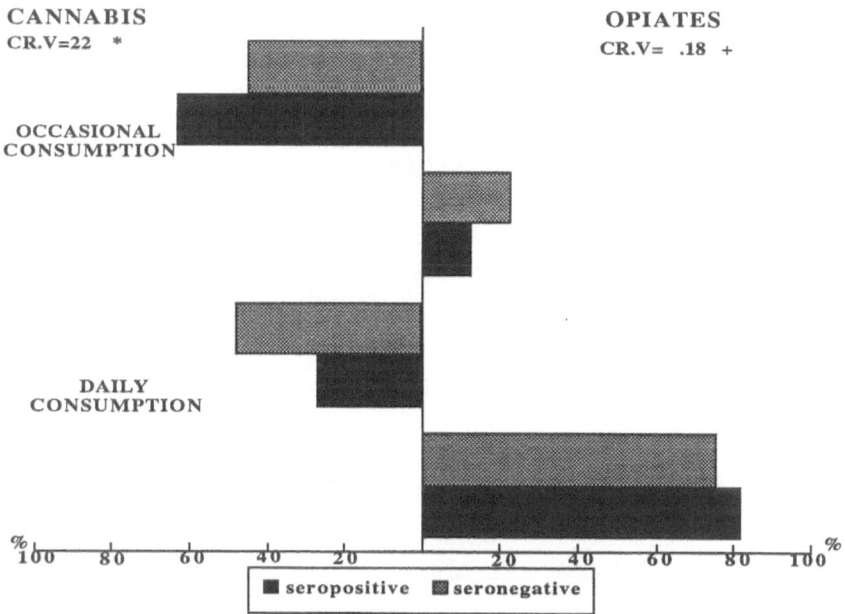

Looking at the way of application of drugs, we see on figure 9, that the seropositive group shows more often the special high-risk behaviour of drug addicts reporting more daily IV-drug use.

Figure 9: Frequency of IV-drug use

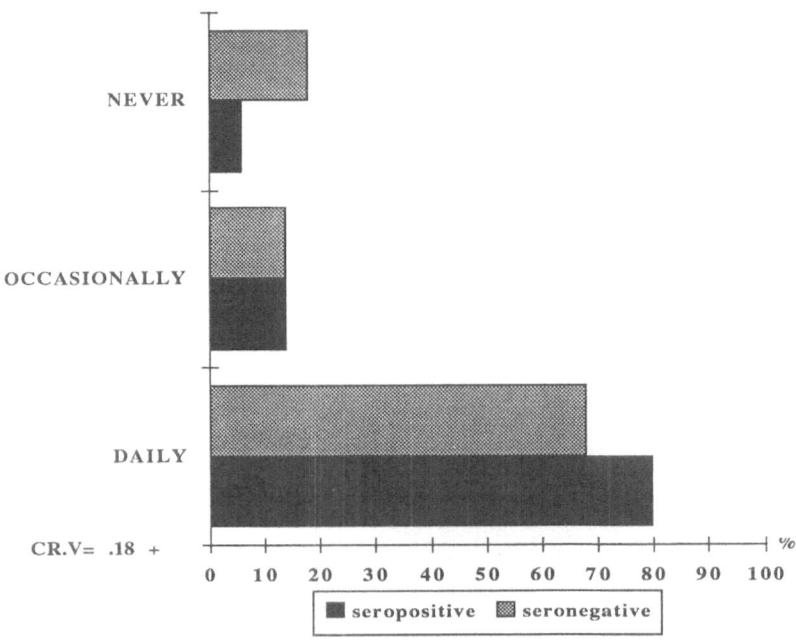

4. CONCLUSIONS AND FINAL REMARKS

There are different studies which show that the risk of acquiring HIV-infection seems to be a product of a complex interaction of drug-use and sexual behaviour, increasing seroprevalence over a time and ethnic background (Schoenbaum EE, Hartel D, Selwyn P, Klein RS, Davenny K, Rogers M, Feiner C, Friedland G, 1989, Des Jarlais DC & Friedman SR, 1988). Especially, members of social groups characterized by high social marginality and lack of material and immaterial ressources are proned to become HIV-seropositive. In this context it seems clear that the social milieu in which drugs are injected is an important predictor. Thus, we can hypothesize that HIV-positive drug-addicts are especially socially isolated and display many characteristics of social marginality, even more than drug-addicts on average. Our analysis of basic-data in a cohort of 250 heroin-addicts - half of which HIV-seropositive and half seronegative - concern the corresponding social mechanisms and follow the question whether or not both subgroups show significant differences in parameters of biographical and current social intergration. Looking for the association between HIV-risk and social integration, we were interested in whether HIV-seropositive drug-addicts disclose more characteristics of social desintegration and less social ressources - currently and in their social background - than their HIV-negative counterparts.

Based on corresponding results we can summarize:

1. Many drug-addicts show poor social integration and family distress in their childhood and youth (Uchtenhagen & Zimmer-Höfler, 1985a; Uchtenhagen & Zimmer-Höfler, 1985b). However, there is no relevant association between such kind of lack of early family ressources and the later HIV-risk.

2. Also in their current structural integration drug-addicts often show many deficiencies: they are often characterized by homelessness and lack of jobs (Zimmer-Höfler D, Dobler-Mikola A, Kaufmann B, in work). This fact seems to be especially true for the HIV-seropositive group of drug-addicts whereas their seronegative counterparts more often have their own accomodation and show a higher degree of job performance.

3. Criminalization of drug-addicts is often observed to be an important obstacle of successfull reintegration of drug-addicts (Uchtenhagen A, 1988b). Based on our results we can see that this kind of negative labelling even more pronounced in the group of HIV-positive drug-addicts: they are especially repeatedly in contact with the law. Looking at the patterns of typical delinquence-behavior, however, there are no differences between the two groups.

4. Drug consumption is generally associated with breakdown of social relationships to family and friends (Zimmer Höfler D, Uchtenhagen A, Christen St, 1983; Uchtenhagen & Zimmer, 1985a,b; Friedman SR, Des Jarlais DC, Sterk CE, 1990). Comparing the two groups in our analysis we see that also this aspect is especially pronounced among the HIV-seropositive subjects. They receive less emotional support from their parents and have less close friends.

5. An association between typical patterns of consumption-behavior and risk to get infec ted is observed by many studies (e.g. Des Jarlais DC & Friedman SR, 1988; Schoenbaum EE, Hartel D, Selwyn PA, Klein RS, Davenny K, Rogers M, Feiner C, Friedland G, 1989; Coleman RM, Curtis D, 1988). Our data confirm this fact: the seropositive subjects disclose daily IV-heroin abuse within the last 12 months more than the seronegative group. Those, however, took more cannabis within the same period.

Thus our data indicate that HIV-seropositive drug-addicts display many characteristics of social marginality, more than their HIV-seronegative counterparts and confirm the hypothesis that they are generally more marginalized than drug-addicts in average. This marginality, however, does not seem to be biographically determined. On the basis of our data we cannot say if the social marginality means a higher risk to become HIV-seropositve or on the contrary. Nevertheless, we assume here a mutual interaction of both factors. We hope to get more information about this process in the future analysis of our follow-up data we are collecting currently. Consequences for therapy would be that a broad variety of efforts for reintegration and support could be a help to stop a vicious circle of ongoing marginalization, enhancing in risktaking-behaviour. The earlier the demarginalization starts the better.

REFERENCES

Bauer G, Heusser R, Kerker M (1990) Epidemiologie von HIV und Aids in der Schweiz. HOSPITALIS 60, Nr. 7:405-410

Coleman RM, Curtis D (1988) Distribution of Risk Behaviour for HIV Infection Amongst Intravenous Drug Users. Br J Addict 83:1331-1334

Des Jarlais DC (1989) AIDS Prevention Programs for Intravenous Drug Users: diversity and evolution. Int Rev Psych 1:101-108

Des Jarlais DC, Friedman SR (1988) HIV and intravenous drug use. AIDS 2(suppl):65-6

Dobler-Mikola A, Zimmer Höfler D (1989) Zur spezifischen Situation drogenabhängiger Frauen. In: H. Jäger (Hrsg) Frauen und AIDS. Springer Verlag, Berlin, Heidelberg, New York:103-115

Friedland GH, Harris C, Butkus-Small C, Shine D, Darrow W, Klein R (1985) Intravenous Drug Abusers and the Acquired Immunodeficiency Syndrome (AIDS)
Arch Intern Med, Vol. 145:1413-1417

Friedman SR, Des Jarlais DC, Sterk CE (1990) AIDS and the Social Relations of Intravenous Drug Users. Milbank Mem Fund Q, Vol. 68, Suppl. 1:85-110

Kaplan HB, Johnson RJ, Bailey CA, Simon W (1987) The Sociological Study of AIDS: A Critical Review of the Literature and Suggested Research Agenda.J Health and Soc Behav, Vol. 28 (June):140-15

McKeganey N, Barnard M, Watson H (1989) HIV-related Risk Behaviour Among a Non-clinic Sample of Injecting Drug Users. Br J Addict, 84:1481-1490

Robertson JR, Skidmore C, Roberts M (1988) HIV-Infection in Intravenous Drug Users: a follow-up study indicating changes in risk-taking behaviour. Br J Addict, 83:387-391

Schoenbaum EE, Hartel D, Selwyn PA, Klein RS, Davenny K, Rogers M, Feiner C, Friedland G (1989) Risk factors for human immunodeficiency virus infection in intravenous drug users. N Engl J Med, No. 13, Vol. 321:874-879

Uchtenhagen A (1988a) AIDS-Epidemiolgie und Prävention bei I.V.-Drogenabhängigen. Sondernummer Epidemiologie und Prävention von AIDS. Soz Praventivmed, 7, Vol. 33:326-330

Uchtenhagen A (1988b) Zum Delinquenzverlauf bei Drogenabhängigen.
In: Jugend und Delinquenz. Schweizerische Arbeitsgruppe für Kriminologie, Reihe Kriminologie Band 3:337-369

Uchtenhagen A, Fuchs W (1989) Drogenabhängigkeit und AIDS. In: H. Jäger (Hrsg) AIDS und HIV-Infektion. ecomed Verlagsgesellschaft mbH, Landsberg, VIII/2.1:1-10

Uchtenhagen A, Zimmer Höfler D (1985a) Heroinabhängige und ihre "normalen" Altersgenossen. Verlag Paul Haupt Bern und Stuttgart

Uchtenhagen A, Zimmer Höfler D (1985b) Psychosocial Development Following Therapeuticand Legal Interventions in Opiate Dependence. A Swiss National Study. Eur J Psychol Educa, Vol. II, 4:443-458

Zimmer Höfler D, Dobler-Mikola A, Harte B (1987) Berufliche Idealvorstellungen Heroinabhängiger und langfristige Integration. In: D. Ladewig (Hrgs) Drogen und Alkohol. ISPA-Press, Lausanne:64-83

Zimmer Höfler D, Dobler-Mikola A, Kaufmann B (in work) Trendtendenzen aus der Drogenszene.

Zimmer Höfler D, Dobler-Mikola A, Uchtenhagen A (in work) Psychosoziale Aspekte der HIV-Infektion und AIDS-Erkrankung bei Heroinabhängigen (1) Erster Bericht an den Schweizerischen Nationalfonds

Zimmer Höfler D, Uchtenhagen A (1990) Forschen nach Mass. Die Verbundforschung therapeutischer Einrichtungen. Die Kette, Nr. 4:26-28

Zimmer Höfler D, Uchtenhagen A, Christen St (1983) The Familiy Situation of Addicts and non Addicts. Proc 7th World Conf Ther Communities, Chicago, May 8-13

Zimmer Höfler D, Uchtenhagen A, Christen St. (1984) From Exclusion to Integration Proc 8th World Conf Therapeutic Communities, Rome, Vol. 2:241-248

Assessment of the Work with Pregnant IV Drug Users in Oslo

B. NILSEN and G. WELLE-STRAND

Municipal Outreach Program, Hegdehaugen, N-0354 Oslo 3, Norway

The Municipal Outreach Program in Oslo is concerned with street work among drifting youth involved with drug addiction. 1000 different youths are in contact with us every year. The mean age of the youngsters are 22 years. The medical service has about 200 different patients every year. 15% of the patients are HIV-positive.

Our objective is to act as an intermediary between the individual in need and necessary resources to meet these needs. During the last 5-6 years the municipal outreach program has had an increased involvement with pregnant IVDU's. Ullevaal hospital in Oslo has a special team to coordinate and advice the municipal work with pregnant drug and alcohol users. In 1990 they reported 61 cases. Of the 38 babies born in 1990, only 11 were kept in custody with their parents shortly after birth. A lot of the women we are in contact with have given birth to children they have lost custody for immediately after birth or after a longer periode.

In Norway there is a common opinion that responsibility for children are incompatible with the abuse of drugs or alcohol. But for a lot of drug abusing women becomming a mother serves as the only visible opportunity to be able to live drug free and "normal".

OBJECTIVES

The objectives of this study is to assess our own work with pregnant drug abusers, and to find out how the situation for the

CASES

Eva

She was about 28 years old when confirmed pregnant during a stay at an acute ward for drug abusers. She had been a heavy intravenous drug addict for several years, mostly heroin. This was also the case for the childs father. Eva is HIV-positive, and was extremely suspicious towards the welfare system and the different service institutions. She would not allow any discussion of her HIV-status, and would not conduct herself to this fact.

Eva was referred to the Ullevaal-team, but due to her suspicion and lack of cooperation with the child care unit it was difficult to come up with any constructive action. During pregnancy she abused drugs. The father of the child died from an overdose of heroin shortly before birth. Due to his death there was a justified fear for an overdose on behalf of Eva.

After birth Eva lost custody of the child immediately. Because of her situation as HIV-positive she was given an opportunity to regain custody if she would refer herself to an institution. She was admitted to an institution and stayed there for 1 1/2 years, and was reported to be well-functioning. Shortly after her baby was 2 years old it was confirmed that he was HIV-negative. Eva was at this point moving out of the institution to an appartment in Oslo. It became too hard for her to stay away from drugs. She lost custody for her child and are now reported as continuously drug abusing.

Marit

Marit was about 26 years old when coincidently confirmed pregnant when she was 23 weeks pregnant. She was a heavy drug addict engaged in contiuous prostitution at the time. Her case was immediately referred to the Ullevaal team and she was admitted to an acute ward for drug abusers for detoxification and assessment. Directly referred to an institution for drug abusers. She is still connected to this institution and is reported well-functioning. The child care unit is following her case closely and in cooperation with the institution. Marit has been at a central child care institution in order to assess her caretaking abilities. The child is now about one years old.

Sissel

Sissel was about 20 years old when pregnant for the first time. Her drug abuse was reported to be alcohol and cannabis. Only a short and supposed terminated intravenous drug abuse. She had a job and her own apartment. She agreed to a reference to the babies and the mothers are after a follow-up period from 6 months to 2 years after birth.

Our aim with this work is either to influence on the possibility for the parents to master the responsibility for the child, or to prepare the parents for loss of custody of the child. Both of these objectives need equal involvement and resources in order to give a decent result. Accordingly we concider other alternatives than continuing the pregnancy, Abortion is always discussed. We also inform about the child care services and how they will work with these cases. These issues are especially difficult when the woman is HIV-positive, because the discussion must include the possible sickness and a possible death for both the mother and the becomming child.

METHOD

We have made a follow-up study of 7 pregnant drug abusers. Three of these will be presented as case-material in this presentation.

RESULTS

The average age of the 7 mothers at the time of birth was 23 years. 4 were less than 20 years old when found pregnant. 6 of the 7 mothers were intravenous drug users at the time of confirmation of pregnancy. Duration of drug abuse varied from 2 months up to ten years of heavy IV drug abuse. One of the 7 women were HIV-positive. 4 out of 7 have been engaged in prostitution. 3 out of 7 women did not have a steady partner at time of birth. 2 out of 4 had a drug abusing partner.

4 out of 7 women were institutionalized after birth; 2 of these in special institutions for drug abusers. 3 out of 7 still have custody for their child. One lost custody of the child at birth, and two lost custody because of drug abuse before the baby was 6 months old. One lost custody after 2 years. In addition one of the 7 mothers have now been informed that she will loose custody for her one year old child in june 1991. 2 out of the 7 women are now pregnant with their second child; one of these lost custody of the first born child.

1 of the 7 women were confirmed pregnant at 6 months pregnancy, for the 6 others pregnancy was confirmed after 2-3 months.

Ullevaal team. Everything seemed to be working very fine, and Sissel appeared to be motivated and with no intake of any drugs. But her urine-screening gave positive test-results conserning several drugs. Confronted with this Sissel denied convincingly any use of drugs. After this Sissel dropped out from her appointments. At birth she lost custody of her child.

Approximately 3 months after this Sissel was again pregnant. This time she would not agree to be referred to the Ullevaal-team, and she would not keep in contact with our program. She was referred to the Ullevaal-team by her social welfare officer. The same story repeated itself with positive urine-screening and denial of any drug intake. After 6 months pregnancy she has now admitted drug abuse as shown by the urine-screening. She is now at an institution for drug abusers hoping to be able to keep her next child.

DISCUSSION

Among drug abusing women contraception is rarely used because many believe that they can not become pregnant. Drug abuse gives a certain reduced fertility as long as the drug abuse continues. These women often come for a test to disconfirm pregnancy. Many of them have longer periods whithout regular menstruation. Concerning abortion it is our experience that if we persuade a woman for an abortion there is a greater chance for a new pregnancy shortly afterwards. The same is true with women who looses custody of the child and denies any drug abuse or any resposibility for this failure at all. It is important not to force any solution on the couples, but work through a realistic judgement on their behalf.

We find it important that even though the mothers will loose custody they need to receive proper handling. Most women experience the loss of custody as a bereavement they need a lot of time to overcome. Years of grief over the lost child is our experience, even though the mother can admit that she was not fully able to handle the responsibility. Combining the efforts to help mothers keeping their child, with the work with mothers who will loose their child may give us important competence in dealing with the total problem. A mother who has lost her child will naturally seek a substitution in a new child. This is something we must take serious and seek to prevent.

CONCLUSION

Pregnancy and becomming a family may in some cases serve as a motivational factor for rehabilitation from drug abuse. Unfortunately this is seldom the case. Even though some women stop taking drugs in a period during pregnancy and early motherhood, we often meet a serious relapse problem which often ends up with a loss of custody. The situation is even more difficult when the mother is HIV-positive; vulnerable periods seem to be when the serostatus of the child is finally confirmed and when the health of the mother is detoriating.

There are a considerable distrust among pregnant IVDU's towards the social service and child care system. Due to a lack of competence and resources the child care system in Oslo works unsystematically and with a great variance depending on the area of town. Also there is a variation in the recognition of the special needs for pregnant IVDU's. There seems to be a general view that the children should be taken from the mothers at once regardless of her need for help.

Pregnancy is an important period for assessing the mother's (and parent's) caretaking abilities and deciding on what kind of support and control the new family will require. Firm control and support is needed for many years when handling pregnant women with a drug problem.

Required action conserning pregnant IVDU's:
1. Immediate intervention strategies and establishing routines for cooperation with the becomming parents.
2. Anamnestic interview and analysis of complete life situation.
3. Establish committing cooperation with different institutions and services, especially with the child care system.
4. Longterm follow-up period (more than two years) based on diagnostic asessment linked with the needs of parents and child.
5. Sentralization of the assessment and treatment of pregnant IVDU's to ensure equal treatment and develop competence.

Treatment of Heroin Abuse and AIDS in Italy

D. Serraino

Epidemiology Unit, Aviano Cancer Centre, I-33081 Aviano, Pordenone, Italy

Introduction

The number of AIDS cases associated with intravenous drug use is substantial in most countries (32% of all cases in Western Europe) (European Centre For The Epidemiological Monitoring Of AIDS, 1990), but the problem is especially serious in Italy, which has one of the highest proportion in the world of cases due to the illicit use of intravenous drugs. As of December, 1990, 8,227 AIDS cases were registered in Italy: 5,424 (66%) occurred among intravenous drug users (IVDUs) (Ministero della Sanità, 1991). Furthermore, 281 out of 514 cases (55%) among Italian heterosexuals were partners of IVDUs and 115 out of 204 (56%) children with AIDS were born from IVDU mothers infected with HIV (Ministero della Sanità, 1991). As a consequence of AIDS, in less than ten years hundreds of studies have focused on drug-using habits, leading to a close identification of the main modes of HIV transmission. Reducing the sharing of injection equipment has been thus recognized as the primary objective of any effort aimed at limiting the diffusion of HIV among IVDUs, and, indirectly, to prevent the further spread of HIV among their sexual partners (for a review, see Des Jarlais and Friedman, 1988). Although there is still debate as to what methods of service provision are most likely to fulfill the prevention objective, drug clinics should be considered an optimal place for integrating the prevention and control of both drug use and HIV transmission. The purpose of this paper is to describe temporal patterns and the geographic distribution of public and private drug clinics in Italy, from the beginning of the AIDS epidemic through 1989.

Methods

Since 1984, the Drug Abuse Surveillance Program of the Italian Ministry of Home Affairs has published quarterly data regarding public drug clinics (PDCs) and private residential therapeutic communities (PRTCs); the number of drug addicts in treatment and the proportion of them in substitution therapy - mainly methadone maintenance programmes (MMPs) (Ministero dell'Interno, 1985-1990). Such information is mandatorily reported by health authorities to the Ministry of Home Affairs every three months (March, 15; June, 15; September, 15 and December, 15), thus ensuring a good completness of the data. To limit a potential bias due to seasonal variability in the frequency of drug clinic attendance, data herein presented are from the December survey of each year.

Comparisons among different geographic areas were made using rates per 100,000 population aged between 15 and 44 years (Istituto Centrale di Statistica, 1986). For the purposes of this study, Italy was divided into five broad geographic areas, according to the criteria of the Ministry of Home Affairs and to the cumulative incidence of AIDS - i.e. Nortwest, Northeast, Central, South and Sardinia.

Results

Four hundred and thirty six public drug clinics (1.8 clinics for 100,000 population) were available in Italy for IVDUs seeking treatment as of December, 1984, - when the first cases of AIDS among IVDUs occurred (Table 1).

Table 1. Distribution of public drug clinics and private residential therapeutic communities, by geographic area. Italy, 1984-1989.

Area	1984		1985	1986	1987	1988	1989		Difference *
	#	( )**	#	#	#	#	#	( )**	%
Public drug clinics:									
Northwest	154	(2.4)	172	175	178	181	181	(2.8)	+ 15
Northeast	91	(2.1)	91	93	94	96	97	(2.2)	+ 7
Central	105	(2.3)	107	110	109	109	112	(2.4)	+ 7
South	81	(1.0)	80	85	87	99	120	(1.5)	+ 48
Sardinia	5	(0.7)	5	5	5	5	5	(0.7)	0
Italy	436	(1.8)	455	468	473	490	515	(2.1)	+ 18
Private residential therapeutic communities:									
Northwest	103	(1.6)	133	136	135	142	164	(2.5)	+ 59
Northeast	51	(1.2)	74	79	85	84	93	(2.2)	+ 82
Central	47	(1.0)	53	59	60	58	72	(1.5)	+ 53
South	17	(0.2)	36	45	56	59	78	(0.9)	+359
Sardinia	4	(0.6)	5	5	6	7	8	(1.2)	+100
Italy	222	(0.9)	301	324	342	350	415	(1.7)	+ 87

*: Relative difference, computed as ((1989-1984)/1984)*100.
**: Number of public drug clinics or private residential therapeutic communities per 100,000 population.

Most of the clinics (56%) were located in Northern Italy, in particular in the Northwest, with a rate that was more than twice that reported in the South, and four times higher than in Sardinia (Table 1). From 1984 to 1989, there was a 18% increase in the number of PDCs, with the highest relative increase seen in Southern Italy (+48%). On a population basis, however, in the North there was still a higher offer of PDCs than in the rest of the country. A similar picture emerged as regards the PRTCs. All over the study period, there was a clear north-south gradient, both in the absolute number of PRTCs and in the number of PRTCs per 100,000 population, with the highest increase seen in Southern Italy (Table 1).
  The number of IVDUs seeking treatment in PDCs steadily increased after the beginning of the AIDS epidemic, in particular from 1986 onwards "Fig. 1". As of Decembre, 1984, 20,847 IVDUs were in treatment in PDCs, 87 per 100,000 population. The rates of IVDUs in treatment increased more markedly in the areas most involved by the AIDS epidemic, and the ranks across areas for AIDS incidence and those for IVDUs in treatment were the same in 1989 (not shown). In absolute terms, 33,904 IVDUs were assisted for heroin addiction as of Decembre, 1989, a 63% relative increase, as compared with 1984.

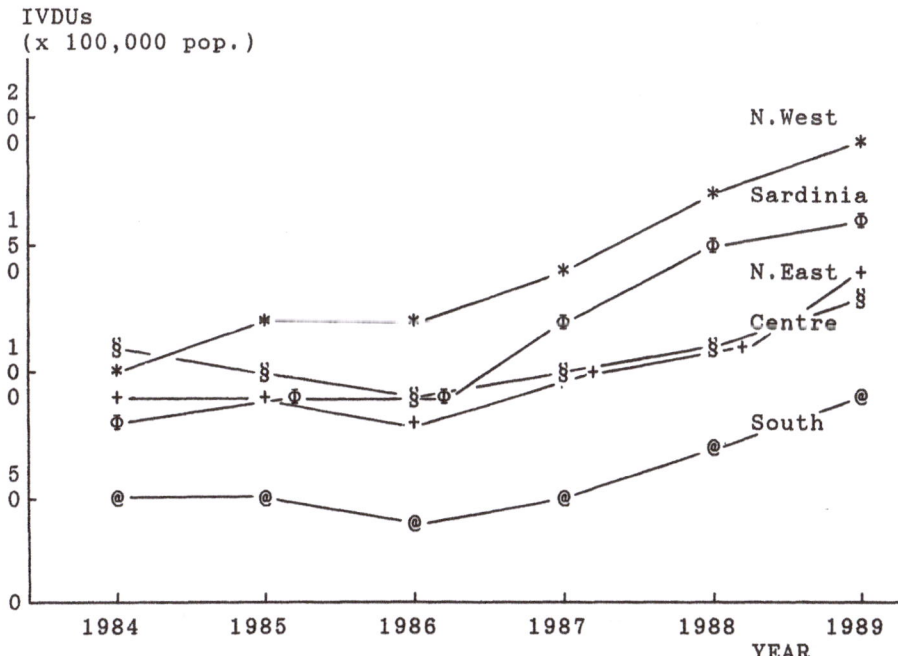

Figure 1. Intravenous drug users attending public drug clinics, per 100,000 population, by geographic area.

The proportion of IVDUs who were enrolled in MMPs is illustrated in "Fig. 2". Apart Sardinia, where almost all

IVDUs in PDCs were always treated with MMPs, a clear
downward trend in the use of such programmes emerged. In
1984, 59% of Italian IVDUs seeking treatment were enrolled
in MMPs: this percentage decreased to 38% in 1989 (test for
trend: p<0.001). The decreasing use of substitution therapy
was more pronounced in Northern regions, with nearly 25% of
IVDUs enrolled in such treatment, than in the rest of the
Country "Fig. 2".

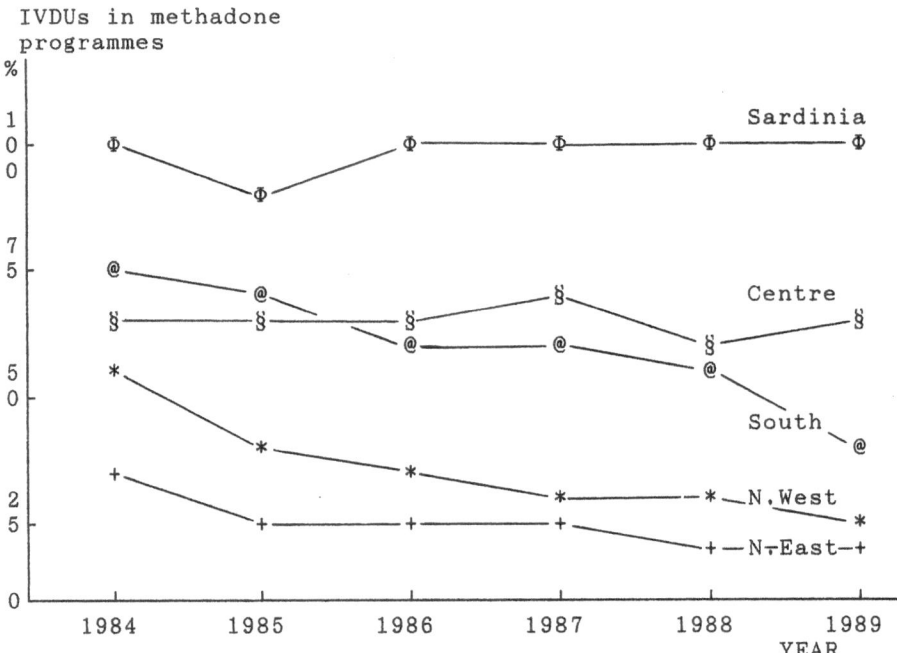

Figure 2. Percent of IVDUs enrolled in methadone
programmes, by geographic area. Italy, 1984-1989.

Discussion

There is little epidemiologic information on the
population of drug addicts in Italy. It is estimated that
between 250,000 and 300,000 persons are regular users of
illicit drugs, mostly living in the Northern part of the
Country (Ministero dell'Interno, 1984). Based on data
deriving from heroin over-dose deaths, men are estimated to
account for nearly 75% of the drug addict population, and
heroin is the drug mostly abused (Ministero dell'Interno,
1985-1990). Although geographic variations in drug using
habits should taken into account (Serraino, 1991; Titti,
1987), such figures are substantially in agreement with the
epidemiology of AIDS and HIV infection in Italy. A clear
North-South geographic gradient exists, both for the number
of AIDS cases (Ministero della Sanità, 1991) and for HIV
seroprevalence rates (Greco, 1988). Approximately 70% of the

cases were registered in the Northern regions, in particular
in the Milan metropolitan area (Ministero della Sanità,
1991), which also showed the highest rates of HIV
seroprevalence among IVDUs (Greco, 1988; Titti, 1987). A
noteworthy exception to such geographic gradient is
represented by Sardinia, where the prevalence of HIV
infection among IVDUs is similar to that reported in the
Northern urban areas (Panichi, 1990).

Although the percentage of Italian IVDUs seeking treatment
seems to be very low (10-15%), the data presented in this
paper show an increased treatment demand as a response of
IVDUs to the AIDS epidemic, in particular in the areas most
affected by AIDS. This finding is in contrast with the
common stereotype of drug-addicts as self-destructive
individuals, unwilling to change risky behaviours that may
treaten their life, and it has positive implications for the
control and the prevention of AIDS in Italy. The AIDS
epidemic, however, does not seem to have influenced the
quantity and the geographic distribution of services in
Italy, although the available information did not allow a
thorough assessment of such topic.

In Sardinia, while the average number of IVDUs per clinic
was constantly and steadily increasing (up to 240 IVDUs per
clinic in 1989), only five PDCs were available to IVDUs from
1984 to 1989. The paucity of therapeutical provisions in
this area is still more alarming when HIV prevalence data
are considered. Despite of its geographic location, 2,314
out of 4,672 (49%) IVDUs tested in Sardinia between 1983 and
1988 were seropositive for HIV antibody (Panichi, 1990).
In South Italy, the lack of public health services for drug
addicts seemed to have been partially counterbalanced by an
increased number of PRTCs. However, because of their
organization, and apart from some very large communities,
the PRTCs can offer hospitality to a limited number of
IVDUs, and, moreover, great variability exists as regards
their rehabilitation objectives and methods.

Among the findings of the study, it is worth noting the
substantial decline in the use of MMPs which emerged in
Italy since the beginning of the AIDS epidemic. This is in
sharp contrast with the evidence showing that many IVDUs
stop injecting drugs when adequate doses of methadone are
given, and which suggests that MMPs may have a critical
role to play in controlling the spread of AIDS (Cooper,
1989). Moreover, such treatment modality has demonstrated
its ability to retain a great proportion of patients in
treatment for a long period of time, especially during
the initial part of treatment (Senay, 1985), which is
critical to the AIDS public health issue. In The
Netherlands and in other North-European countries, a wide
use of MMPs and a well-structured health facilities for drug
addicts have been implemented well before the AIDS epidemic
(Blix, 1988; Hoek, 1989), and, in such Countries, less than
10% of AIDS cases have been registered among IVDUs.
Notwithstanding the positive data, in Italy the general
opinion remains negative about MMPs, even if a large-scale
AIDS prevention programme is far to be implemented.

In conclusion, the data herein presented seems to suggest that the use of public and private drug clinics by IVDUS increased after AIDS, although it is not possibile from the available information to state whether such increase is totally demand driven. Such finding has important positive implications for the control of HIV spread in Italy and it stresses the urgent need for a global intervention programme, aimed at integrating the treatment of heroin addiction with the prevention and control of HIV spread.

This work was supported by a grant from the Italian Ministry of Health - Istituto Superiore di Sanità, Progetto AIDS 1989-90, Sottoprogetto Epidemiologia 420/05/03 - Rome, Italy.

References

Blix O, Gronbladh L (1988). AIDS and IV heroin addicts: the preventive effort of methadone maintenance in Sweden. Fourth International Conference on AIDS, June 1988, Stockolm, Sweden, Abstract No. 8548.

Cooper JR (1989). Methadone treatmnet and acquired immunodeficiency syndrome. JAMA 262:1664-1668.

Des Jarlais DC, Friedman SR (1988). HIV and intravenous drug use. AIDS 2 (suppl 1): S65-S69.

European Centre for the Epidemiological Monitoring of AIDS (1991). AIDS Surveillance in Europe, Quarterly Report No. 28. Paris, France.

Greco D, Luzi S (1988). L'infezione da HIV-1 in Italia al 31 agosto 1988. Epidemiologia e Prevenzione 37:26-31.

Hoek JAR van den, Haastrecht HJA van, Coutinho RA (1989). Risk reduction among intravenous drug users in Amsterdam under the influence of AIDS. Am J Public Health 79:1355-1357.

Istituto Centrale di Statistica (1986). Annuario statistico Italiano: popolazione residente al 12° censimento generale. Rome, Italy.

Ministero della Sanità (1991). Istituto Superiore di Sanità. Aggiornamento dei casi di AIDS conclamato notificati in Italia al 31 Dicembre 1990. Rome, Italy.

Ministero dell'Interno (1984). Diffusione delle Tossicodipendenze. Quantità e qualità degli interventi pubblici e privati in Italia. Rome, Italy.

Ministero dell'Interno (various issues, 1985-1990): "Osservatorio permanente sul fenomemo droga". Rome, Italy.

Panichi G, Babudieri S, Manconi PE, and HIV Sardinia Group (1990). Epidemiology of HIV-1 infection in the island of Sardinia. (Letter). AIDS 4:167-170.

Senay EC (1985). Methadone maintenance treatment. Int J Addict 20:803-821.

Serraino D, Franceschi S, Vaccher E et al (1991). Risk factors for human immunodeficiency virus infection in 581 intravenous drug users, Northeast Italy, from 1984 to 1989. International Journal of Epidemiology, in press.

Titti F, Lazzarin A, Costigliola P (1987). Possibile storia naturale dell'infezione da HIV in tossicodipendenti in Italia. In: Ministero della Sanità, Istituto Superiore di Sanità: AIDS e Sindromi Correlate, Rome, Italy.

Neuropsychiatric Problems and Psychotropic Medication in Patients with AIDS. Data from Warsaw

T. Nasierowski[1], H. Matsumoto[1], E. Kamińska-Kopicz[2], and L. Babiuch[2]

[1] Warsaw Medical Academy, Department of Psychiatry
[2] AIDS Hospital Department, Warsaw, Poland

AIDS in Poland

If we accept that the beginning of the history of AIDS in Poland was the first observed case in USA citizen of Polish extraction, than we may state that AIDS appeared in this country in 1986, that is 5 years after observation of the first case in the world [8]. One might think that we had received as a gift 5 years for preparing ourselves for the advent of HIV pandemia. However, were this true we should have been exceptionally reasonable and well-off population, and most of us, or at least the medical professionals should overcome all fears and aversion appearing in contact with HIV carriers and with AIDS patients. On the other hand, if the beginning of the history of AIDS in Poland is the time when blood tests have been introduced in 1985 [7], then the difference between our country and the West European states appears as only quantitative, that is economic-organizational. We must admit that as yet we have not evolved efficient organization of AIDS control, and have not prepared the population for the contact with this disease. An evident example of this situation is the lack of sufficient number of outpatient clinics for HIV carriers and AIDS patients (only one of such clinic is presently available), although we have 9 hospital departments for these patients.

An additional difficulty is the fact that the main risk group in Poland are intravenous drug abusers (IV DAs) who are not accepted by the people because of addiction. The first case of HIV seropositivity in drug addict was recorded in Poland only in 1988 [8], but to the end of January 1991 since the beginning of blood tests, 1488 HIV carriers were found in Poland, and 1065 (72%) of them were IV DAs. Among 51 cases of AIDS recorded in Poland since 1986 there were 11 cases of IV DAs (21%), 34 homosexuals (67%) and 6 (12%) heterosexuals [9].

Data on HIV seropositive patients admitted to AIDS
Hospital Department, Warsaw Medical Academy, in 1990

Material of this study consists of data collected during treatment of HIV infected patients
admitted to AIDS Hospital Department in Warsaw in 1990. The department was founded in May
1990 as a part of the Department of Hepathology which in 1988 was separated and destined for
AIDS patients. This was the first, and for nearly 2 years, the only hospital department in Poland,
where these patients were treated.

Already in the first patient with AIDS, treated in the department in February 1987, psychic
disturbances appeared. The ever increasing number of admissions of these patients and the growing
need for psychiatric interventions caused that the psychiatrist was in 1989 employed as a part of staff.

In 1990 the department admitted 89 HIV seropositive patients whose characteristics are shown
in Fig.1 and Fig.2.

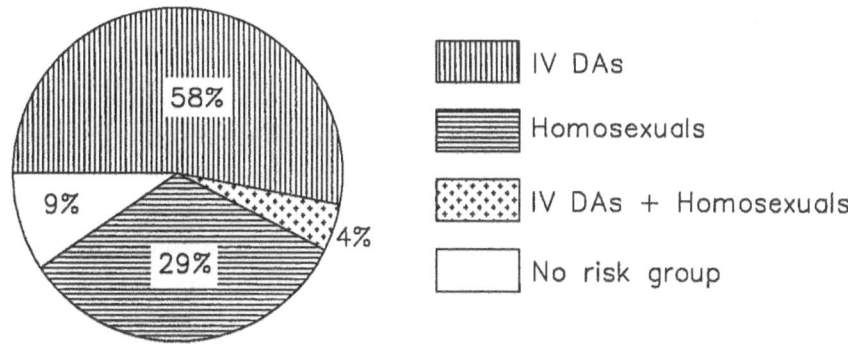

Fig. 1 Risk groups among HIV seropositives

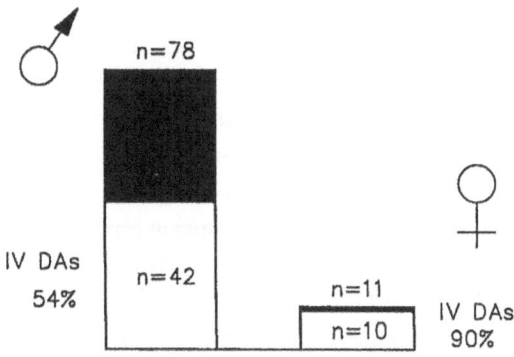

Fig. 2 IV DAs among HIV+ male and female patients

Neuropsychiatric disorder in patients with fully developed AIDS. Case reports.

In six of 12 patients with AIDS diagnosis (50%) neuropsychiatric disorders were stated: depressive syndromes, dementia syndromes with severe neurological symptoms and delirium syndromes (Fig.3).

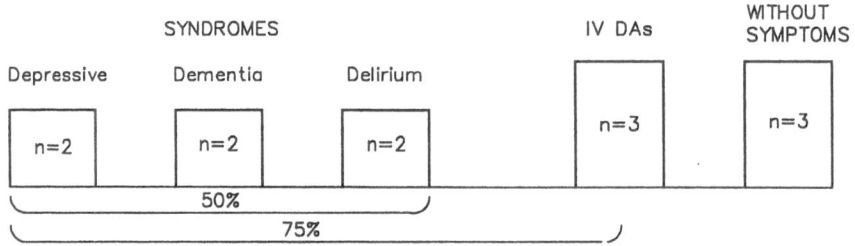

Fig. 3 Spectrum of neuropsychiatric diagnoses in AIDS patients

1. Depressive syndromes

1.1. Male patient W.O., aged 51, bisexual, with the history of HIV infection acquired in 1982, with paranoid personality features before the disease, was admitted to hospital with deterioration of physical status and increasing symptoms of depressive syndrome. Worsening of the mental state was noted at the time when he lost his job. In the hospital the patient showed profound mood depression, psychomotor sluggishness, sleep disorders, depressive delusions of hypochondrial type. He was treated initially with Sinequan in doses up to 200 mg daily, without detectable effect. Then he was changed over to Azaphen 100 mg daily and Chlorprotixen 50 mg daily with good result. His emotional status improved greatly, but his physical condition deteriorated steadily till death. He was not treated with AZT because he had gastrointestinal bleeding. Three weeks before his death the T_4/T_8 ratio was 0.49 and the T_4 count was 46/mm^3. On autopsy miliary tuberculosis of haematogenous origin was found (not recognized during his life) and adrenal atrophy.

1.2. Male patient T.G., aged 59 years, homosexual, with HIV infection diagnosed in 1986, was admitted to hospital with poor physical condition and increasing sleep disorders. In childhood he had received psychiatric treatment for anxiety neurosis. Before admission to hospital he received Sinequan and hypnotics. During his stay in hospital mood depression kept progressing, with tearfulness, despondency, guilt and sin feeling (the patient was a clergyman). Anxiety increased, sleep disturbances were refractory to treatment, slowness of psychomotor functions progressed. The patient became ever secluded, became mutistic, periodically refused taking of all drugs. Initially he was treated with Azaphen (up to 100 mg daily), and then with Sinequan, without effect. At times he was given benzodiazepines (diazepam, alprazolam, clorazepate). No improvement of his depression was obtained. Several days prior to his death the T_4/T_8 ratio dropped to 0.18 and leucocyte count was 600/mm^3. During about one year the patient received AZT 600 mg daily.

2. Dementia with associated neurological changes

2.1. Male patient A.C., aged 48, homosexual, with antibodies to HIV demonstrated in 1987, was admitted to hospital with recurrence of Pneumocystis carinii infection and initial symptoms of dementia. During 6 weeks of hospital stay mental deterioration progressed, with difficulties in orientation in time, attention concentration, memory loss and loss of ability of logical thinking. At the end of his stay confabulations appeared. Prior to discharge the T_4/T_8 ratio was 0.40 and the T_4 count was 120/mm^3. After about one month the patient was readmitted with severe dementia. Neurological examination demonstrated signs of cerebellar syndrome. After several days a meningeal syndrome developed with paresis of three extremities (both lower extremities and right upper extremity). Cerebrospinal fluid examination showed presence of Toxoplasma gondii, cytomegalovirus and herpes virus. The protein level was 110 mg/100 ml, and cell count was 2. CT demonstrated a small focus in the left cerebellar hemisphere. After 2 weeks the patient died. Autopsy demonstrated pulmonary artery inbolism. During both hospital stay the patient received no AZT or psychotropic agents.

2.2. Male patient R.Z., aged 25 years, homosexual, had presence of HIV antibodies demonstrated immediately before admission to hospital with sudden deterioration of his general condition (lymphadenopathy, fever since several weeks, herpes stomatitis). Some days later herpes meningoencephalitis developed, and was treated successfully with acyclovir (Zovirax). One month after admission the patient became irritable, had emotional outbursts, affect lability, loss of interests, memory disorders. Sporadically he experienced anxiety and bizarre behaviour. He expressed delusion-like phantasies. Extrapyramidal signs appeared. The patient was treated at the time with hydroxyzine. The condition of the patient was continuously downhill, he became passive, apathetic, memory disorders increased, his speech became blurred, dysphagia and sleep disturbances appeared. Neurological examination revealed disseminated signs indicating multifocal lesions. Cerebrospinal fluid contained again herpes virus. CT of brain showed no pathological changes. Acyclovir was given again. Besides that, the patient received haloperidol three drops thrice daily. AZT was never given. The patient died 4 month after admission. One month prior to his death his T_4/T_8 ratio was 0.48 and the total count of lymphocytes T_4 was 133/mm^3. Autopsy revealed miliary tuberculosis.

3. Delirium syndromes

3.1. Male patient A.G., aged 46, not belonging to risk groups, with a history of HIV infection in years 1981-83, was admitted with poor general condition (hepatocellular damage, bone marrow depression, adrenal failure). During the hospital stay the patient had a two-day episode of delirium associated with fever. The most spectacular behaviour was reading from a blank sheet of paper names of persons to whom he owed money. During this delirium the patient had an episode of gastrointestinal haemorrhage, perhaps related to administration of AZT with Fansidar. After transfusion of the first 500 ml of blood delirium regressed. Immediately after admission his T_4/T_8 ratio was 0.59 and his T_4 count was 200/mm^3.

3.2. Male patient W.C., aged 51, with HIV antibodies found in 1990. Promiscuity was the probable cause of infection. He was admitted with extreme cachexia and persistent fever. During his hospital stay delirium persisted for 2 weeks and regressed parallelly with general improvement. At admission his T_4/T_8 ratio was 0.13 and his T_4 cell count was 51/mm^3.

Table 1. Clinical and anatomopathological diagnoses of two patients with AIDS

Patients initials and age	Clinical diagnosis		Results of brain autopsy	
	somatic	psychiatric	Anatomic diagnosis	Histopathological diagnosis
N.O. aged 51	pneumonia, circulatory failure, gastrointestinal bleeding	depressive syndrome	Oedema cerebri Atrophia cerebri	HIV encephalophatia micronodularis
R.Z. aged 25	cerebral and spinal meningitis, Herpes simplex, bilateral pneumonia	dementia syndrome	Hyperaemia cerebri	Encephalitis micronodularis

Our case reports are similar to those described by other authors [1, 4-6, 10].

4. Intravenous drug abusers (IV DAs) with AIDS

Three of 12 patients with AIDS diagnosis were IV DAs. Available information on their case was very poor, probably because of short hospital stays.

4.1. Female patient N.N., aged 24, during her stay in the department viral hepatitis B and left-side pneumonia was found and severe thoracic empyema developed. Very poor physical condition of the patient caused that the opiate abstinency syndrome symptoms were not recognized.

4.2. Female patient Z.S., aged 34. In 1990 treated in the department three times because of interstitial pneumonia. Always, during her hospital admissions she was in the state of so called narcotic hangover. After the last discharge from hospital she appeared again in the department with narcotics to sell.

4.3. Male patient G.G., aged 27 years, was admitted to hospital in preagonal state, with massive gastrointestinal haemorrhage. In the case record there was information on his endocarditis. The patient died one day after admission. Table 2 summarized his clinical and anatomopathological diagnosis.

Table 2.   Clinical and anatomopathological diagnosis of an intravenous drug abuser

Patients initials and age	Clinical diagnosis	Results of brain autopsy	
		Anatomic diagnosis	Histopathological diagnosis
C.G. aged 27	AIDS, circulatory failure, Pneumocystis carinii pneumonia, hepatosplenomegalia, gastrointestinal bleeding	Ofuscationes leptomeninguum, Perivasculares oedema cerebri	Cryptococcosis cerebri

Difficulties in the diagnosis of neuropsychiatric symptoms in intravenous drug abusers infected with HIV

The differential diagnosis of neuropsychiatric disturbances in IV DAs, both, in so called asymptomatic carriers and in AIDS patients is very difficult. Many clinical manifestations and prodromata of HIV infection, such as weight loss, night sweats, fever, diarrhoea, lymphadenopathy, skin eruptions, respiratory symptoms and signs, as well as psychoneurological abnormalities, occur in drug abusers even without HIV infection. Neuropsychiatric symptoms and signs observed in IV DAs are viewed usually not treated as an expression of HIV infection [2, 3]. This attitude is reflected in the documentation of the cases. Correct diagnosing of neuropsychiatric problems in HIV seropositive drug abusers requires a proper training and the availability of greater number of laboratory investigations than in dealing with non-addicts. These investigations are not always available.

The separate problem is the pharmacological treatment of HIV seropositive IV DAs in view of:
- possible various drug interactions
- changed pharmacokinetics of the drugs and distorted metabolism in drug addicts.

Many side effects resulted from the above factors may manifest themselves with neuropsychiatric disturbances.

The treatment of diseases caused by HIV infection in IV DAs should not take place during intense withdrawal symptoms (including neuropsychiatric ones). Methadone used recommended for the substitutive and maintenance treatment of HIV infected IV DAs [2, 3] is waiting as yet in

Poland for registration, and is to be introduced for experimental purposes in 1-2 centres treating drug addicts. In AIDS Hospital Department in Warsaw till now IV DAs patients do not maintain abstinence because of lack of conditions for alternative pharmacological treatment.

Conclusions

1. On the ground of follow-up analysis in 1990 in the AIDS Hospital Department in Warsaw neuropsychiatric disturbances were found in 50% of AIDS patients, apart from IV DAs (25%). This indicates the necessity of paying particular attention to the possibility of development of these disturbances during AIDS, and, consequently, the necessity of careful observation of the patients for these signs, and gathering of information on the clinical manifestations and the used psychotropic medication.
2. Particular problems are encountered in the diagnosis and the treatment of neuropsychiatric disturbances in HIV-infected persons and AIDS patients who are drug abusers. The medical staff should be properly trained for dealing with these patients.
3. In future, the number of IV DAs among AIDS cases in Poland will be growing up.

References

1. Baer J.W. (1989) Study of 60 patients with AIDS or AIDS-related complex requiring psychiatric hospitalization. Am. J. Psychiatry 146: 1285-1288.
2. Bridge P.T., Mirsky A.F., Goodwin F.G. (eds) (1988) Psychological, neuropsychiatric, and substance abuse aspects of AIDS. Raven Press, New York.
3. Flegg P. (1989) Injection drug abuse and HIV infection. Transcript 8: 7-10.
4. Hinz S., Kuck J., Peterkin J.J., Volk D.M., Zisook S. (1990) Depression in the context of human immunodeficiency virus infection, implication for treatment. J. Clin. Psychiatry, 12: 497-501.
5. Perry S.W. (1990) Organic mental disorders caused by HIV: up-date on early diagnosis and treatment. Am. J. Psychiatry 147: 696-710.
6. Report of the consultation on the neuropsychiatric aspects of HIV infection (1988), WHO, Geneva, 14-17 March.
7. Szata W. (1989) Rozpowszechnienie zakażeń wirusem HIV w 1987 r. - sytuacja w Polsce na tle sytuacji w świecie. Przegl. Epid. 43: 115-123.
8. Szata W. (1990) AIDS i zakażenie HIV - 1988 rok. Przegl. Epid. 44: 130-133.
9. Szata W. (1991) Communication on HIV infection and AIDS cases registration in Poland. January 31, National Institute of Hygiene, Dep. Epidemiology.
10. Wolcott D.L., Dilley I.W., Mitsuyasu R.T. (1989) Psychiatric aspects of acquired immune deficiency syndrome. In: Kaplan M.I., Sadock B.I., (eds) Comprehensive text-book of psychiatry. Williams & Wilkins, London, Sidney, 1297-1316.

Neopterin to Predict Disease Progression in Intravenous Drug Users Infected with HIV-1

R. Zangerle[1], D. Fuchs[2], G. Reibnegger[3], P. Fritsch[3], H. Wachter[2]

The AIDS Unit, Department of Dermatology and Venereology, [2] Institute of Medical Chemistry and Biochemistry, University of Innsbruck, and [3] Ludwig Boltzmann Institute of AIDS Research, Innsbruck, Austria

Most of our knowledge about the natural history of HIV infection comes from cohorts of homosexual men and men with hemophilia. The natural history of Human Immunodeficiency Virus (HIV) infection in intravenous drug users (IVDUs) is different from other people at risk in as far as some diseases, such as bacterial pneumonia or endocarditis, contribute to morbidity and mortality (Moss 1989); however, these diseases related to drug intake are not listed in the existing HIV staging classifications nor in the AIDS definition. A staging system for HIV infection should be easily capable of determining individual prognosis for all people at risk, but such a system is still lacking (Chaisson 1990). Therefore, the identification of factors correlated with and possibly contributing to the outcome of infection with HIV is important for our understanding of the pathogenesis and natural history of HIV infection and in designing therapeutic trials. Many reports address the possibility of early prediction of HIV-1 related disease progression. Low numbers of CD4+ T cells and low ratios of CD4+/CD8+ T cells were shown to be associated with a more unfavourable disease course (Polk 1987, Moss 1988, Eyster 1989, Fahey 1990, Fernandez-Cruz 1990). Additionally, HIV-1 p 24 antigenaemia (de Wolf 1988), increased concentrations of ß2-microglobulin in serum (Moss 1988, Anderson 1990) and increased urinary and/or serum concentrations of neopterin

(Fahey 1990, Fuchs 1988, Fuchs 1989) indicated more rapid progression of the disease. However, the question remains whether these data, which were raised mainly from cohorts of homosexual men and men with haemophilia, also are valid for people with intravenous drug use. The aim of our study was to investigate the power of urinary neopterin to predict the development of AIDS or Walter Reed stage 5 (oral candidiasis in combination with a CD4 T cell count below 400 x 10^{-6}/liter).

MATERIAL AND METHODS

Patients: This retrospective study comprised a population of 47 IVDUs out of 121 HIV-1 infected IVDUs at our AIDS Outpatient clinic. The selection was made by the requirement of a complete clinical examination in combination with measurement of urinary neopterin and T cell subsets in 1989/1990, a follow-up of at least 3 months and absence of HIV-1 related symptoms at entry into the study. The mean observation period was 48 months (range 3-82 months). Mean age of the 30 men and 17 women was 25 years (range 18-36 years). All were persistent IVDUs and 16 were enrolled in late 1988 in the newly established methadone maintenance treatment programme (median duration of these participants in the programme was 11 months) and none of them received ziduvudine or inhaled pentamidine before the end point of the observation period, which was determined by either the last visit, or the development of AIDS, or diagnosis of oral candidiasis in combination with a CD4 T cell count below 400 x 10^{-6}/liter (WR 5). AIDS was diagnosed on the basis of the revised CDC definition of 1987 and oral candidiasis was diagnosed when in the presence of characteristic intraoral lesions, the examination of scrapings by potassium hydroxide revealed fungal forms. Other possible causes for the oral candidiasis were excluded in all patients. HIV-1 antibody status was determined by enzyme linked immunosorbent assay (Abbott) and confirmed by Western blot analysis (DuPont) and was available at the initial visit. In some subjects the first HIV test was done with a sample from frozen serum stored before HIV testing was available.

Assay Methods: Neopterin was determined in early morning urine specimens by reversed phase high performance liquid chromatography (HPLC) method described elsewhere, which allows simultaneous determination of urinary creatinine (Wachter 1989). Neopterin concentrations were related to creatinine values to compensate for physiological variations of analyte concentrations in urine.

Statistical Analysis: Cumulative incidence of AIDS and oral candidiasis in combination with a CD4+ T cell count below 400 x 10^{-6}/liter were computed by the product limit approach (Kaplan-Meier) and separately for subgroups of patients. These subgroups were defined by dichotomizing the patients at the first quartile (25th percentile). Significance of differences of incidences between subgroups of patients was assessed by Mantel-Cox test. Comparison of paired samples was done by the paired Wilcoxon-Rank sum test.

RESULTS

Table 1 shows the results of measurement of urinary neopterin at the initial visit in comparison to the last visit. During the observation period the concentrations of urinary neopterin increased significantly.

TABLE 1 - MEASUREMENTS OF URINARY NEOPTERIN

	First visit*	Last visit*
median	407**	464
minimum	183	134
maximum	900	5668
1st quartile (25th percentile)	313	287
3rd quartile (75th percentile)	511	863
normal range	<195	<195
% outside normal range	98%	91.5%

* significance of difference (p=0.007, Wilcoxon rank test)
** μmol/mol creatinine

Of the 47 IVDUs enrolled in this study, 5 (11%) developed WR 5 (oral candidiasis in combination with a CD4+ T cell count below 400 x 10^{-6}/l) and 6 (13%) AIDS (Table 2). One patient died during follow up due to suicide. Two of 5 patients with WR stage 5 and one of the 6 AIDS patients were female. From the 31 patients who were initially enrolled to WR stage 1 or 2, 71% remained in this stage, 20% reached WR 3 or 4, 6% WR stage 5 and 3% WR stage 6.

TABLE 2 - DISEASE PROGRESSION ACCORDING TO WR STAGE

WR stage initial	WR stage at follow-up			
	WR 1/2	WR 3/4	WR 5	WR 6
All (n = 47)*	53%	23%	11%	13%
WR 1/2 (n = 31)	71%	20%	6%	3%
WR 3/4 (n = 7)	–	71%		29%

*The CD4+ T cell count was not available for 9 subjects and they were therefore initially classified as WR stage 1-4.

The mean time to disease progression was 35 months (range 3-67 months). The relation of this disease progression to the concentrations of urinary neopterin is illustrated in Figure 1 of a Kaplan-Meier plot of the cumulative incidence of the development of AIDS or WR 5 (oral candidiasis in combination with a CD4+ T cell count below 400 x 10^{-6}/l).

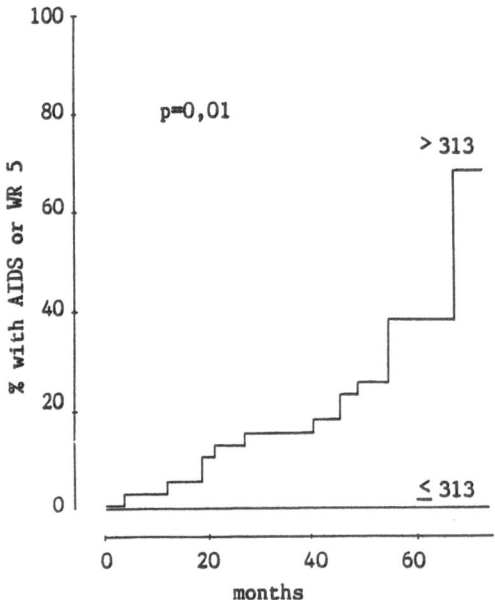

Figure 1. The HIV-1 positives were divided into two groups: the 75 percent (n=35) with the most abnormal values versus the remaining subjects (n=12). Of 35 subjects, having urinary neopterin concentrations higher than 313 umol/mol creatinine at study entry, 11 progressed either to AIDS or WR 5.

DISCUSSION

The clinical diagnosis of AIDS, as well as, oral candidiasis in combination with a CD4+ T cell count below $400 \times 10^{-6}/1$ (WR stage 5), were the two defined endpoints for progression of HIV disease in this study. We did this for two reasons: first, it has been shown that oral candidiasis in combination with a low CD4+ T cell count ultimately leads to AIDS (MacDonald 1988). Secondly, since zidovudine is given to many patients with oral candidiasis, who have a low CD4+ T cell count, this therapeutic intervention would influence the rate of disease progression (Gail 1990).

As this study shows, reliable predictive information on HIV-related disease can be obtained by measuring urinary neopterin. IFN-gamma induces the production of neopterin by macrophages in vitro (Huber 1984). Serum concentrations of IFN-gamma correlate to neopterin concentrations in HIV infection (Fuchs 1989). Therefore, it is likely that IFN-gamma is the immediate cause of the increased level of urinary neopterin.

Therefore increased levels of urinary neopterin indicate chronic immune activation. Immune activation occurs very early in HIV-1 infection and evidence of it can be found in the period during and after acute HIV-1 infection as was shown by monitoring those patients (Sonnerborg 1989). In our study, almost all of the asymptomatic HIV-1 infected IVDUs presented with increased concentrations of urinary neopterin.

Urinary neopterin is of additional interest because recent studies have demonstrated that they can predict the future rate of decrease in CD4+ T cells for at least 2 or 3 years (Melmed 1989). Therefore it seems justified that an immune activation marker, such as urinary neopterin, should be included into a staging classification.

In our experience the variability of repeated measuring of urinary neopterin in the same patients is low. Concentrations of urinary neopterin are increasing along the progression of HIV disease, interestingly urinary neopterin declined in 3 IVDUs to a normal level. These 3 patients entered our methadone maintenance programme in 1988. The observed decrease of neopterin may indicate that methadone treatment contributed to immunological improvement. However, the follow up in the methadone maintenance programme was short and the number of those who entered this programme was too small for a final conclusion.

The levels of immune activation markers seem to be higher in IVDUs compared to homosexual men at a given timepoint in the course of HIV-1 infection (Gorter 1990). The degree of immune activation is possibly related to the frequency and/or unsterility and/or coinfection with other microorganisms of injecting drugs, but not to a distinct drug. High frequency of injecting drug is associated with a decline in CD4+ T cells (Des Jarlais 1987). Whether this higher level of immune activation in IVDUs could be the cause of a faster disease progression or if the immune activation markers are just not as good predictors as in homosexuals, cannot be definitively answered at the moment. However, neopterin is a good prognostic marker in IVDUs and its use is recommended since it is relatively inexpensive compared to e.g. cell counting. It is of particular advantage to use urine samples because it may be cumbersome to draw blood from intravenous drug users. Furthermore, in most methadone maintenance treatment programmes, urine specimens are regularly collected.

REFERENCES

ANDERSON RE, LANG W, SHIBOSKI S, ROYCE R, JEWELL N, WINKELSTEIN W Jr (1990) Use of beta 2-microglobulin level and CD4 lymphocyte count to predict development of acquired immunodeficiency syndrome in persons with human immunodeficiency virus infection. Arch Intern Med 150:73-77.

CHAISSON RE, VOLBERDING PA (1990) Clinical manifestations of HIV infection In Principles and Practice of Infectious Diseases, 3rd Edition edited by Mandell GL, Douglas RG Jr, Bennett JE. New York: Churchill Livingstone pp 1059-1092.

DES-JARLAIS DC, FRIEDMAN SR, MARMOR M et al (1987) Development of AIDS, HIV seroconversion, and potential co-factors for T4 cell loss in a cohort of intravenous drug users. AIDS 1:105-111.

DE WOLF F, LANGE JMA, HOUWELING JTM et al (1988) Numbers of CD4+ cells and the levels of core antigens of an antibodies to the human immunodeficiency virus as predictors of AIDS among seropositive homosexual men. J Infect Dis 158:615-621.

EYSTER ME, BALLARD JO, GAIL MH, DRUMMOND JE, GOEDERT JJ (1989) Predictive markers for the acquired immunodeficiency syndrome (AIDS) in hemophiliacs: persistence of p24 antigen and low T4 cell count. Ann Intern Med 110:963-969.

FAHEY JL, TAYLOR JM, DETELS R et al (1990) The prognostic value of cellular and serologic markers in infection with human immunodeficiency virus type 1. N Engl J Med 322:166-172.

FERNANDEZ-CRUZ E, DESCO M, MONTES MG, LONGO N, GONZALEZ B, ZABAY JM (1990) Immunological and serological markers predictive of progression to AIDS in a cohort of HIV-infected drug users. AIDS 4:987-994.

FUCHS D, HAUSEN A, REIBNEGGER G, WERNER ER, DIERICH MP, WACHTER H (1988) Neopterin as a marker for activated cell-mediated immunity: application in HIV infection. Immunol Today 9:150-155.

FUCHS D, SPIRA TJ, HAUSEN A et al (1989) Neopterin as a predictive marker for disease progression in human immunodeficiency virus type 1 infection. Clin Chem 35:1746-1749.

FUCHS D, HAUSEN A, REIBNEGGER G et al (1989) Interferon-gamm concentrations are increased in sera from individuals with human immunodeficiency virus type 1. J Acquir Immune Defic Syndr 2: 158-162

GAIL MH, ROSENBERG PS, GOEDERT JJ (1990) Therapy may explain recent deficits in AIDS incidence. J Acquir Immune Defic Syndr 3: 296-306.

GORTER RW, VRANIZIAN K; MOSS AR, BRODIE B, WOLFE H (1990) Progression of HIV disease in intravenous drug users. Sixth International Conference on AIDS, San Francisco, June 22-24, Th. C. 644

HUBER C, BATCHELOR JR, FUCHS D et al (1984) Immune response associated production of neopterin release from macrophages primarily under control of interferon-gamma. J Exp Med 160: 310-316.

MACDONALD KB, CHMIEL JS, GOLDSMITH J et al (1988) Prognostic usefulness of the Walter Reed Staging Classification for HIV infection. J Acquir Immune Defic Syndr 1:367-374.

MELMED RN, TAYLOR JM, DETELS R, BOZORGMEHRI M, FAHEY JL (1989) Serum neopterin changes in HIV-infected subjects: indicator of significant pathology, CD4 T cell changes, and the development of AIDS. J Acquir Immune Defic Sndr 2:70-76.

MOSS AR, BACCHETTI P, Osmond D et al (1988) Seropostivity for HIV and the development of AIDS or AIDS related condition: three year follow up of the San Francisco General Hospital cohort. Br Med J 296:745-750.

MOSS AR, BACCHETTI P (1989) Natural history of HIV infection. AIDS 3:55-61.

POLK BF, FOX R, KANCHANARAKSA S et al (1987) Predictors of the acquired immunodeficiency syndrome developing in a cohort of seropositive homosexual men. N Engl J Med 316:61-66.

SONNERBORG AB, VON STEDINGK LV, HANNSON LO, STRANNEGARD OO (1989) Elevated neopterin and beta 2-microglobulin levels in blood and cerebrospinal fluid occur early in HIV-1 infection. AIDS 3:277-283.

WACHTER H, FUCHS D, HAUSEN A, REIBNEGGER G, WERNER ER (1989) Neopterin as a marker for activation of cellular immunity: immunologic basis and clinical application. Adv Clin Chem 27:81-141.

ACKNOWLEDGEMENT

This work was supported by the Austrian funds "Zur Förderung wissenschaftlicher Forschung", Projekt P 7910

Spect and Transcranial Doppler Sonography for the Assessment of Cerebral Perfusion in Intravenous Drug Users with AIDS Encephalopathy

P. Pohl[1], J. Bangerl[2], E. Milly[2], G. Kemmler[3], H. Rössler[4], F. Deisenhammer[1], E. Schmutzhard[1]

[1] Departments of Neurology, [2] Nuclear Medicine, [3] Biostatistics and [4] Psychiatry, University and University Clinic of Innsbruck, A-6020 Innsbruck, Austria

Introduction

Infection with human immunodeficiency virus type 1 (HIV-1) can lead to a variety of central nervous system (CNS) manifestations [5]. AIDS encephalopathy (AE), considered as a primary HIV-1-induced CNS affection, has been recognized as the most common cause of neurological dysfunction [12]. The diagnosis of AE is mainly based on neuropsychiatric features. Computerized tomography (CT), magnetic resonance imaging (MRI), and cerebrospinal fluid analysis are useful for ruling out other manifestations and for supporting the diagnosis of AE. More sensitively than CT and MRI, functional imaging methods like positron emission tomography (PET) and single photon emission computed tomography (SPECT) show pathological changes even in early stages of the disease [3,6,10,11,13,15]. The pathogenesis of AE has not been clearly defined. Besides mechanisms like neuropathological changes following infection of monocytes/macrophages and related microglia, alterations of regional cerebral blood flow (rCBF) can be considered as an additional pathogenetic factor. This suggestion is supported by a series of recent findings:

microvascular changes of small brain vessels [2,8,14];

microscopically noted cerebral infarcts [4,8];

presence of HIV-1 antigens in brain endothelial cells [16];

perivascular localization and occasional vasculitic appearance of HIV-1-related multifocal giant cell encephalitis [1];

interference of HIV-1 envelope proteins with physiological regulation mechanisms of rCBF [9];

previous SPECT studies demonstrating focal or multifocal reduction of rCBF in almost all of the patients with AE [3,6,10,11,15].

In the past few years transcranial Doppler (TCD) sonography has proved to be a useful method for the evaluation of intracranial hemodynamics. The objective of the present study was to evaluate cerebral perfusion by means of ^{99m}Tc-HMPAO-SPECT and TCD in HIV-1-negative and HIV-1-positive iv. drug users (IVDUs) with and without AE.

Patients and methods

Patient population

Three groups of IVDUs were studied (mean age $\pm$ SD: 29.5 $\pm$ 5.5 years): (i) 8 patients with AE; (ii) 14 HIV-1-positive patients without CNS disease; (iii) 16 HIV-1-negative drug users. Twenty HIV-1-negative, healthy volunteers aged 24.3 $\pm$ 4.7, who did not have a history of neurological disease or substance abuse served as control group. All patients and control persons underwent neurological examination and psychiatric evaluation prior to CT, MRI, duplex scanning, TCD, and SPECT. The diagnosis of AE was established if the neurologic and psychiatric signs and symptoms were sufficient and other CNS manifestations were excluded.

SPECT methods

SPECT imaging was performed with a rotating single-head gamma camera (Siemens ZLC 37 Digitrac) with Microdelta system and an identical image reconstruction program. A dose of 555 MBq ^{99m}Tc-HMPAO was administered intravenously in a quiet room with dimmed lights. The patients were positioned supine. Data acquisition was started about 10 minutes after administration of the radiopharmaceutical. The acquisition time was 25 sec per projection. Transverse, coronal, and sagittal slices were processed routinely (slice thickness 6 mm). Brain SPECT scans were evaluated by the staff of the department of nuclear medicine being unaware of the patient's clinical state.

TCD methods

Transcranial Doppler sonography of the middle cerebral artery (MCA), the anterior cerebral artery (ACA), the posterior cerebral artery (PCA), and the basilar artery (BA) was performed by means of a 3-dimensional TCD scanner (Trans-Scan, EME, Überlingen, FRG) using a 2 MHz probe and a spectral analyzer. For each artery the systolic, diastolic, and mean flow velocity (MFV) were measured, and both the pulsatility index and the pulsatility transmission index were calculated. A MFV higher or lower than x $\pm$ 2SD of the reference sample of normal subjects were considered abnormal. The interhemispheric asymmetry index (AI) was calculated for the MCA, ACA, and PCA according to the formula given by Zanette et al. [17]. An AI higher than x + 3SD of the reference sample was considered beyond normal limits.

Results

SPECT results

Pathological uptake defects detected by ^{99m}Tc-HMPAO-SPECT were present in all patients with AE, in 3/14 HIV-1-positive patients without CNS disease, and in 2/16 HIV-1-negative drug users. Multiple focal uptake defects were detected in 6 patients with AE, and in 1 HIV-1-positive patient without brain dysfunction. All other subjects revealed single perfusion deficits.

TCD results

The MFV interhemispheric asymmetry indices of the MCA, ACA, and PCA of the different groups are summarized in table 1. In the AE group 7 of 8 patients showed reduced MFV values in at least one artery (most commonly in the MCA), and an interhemispheric asymmetry of the MFV between the MCA's in all cases (100%), between the ACA's in 6/8 (75%), and between the PCA's in 4/8 cases (50%). In comparison with all other groups, patients with AE demonstrated a highly significant elevation of the asymmetry indices of the MCA, ACA, and PCA (p < 0.0001 for each artery).

TABLE 1
INTERHEMISPHERIC ASYMMETRY INDICES (AI) OF THE MEAN FLOW
VELOCITIES OF THE MCA, ACA, AND PCA

	AE	HIV-positives without CNS disease	HIV-negatives	Normal subjects
	N=8	N=14	N=16	N=20
MCA	33.8 + 7.7	4.6 + 3.9	5.0 + 4.1	3.9 + 3.3
ACA	35.0 + 19.8	5.2 + 3.2	4.8 + 3.0	3.7 + 3.5
PCA	40.7 + 25.2	5.1 + 3.6	6.4 + 3.7	7.7 + 8.6

Comparison of SPECT and TCD

Both TCD and SPECT exhibited reduced cerebral perfusion most commonly in the MCA territory. However, in contrast to transcranial Doppler sonography ^{99m}Tc-HMPAO-SPECT imaging revealed perfusion deficits in additional territories or in regions which exceeded the circulation areas of the arteries with reduced MFV (Fig. 1 and 2).

Other results

In 3 of 8 patients with AE cerebral CT scans revealed diffuse cortical atrophy of various degrees, in one of these patients, atrophy was combined with an attenuation of the periventricular white matter. In two patients MRI showed white matter lesions on

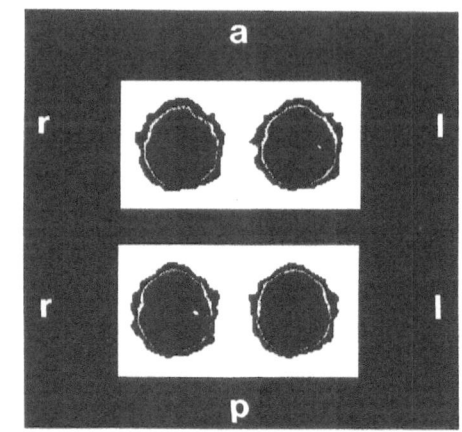

FIGURE 1:
^{99m}Tc-HMPAO-SPECT of an IVDU with AIDS
encephalopathy: extensive uptake defect in the
right hemisphere

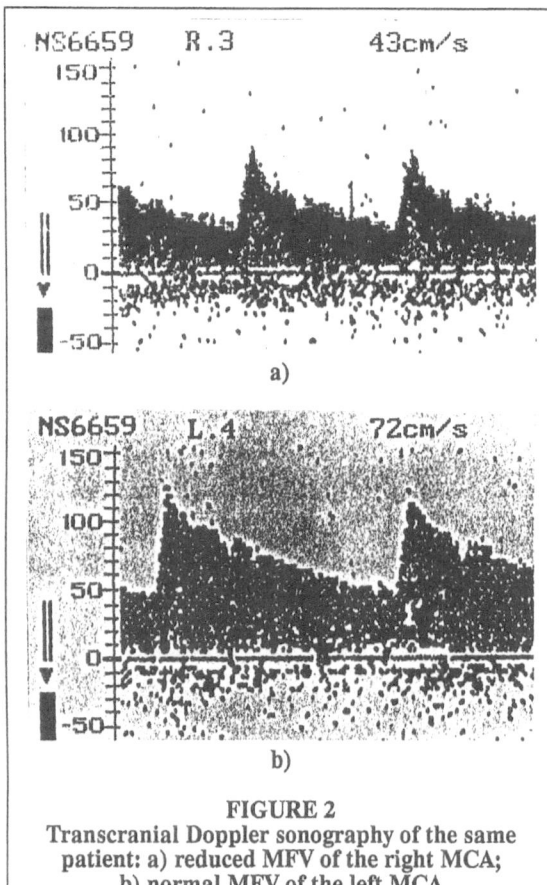

FIGURE 2
Transcranial Doppler sonography of the same
patient: a) reduced MFV of the right MCA;
b) normal MFV of the left MCA

T2-weighted images. None of the patients exhibited cerebral mass lesions. Cortical atrophy was observed in 2 of the 14 HIV-1-positives without CNS disease. In HIV-1-negative iv. drug users CT revealed normal findings. Duplex scanning of the extracranial carotid and vertebral arteries showed normal results in all groups.

Discussion

AIDS encephalopathy is the most common neurological disorder in all risk groups of HIV-1 infected subjects. This HIV-1-related CNS disorder characteristically manifests with progressive cognitive dysfunction accompanied by motor impairment and has not been found in other immunosuppressed states [12]. In a number of previous SPECT studies perfusion deficits were common findings in patients with AE [3,6,10,11,15]. These findings are in general agreement with recent neuropathological findings which revealed microvascular changes of brain vessels in HIV-1 infected individuals [2,8,14]. Since it may be difficult to differentiate AE from toxic effects of psychotropic drugs in IVDUs, we performed the cerebral perfusion studies in individuals with and without AE as well as in those without HIV-1 infection.

Our TCD results showed reduced MFV (most commonly in the MCA) and a significant interhemispheric asymmetry of the MFV in all patients with AE but not in the other groups. SPECT scans exhibited that perfusion changes occur more frequently in IVDUs suffering from AE than in drug users without AE or without HIV-1 infection. Compared with TCD ultrasound ^{99m}Tc-HMPAO-SPECT either revealed areas of reduced perfusion which exceeded the territories of the brain arteries with lowered MFV, and/or exhibited additional regions with hypoperfusion.

It was shown by recent TCD sonography studies, that a reduction and interhemispheric asymmetry of the MFV of the MCA correlate with angiographically proven occlusions of peripheral MCA branches [7,17]. Since angiography of our AIDS patients was not possible for many reasons, we hypothesize that our TCD data indicate pathological changes in distal branches of cerebral arteries of AE patients. Both TCD ultrasound and ^{99m}Tc-HMPAO-SPECT neuroimaging may represent the functional effect of recently described cerebrovascular changes in AE. The present study confirms previous findings that hypoperfusion is a common feature in patients with AE and therefore can be regarded at least as a cofactor in the pathogenesis of this disorder.

References

1. Budka H, Costanzi G, Cristina S, Lechi A, Parravicini C, Trabattoni R, Vago L (1987) Brain pathology induced by infection with the human immune deficiency virus (HIV). A histological, immunochemical, and electron microscopical study of 100 autopsy cases. *Acta Neuropathol (Berlin)* 75:185-198

2. Cho E-S, Sharer LR, Reress NS, Little B (1987) Intimal proliferation of lepto-menigeal arteries and brain infarcts in subjects with AIDS. *J Neuropathol Exp Neurol* 46:385

3. Ell PJ, Costa DC, Harrison M (1987) Imaging cerebral damage in HIV infection. *Lancet* ii:569-570

4. Engstrom JW, Lowenstein DH, Bredesen DE (1989) Cerebral infarctions and transient neurologic deficits associated with acquired immunodeficiency syndrome. *Amer J Med* 86:528-532

5. McArthur JC (1987) Neurologic manifestations of AIDS. *Medicine* 66:407-437

6. Maini CL, Pigorini F, Pau FM, Narciso P, Rosci MA, Galgani S, Volponi V, Leonetti C, Atzei G (1990) ^{99m}Tc-HM-PAO brain SPECT in acquired immune deficiency syndrome (AIDS). In: Schmidt HAE, Chambron J (eds) *Nuclear Medicine. Quantitative analysis in imaging and function.* European Nuclear Medicine Congress, Straßbourg, August 28 - September 1, 1989. Schattauer, Stuttgart - New York, pp 334-336

7. Mattle H, Grolimund P, Huber P, Sturzenegger M, Zurbruegg HR (1988) Trans-cranial Doppler sonographic findings in middle cerebral artery disease. *Arch Neurol* 45:289-295

8. Mizusawa H, Hirano A, Llena JF, Shintaku M (1988) Cerebrovascular lesions in ac-quired immune deficiency syndrome (AIDS). *Acta Neuropathol (Berlin)* 76:451-457

9. Pert CB, Smith CC, Ruff MR, Hill JM (1988) AIDS and its dementia as a neuro-peptide disorder: role of VIP receptor blockade by human immunodeficiency virus envelope. *Ann Neurol* 23(suppl):S71-S73

10. Pohl P, Vogl G, Fill H, Roessler H, Zangerle R, Gerstenbrand F (1988) Single photon emission computed tomography in AIDS dementia complex. *J Nucl Med* 29:1382-1386

11. Pohl P, Gerstenbrand F, Riccabona G, Bangerl I, Vogl G, Pallua AK, Fill H (1990) Single photon emission computed tomography as a diagnostic tool in patients with AIDS dementia complex. In: Battistin L , Gerstenbrand F (eds): *Aging brain and dementia. New trends in diagnosis and therapy.* Wiley-Liss, New York, pp 439 451 (Neurology and Neurobiology Vol 54)

12. Price RW, Brew BJ, Rosenblum M (1990) The AIDS dementia complex and HIV-1 brain infection: a pathogenetic model of virus-immune interaction. In: Waks-

man BH (ed); *Immunologic mechanisms in neurologic and psychiatric disease.* Raven Press, New York, pp 269-290

13. Rottenberg DA, Moeller JR, Strother SC, Sidtis JJ, Navia BA, Dhawan V, Ginos JZ, Price RW (1987) The metabolic pathology of the AIDS dementia complex. *Ann Neurol* 22:700-706

14. Smith TW, DeGirolami, Henin D, Bolgert F, Hauw J-J (1990) Human immunodeficiency virus (HIV) leukoencephalopathy and the microcirculation. *J Neuropathol Exp Neurol* 49:357-370

15. Tatsch K, Schielke E, Einhäupl KM, Bauer M, Markl A, Kirsch CM (1990) ^{99m}Tc-HMPAO-SPECT in patients with HIV-infection: a comparison with neurological, CT and MRI findings. In: Schmidt HAE, Chambron J (eds) *Nuclear Medicine. Quantitative analysis in imaging and function.* European Nuclear Medicine Congress, Straßbourg, August 28 - September 1, 1989. Schattauer, Stuttgart - New York, pp 340-342

16. Wiley CA, Schrier RD, Nelson JA, Lampert PW, Oldstone MBA (1986) Cellular localization of human immunodeficiency virus infection within the brains of acquired immune deficiency syndrome patients. *Proc Natl Acad Sci USA* 83:7089-7093

17. Zanette EM, Fieschi C, Bozzao L, Roberti C, Toni D, Argentino C, Lenzi GL (1989) Comparison of cerebral angiography and transcranial Doppler sonography in acute stroke. *Stroke* 20:899-903

The Treatment with Dextromethorphan of Heroin Addicts

H. Koyuncuoğlu

Istanbul Faculty of Medicine, Department of Pharmacology and Clinical Pharmacology, 34390 Çapa-Istanbul, Turkey

In our previous studies, L–aspartic acid (L–ASP) was found to antagonize the inhibitory effects of acute and chronic morphine (M) administration on brain L–asparaginase activity, the developement of physical dependence on M and the manifestation of M abstinence syndrome (19, 21, 24, 26). As a result of these experimental data, we hypothesized that the mechanisms underlying the development of physical dependence on opiates and the abstinence syndrome upon withdrawal from opiates are the inhibition by opiates of the brain L–asparaginase and glutaminase activities, and the disequilibrium due to the inhibitory effect of opiates between L–asparaginase and asparagine synthetase +L–glutaminase and glutamine synthetase (14, 20, 40). As a consequence, the inhibition of the brain L–asparaginase and glutaminase activities, and the subsequent relative hyperactivities of asparagine and synthetases result in less production of the excitatory neurotransmitter amino acids (EAAs), namely ASP and L–glutamic acid (L–GLU), and prompt adaptation of the organism to this newly created state. The similar effects of another L–asparaginase inhibitor D–ASP (30) to those of M (15, 17), the intensification or attenuation by D–ASP administered at the beginning of the M physical dependence development or just before the naloxone precipitated abstinence syndrome (22), and the successful treatment with L–ASP (14, 40) of opiate addicted people have been considered to be supporting evidence for the hypothesis.

On the other hand, nonnarcotic antitussive dextromethorphan (DM), which lacks addiction liability (9, 10, 32) has recently been reported to noncompetitively bind at the ionophor component of the ASP/GLUergic receptors, especially N–methyl–D–aspartate (NMDA) subtype and to prevent the NMDA receptor–mediated neurotoxicity (2, 4, 7, 8). The intratechally administered NMDA–induced behavioural changes and nociceptive action have been shown to be antagonized by opioid mu and to some extent sigma receptor agonists (1). The acetylcholine release evoked by GLU from rat striatal slices was significantly inhibited by mu opiate agonists M and [D–Ala^2, Gly(ol)^5]–enkephalin (DAGO) and delta–opiate agonists [D–Ala^2, D–Leu^5]–enkephalin (DADLE) and [D–Pen^2–D–Pen^5]–enkephalin (DPDPE). This effect was completely blocked by naloxone at one tenth concentration of M, DAGO and DADLE, and equal concentration of DPDPE (3). The addition of 1 microM–1mM methadone, 100 microM–3mM M fentanyl, codeine, meperidine, dextropropoxyphene and naltrexone to the bathing

1) <u>NORMAL</u>

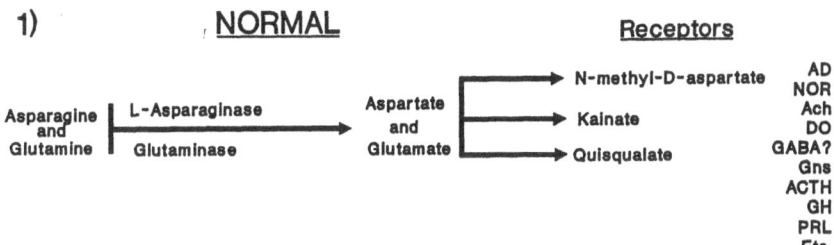

2) <u>OPIATE INTAKE</u>

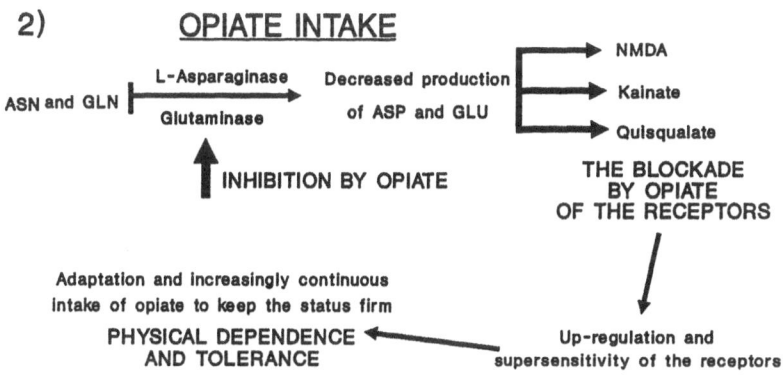

3) <u>WITHDRAWAL</u>

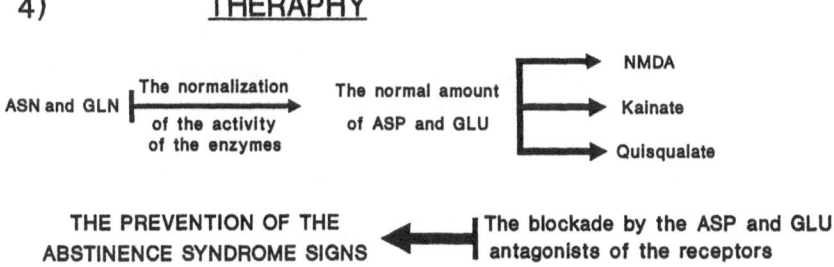

4) <u>THERAPHY</u>

medium of murine cortical cell culture were found to produce a concentration-dependent reduction in the neurotoxicity of exogenously applied NMDA. This neuron-protective action of opioids was claimed not to be mediated by conventional opioid receptors; the non-opioid enantiomers of methadone and M exhibited a potency equal to or greater than those of the opioid enantiomers, and 1mM naloxone did not act as an antagonist (6). On the basis of the experimental results given above, the hypothesis can be briefly reformed as follows. The physical dependence on opiates is the result of the inhibition by opiates of the enzymes, producing neurotransmitters L-ASP and GLU from asparagine and glutamine within the ASP/GLUergic system (4, 37), the blockade by opiates of the ASP/GLUergic system receptors, and the most probable upregulation and supersensitivity of the receptors. In the case of withdrawal from opiates the inhibition of L-asparaginase and glutaminase disappears and the production and release of L-ASP and GLU normalizes. The upregulated and supersensitive ASP/GLUergic receptors which are not blocked by opiates anymore respond to the EAAs stronger than normal. These will cause the release of some neurotransmitters such as norepinephrine (11, 28, 42), dopamine (12, 36, 38), acetylcholine (36, 38) and the release of some pituitary hormones such as growth hormone, luteinizing hormone, follicle-stimulating hormone etc (31, 34). The results of the experiments performed on rats implanted with M containing pellets and injected with opioid antagonist naloxone three days after implantation (23), and the successful treatment with DM of heroin addicts in the clinic (16) are supporting evidence for this hypothesis.

Since the aim of the previous double-blind clinical trial (16) was to show the difference between DM and chlorpromazine (CPZ) in the treatment of heroin addicts, and the markedly causal efficiacy of the DM administration no additional helper drug such as nonnarcotic analgesic, anticholinergic etc could be combined with DM. Instead the goal of the present study was to show whether the treatment of heroin addicts with DM combined with nonnarcotic analgesic, anticholinergic, CPZ and diazepam (DIA) could be possible on ambulatory basis which might provide some advantages.

Patients and Methods

Fourty-eight males and eight females (totally fifty-six addicts) were the subjects of the present study. Some information about the patients are shown in Table 1. The duration of heroin intake, the average amount of daily heroin intake and the mean number of the previous heroin addiction withdrawal treatment in a psychiatry clinic were obtained directly from patients. Before the patients had started having the treatment they had a general medical control to find out any probable clinico-pathological inconvenience for the treatment. After having given the necessary information in relation to the treatment, their verbal consensus was obtained. The patients started taking the treatment always on Mondays in order to be able to follow the patients in the critical period during working days.15 mg DM containing dragees (Romilar) were donated by Roche (İstanbul/Turkey) with the permission of Turkish Ministry of Health, 25 mg CPZ containing dragees (Largactil), 5 mg diazepam (DIA) containing capsules (Diazem) and 10 mg hyoscine-N-butylbromide + 250 mg dipyrone containing dragees (Buscopan compositum) were purchased from Eczacıbaşı, Deva and Boehringer Ingelheim (İstanbul/Turkey), respectively.

Table 1 : Some information about the patients

Total Number	Sex	Duration of Heroin Intake	Daily Heroin Intake (mg)	Route of Heroin Intake	Age	Mean Previous Treatment
56	48 males 8 males	2.73 years	62.7	24 IV 32 Nose	26.3	1.4

The patients who had had the morning first usual heroin dose came to the Department at around 10 o'clock and immediately began receiving 15 mg DM every hour, 25 or 50 mg CPZ in accordance with their daily heroin intake and the duration of heroin intake every six hours. In addition to these, the patients had 10 mg DIA + one dragee of Buscopan compositum every six hours provided they were taken three hours following CPZ (Fig.1). On the 0. and 1. days the patients were kept under a strict observation and control for about four hours to estimate the severity of their abstinence syndrome. Then, appropriate dose of CPZ was estimated at the individual level. The following days the observation

Figure 1

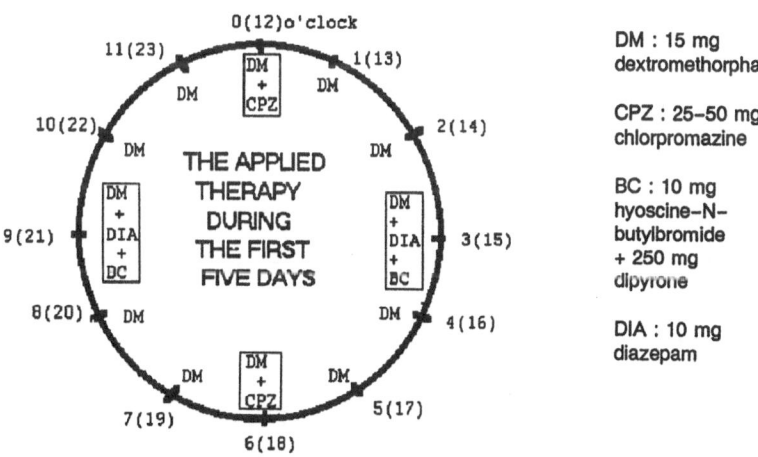

DM : 15 mg dextromethorphan

CPZ : 25–50 mg chlorpromazine

BC : 10 mg hyoscine–N–butylbromide + 250 mg dipyrone

DIA : 10 mg diazepam

period reduced from four hours to two or three hours according to the intensity of the abstinence syndrome signs. From the end of the fourth day till the eigth day, 10 mg DIA giving twice during daytime was decreased to 5 mg DIA; 25–50 mg CPZ taking during daytime was stopped; and 15 mg DM every hour was not given while the patients were sleeping. For the patients who continued coming to the Department after the eighth day of the treatment, the dose of DM was gradually decreased in the first fifteen days and then DM administration was completely stopped. In the meantime they were also given CPZ and DIA in appropriate doses especially against insomnia and restlessness.

To follow the overall intensity of abstinence syndrome and its course yawning, lacrimation, rhinorrhoea, perspiration, goose flesh (piloerection), muscle tremor, dilated pupils, anorexia, joint and muscle aches, restlessness, insomnia, emesis, diarrhoea, craving and rejection of smoking were strictly observed and/or questioned as they were done in the previous trial (16). The signs were ranked mild, bearable and severe and given 1,2 and 3 points, respectively.

Results

The mean values of the points given to the abstinence syndrome signs according to their severity are shown in Table 2. From fifty–six patients participated in the present study on the first day

TABLE 2:
The mean values of the points given to the abstinence syndrome signs
according to their intensity

DAYS	0.	1.	2.	3.	4.	5.	6.	7.	8.
No of Patients	56	45	39	38	38	38	38	38	38
Yawning	0.14	0.48	0.46	0.34	0.05	0.05	0	0	0
Lacrimation	0.05	0.44	0.46	0.34	0.13	0.05	0	0	0
Rhinorrhoea	0.05	0.26	0.23	0.10	0.07	0	0	0	0
Perspiration	0	0.13	0.10	0.08	0.05	0	0	0	0
Goose Flesh (Piloerection)	0	0.13	0.13	0.13	0	0	0	0	0
Muscle Tremor	0	0.40	0.36	0.38	0.05	0	0	0	0
Dilated Pupils	0.16	1.78	2.12	2.16	2.16	2.16	2.16	1.97	1.97
Anorexia	0.44	2.40	1.84	1.52	0.52	0.23	0.21	0.13	0
Joint and Muscle Aches	0.13	0.92	1.23	1.10	0.31	0.16	0	0	0
Restlessness	0.25	1.24	1.10	0.57	0.16	0.16	0.16	0.16	0.16
Insomnia	0	1.60	1.23	1.23	0.45	0.45	0.45	0.34	0.34
Emesis	0	0.40	0.41	0.31	0.10	0	0	0	0
Diarrhoea	0	0.31	0.30	0.16	0.05	0	0	0	0
Craving	0.85	1.08	0.41	0.34	0.07	0	0	0	0
Rejection of Smoking	0.34	1.60	1.23	1.07	0.08	0	0	0	0

of the abstinence syndrome eleven patients, on the second day six patients and on the third day one patient started taking heroin again when the intensity of the abstinence syndrome signs was at the relatively highest degree. Following days the intensity appeared to be gradually faded. On the fourth day the majority of the patients felt extremely well except three ones whose restlessness continued as mild, bearable and severe, respectively. From the fourth day on, the common complaint was insomnia which lasted to be a major discomfort at least 3–4 weeks. Dilated pupils were still existing on the eighth day and it was observed in the patients who regularly came to our Department for about 4–6 weeks decreasing gradually.

In Figure 2 it can be seen the sum of the total mean values in each day which was depleted with or without the mean value of the points given to dilated pupils during the study.

Figure 2

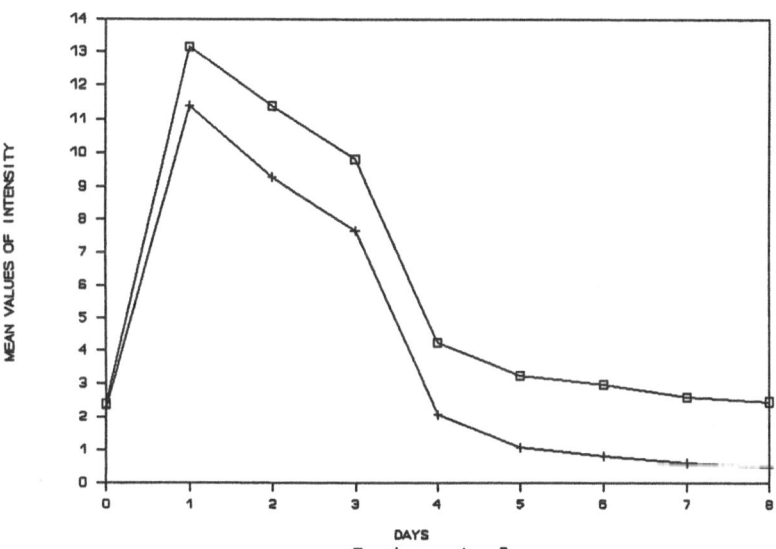

A:Mean Values of All Abstinence Syndrome Signs,
B: Mean Values of 14 Abstinence Syndrome Signs

Discussion

The diagnosis of heroin addiction in the patients taken part in the present study was made on the ground of the information given by patients and obtained from their relatives by using the DSM-III-R criteria. As the information about duration of heroin intake, daily heroin intake, and mean previous treatment were obtained from the patients and/or their relatives one cannot rely on them. Especially daily heroin intake is generally expressed less then real daily heroin intake. On the other hand, the amount of daily heroin intake shown in Table 1 cannot be considered as the real amount of heroin taken by the patients, since the heroin content of the mixture used by the patients varies in accordance with the sources, the availability of heroin,increased control of police, economic conjonctures of the country and/or neighbouring countries etc. The amount of heroin intake was estimated with the aid of the information expressed by the patients following the determination of the heroin content of nine specimens given by the police to us during the present study. However, on the basis of our previous personal experiences, it is possible to say that the amount of daily heroin intake shown in Table 1 might be considerably higher.

The goal of the CPZ combination was to utilize from its well-known anticholinergic, antiadrenergic, antidopaminergic, antiserotonergic and sedative effects. The addition of DIA, hyoscine-N-butylbromide and analgesic dipyrone was to respectively provide anxiolytic, anticholinergic, analgesic supports.

The results of the present study which are very similar to those of the previous one (16) can also be considered supporting evidence for the hypothesis implying the blockade by opiates of NMDA receptors in the development of physical dependence on opiates. Moreover, the attenuation by another noncompetitive NMDA antagonist MK-801 of naloxone-precipitated abstinence syndrome in rats (41) can be in favour of the hypothesis.

The decrease of the number of the patients participated in the present study and the intensity of the abstinence syndrome signs are parallel to each other. Once patients reach the third day of the abrupt withdrawal they continued having the treatment due to the beneficial effects of the treatment. In fact, on the fourth day a drastic well feeling was observed. Even though the mean daily heroin intake (62.7 mg) was markedly higher than that of the patients taken in the double blind clinical trial (23.9 mg) (16) the course of the first most stormy period which was about four day did not show a marked change. Instead dilated pupils and anorexia appeared to be slightly increased, joint and muscle aches, emesis, diarrhoea, craving showed a considerable decrease in comparison to those of the patients taken part in the previous double-blind clinical trial (16).

REFERENCES

1. Aanonsen LM, Wilcox GL (1987) Nociceptive action of excitatory amino acids in the mouse; effects of spinally administered opioids, phencyclidine and sigma agonists. J Pharmacol Exp Ther 243: 9-19

2. Anis NA, Berry SC, Burton NR, Lodge D (1983) The dissociative anesthetics, ketamine and phencyclidine, selectively reduce excitation of central mammalian neurons by N-methyl-L-aspartate. Br J Pharmacol 71: 565-575

3. Arenas E, Alberch J, Arroyos RS, Marsal J (1990) Effects of opioids on acetylcholine release evoked by K or glutamic acid from rat neostriatal slices. Brain Res 523: 51-56

4. Bielarczyk H, Lysiak W, Szutowicz A (1986) Synthesis of glutamate and aspartate in rat brain synaptosomes. Acta Biochim Pol 33: 239–251

5. Choi DW, Peter S, Viseskul V (1987) Dextrorphan and levorphanol selectively block N–methyl–D–aspartate receptor–mediated neurotoxicity on cortical neurons. J Pharmacol Exp Ther 242: 713–720

6. Choi DW, Viseskul V (1988) Opioids and non–opioid enantiomers selectively attenuate N–methyl–D– aspartate neurotoxicity on cortical neurons. Eur J Pharmacol 155: 27–35

7. Ferkany JW, Borosky SH, Clissold DB, Pontecorvo MJ (1988) Dextromethorphan inhibits NMDA induced convulsions. Eur J Pharmacol 151: 151–154

8. George CP, Goldberg MP, Choi DW, Steinberg GK (1988) Dextromethorphan reduces neocortical ischemic damage in vivo. Brain Res 440: 375–379

9. Isbell H, Fraser HF (1953) action and addiction liabilities of dromoran derivatives in man. J Pharmacol Exp Ther 107: 524–530

10. Jasinski DR, Martin WR, Mansky PA (1971) Progress report on the assessment of the antagonists nalbuphine and GPA–2087 for abuse potential and studies of the effects of dextromethorphan in man. Presented at 33rd Meeting of Committee on Problems of Drug Dependence, National Research Council, Toronto, Ontario, Canada

11. Jones SM, Snell LD, Johnson KM (1987) Phencyclidine selectively inhibits N–methyl–D–aspartate– induced hippocampal [H]–norepinephrine release. J Pharmacol Exp Ther 240: 492–497.

12. Jones SM, Snell LD, Johnson KM (1987) Inhibition by phencyclidine of excitatory amino–acid–stimulated release of neurotransmitter in the nucleus accumbens. Neuropharmacol 26: 173–179.

13. Klein M, Paturzo JJ, Musacchio JM (1989) The effects of prototypic ligands on the binding of [H] dextromethorphan to guinea pig brain. Neurosci Lett 97: 175–180

14. Koyuncuoğlu H (1983) The treatment with L–aspartic acid of persons addicted to opiates. Bull Narcotics 35: 11–15

15. Koyuncuoğlu H, Berkman K (1982) Effect of D– and/or L–aspartic acids on feeding, drinking, urine outflow and core temperature. Pharmacol Biochem Behav 17: 1265–1269.

16. Koyuncuoğlu H, Saydam B (1990) The treatment of heroin addicts with dextromethorphan: A double blind comparison of dextromethorphan with chlorpromazine. Int J Clin Pharmacol Ther Toxicol 28: 147–152.

17. Koyuncuoğlu H, Berkman K, Sabuncu H (1984) Feeding, drinking, urine osmolality in Brattleboro rats: Changes by morphine, naloxone, D–amino acids, PLG. Pharmacol Biochem Behav 20: 29–34.

18. Koyuncuoğlu H, Berkman K, Wildmann J, Matthaei H (1982) Antagonistic effect of L–aspartic acid on decrease in body weight, food and fluid intake, and naloxone reversible rectal temparature caused by D–aspartic acid. Pol J Pharmacol Pharm 34: 333–337.

19. Koyuncuoğlu H, Genç E, Güngör M, Eroğlu L, Sağduyu H (1977) The antagonizing effect of aspartic acid on the brain levels of monoamines and free amino acids during the development tolerance and physical dependence on morphine. Psychopharmacology (Berlin) 54: 187–191.

20. Koyuncuoğlu H, Güngör M, Enginar N, Hatipoğlu İ, Hızal A (1986) Brain asparaginase, ACE activity and plasma cortisol level in morphine dependent rats: Effect of aspartic acid and naloxone. Pharmacol Biochem Behav 25: 953–957

21. Koyuncuoğlu H, Güngör M, Eroğlu L, Sağduyu H 1979 (a) The antagonizing effect of aspartic acid on morphine withdrawal and levallorphan precipitated abstinence syndrome signs and on associated changes in brain levels of free amino acids in the rat. Psychopharmacology (Berlin) 62: 89–95

22. Koyuncuoğlu H, Güngör M, Sağduyu H, Arıcıoğlu F (1990) Intensification and attenuation of morphine dependence by D–aspartic acid and PLG. Pharmacol Biochem Behav 35: 47–50

23. Koyuncuoğlu H, Güngör M, Sağduyu H, Arıcıoğlu F (1990) Suppression by ketamine and dextro-methorphan of precipitated abstinence syndrome in rats. Pharmacol Biochem Behav 35: 829–832

24. Koyuncuoğlu H, Güngör M, Sağduyu H, Eroğlu L (1974) The antagonistic effects of aspartic acid on some effects of morphine on rats. Eur J Pharmacol 27: 148–150

25. Koyuncuoğlu H, Keyer–Uysal M, Berkman K, Güngör M, Genç E (1979) The relationship between morphine, aspartic acid and L–asparaginase in rats. Eur J Pharmacol 60: 369–372

26. Koyuncuoğlu H, Güngör M, Sağduyu H, Eroğlu L, Genç E (1977) Antagonizing effect of aspartic acid on the development of physical dependence on and tolerance to morphine in the rats. Drug Res 27: 1676–1679

27. Koyuncuoğlu H, Wildmann J, Berkman K, Matthaei (1982) The effects of D– and/or L–aspartic acid on the total weight of body and the weights of certain organs, and their protein, triglyceride and glycogen contents. Drug Res 32: 738–741

28. Lalies M, Middlemiss DN, Ransom R (1988) Stereoselective antagonism of NMDA–stimulated noradrenaline release from rat hippocampal slices by MK–801. Neurosci Letts 91: 339–342

29. Lehmann J, Scatton B (1982) Characterization of the excitatory amino acid receptor–mediated release of [H]–acetylcholine from rat striatal slices. Brain Res 252: 77–89

30. Lerman MI, Verevkina IV (1962) The inhibition of asparaginase from the blood serum of guinea pigs. Biokhimiya 27:556–561

31. Mason GA, Bisette G, Nemeroff CB (1983) Effects of excitotoxic aminoacids on pituitary hormone secretion in the rat. Brain Res 289: 366–369

32. Mansky PA, Jasinski DR (1970) Effects of dextromethorphan (D) in man. Pharmacologist 12: 231

33. Massachio JM, Klein M, Santiago LJ (1988) High affinity dextromethorphan binding sites in guinea pig brain: further characterization and allosteric interactions. J Pharmacol Exp Ther 247:424–431

34. Price MT, Olney JW, Mitchell MV, Fuller T, Cicero TJ (1978) Luteinizing releasing action of N–methyl aspartate is blocked by GABA or taurine but not by dopamine antagonists. Brain Res 158:461–465

35. Price MT, Olney JW, Anglim M, Buchsbaum S (1979) Reversible action of N–methyl aspartate on gonadotropin neuroregulation. Brain Res 176: 165–168

36. Ransom RW, Deschenes NL (1989) Glycine modulation of NMDA–evoked release of [H]–acetylcholine and [H]–dopamine from rat striatal slices. Neurosci Lett 96: 323–327

37. Reubi JC, Toggenburger G, Cuenod M (1980) Asparagine as precursor for transmitter aspartate in corticostriatal fibers. J Neurochem 34: 1015–1017

38. Snell LD, Johnson KM (1985) Antagonism of NMDA–induced transmitter release in the rat striatum by phencyclidine–like drugs and its relationship to turning behavior. J Pharmacol Exp Ther 235:50–57

39. Snell LD, Johnson KM (1986) Characterization of the inhibition of excitatory amino acid–induced neurotransmitter release in the rat striatum by phencyclidine–like drugs. J Pharmacol Exp Ther 238: 938–946

40. Şener Al, Ceylan ME, Koyuncuoğlu H (1986) Comparison of the suppressive effects of L–aspartic acid and chlorpromazine + diazepam treatments on opiate abstinence syndrome signs in men. Drug Res 36: 1684–1686

41. Trujillo KA, Akil H (1991) Inhibition of morphine tolerance and dependence by NMDA receptor antagonist MK–801. Science 251: 85–87

42. Vezzani A, Wu HQ, Samanin R (1987) [H]–norepinephrine release from hippocampal slices is an in vitro tool for investigating the pharmacological properties of excitatory amino acids. J Neurochem 49: 1438–1432

Buprenorphine: An Opioid Mixed Agonist-Antagonist as Possible Antidote for Acute Cocaine Toxicity

M. Bansinath[1], V. K. Shukla[1], L. R. Goldfrank[2], and H. Turndorf[2]

[1] Department of Biophysics, Panjab University, Chandigarh, India-160 014,
[2] Departments of Anesthesiology and Emergency Medicine, School of Medicine, New York University Medical Center, 550 First Avenue, New York, NY 10016, USA

Abstract. In the patients presenting to the emergency departments, cocaine toxicity has become most common cause. Since heroin abuse among cocaine addicts is frequent, treatment strategies in the emergency medical management of intoxicated patients often include opiate antagonist naloxone. The mixed action opioid, buprenorphine offers several therapeutic advantages for the treatment of heroin abuse, because of its unique pharmacology. Furthermore, buprenorphine decreases cocaine craving. Therefore in this study, the effect of buprenorphine on acute cocaine toxicity was assessed in male Swiss Webster (SW) mice (20-24 g). Buprenorphine in dose dependent manner protected against cocaine-induced toxicity and increased ($p < 0.05$) the LD_{50} and decreased the potency ratio of cocaine. However, neither naloxone nor naltrexone altered the lethality of cocaine (100 mg/kg). Buprenorphine pretreatment also significantly ($p < 0.05$) attenuate cocaine-induced (80 mg/kg) increase in plasma lactate dehydrogenase (LDH) activity. The results indicate that buprenorphine could be of potential advantage over naloxone in the management of "speed ball" toxicity.

Introduction. In the past few years as a result of cocaine intoxication, there has been a dramatic increase in the number of patients presenting to the emergency medicine departments in the United States[31]. Even though different body systems are implicated, the mechanisms involved in the lethal effects of cocaine are not well known[43].

The treatment modalities of the acute cocaine intoxication are selected empirically to antagonize cocaine-induced signs and symptoms[41]. From the last so many years different workers employed different types of drugs experimentally and clinically in cocaine-induced toxicity and got different results (Table 1).

Currently, two major problems encountered in treating cocaine abuser are: to reverse or treat toxic effects of drug overdose and to develop methods for dealing with the drug craving[21]. Moreover it is common practice in drug abuse to combine opioid agonist with cocaine (speed balling). Opiate antagonist naloxone is often used to treat the opioid toxicity[41]. Recently, chronic administration of buprenorphine, opioid mixed agonist-antagonist has shown to suppress cocaine self-administration in Rhesus monkeys[46,47] suggesting that buprenorphine may be an effective pharmacotherapy for the treatment of cocaine abuse as well as dual abuse of cocaine plus heroin. Therefore in this study, the effect of buprenorphine on cocaine-induced acute toxicity was studied.

Material and Method. Male SW mice weighing 25-30 g (Taconic farm) were housed five per cage in a room with controlled temperature ($22\pm2C$), humidity and artificial light (06:30-19:00 hr). The animals had free access to food and water and were used after minimum of four days acclimation to the housing condition. Cocaine hydrochloride (Sigma Chemicals, St Louis, MD, USA) in the dose of 60, 80, 100, 120 and 140 mg/kg was injected intraperitoneal (ip) to groups of mice (n>20) pre-treated 30 mins before either with vehicle (0) or buprenorphine hydrochloride (Reckitt & Colman, Kingston-upon-Hull, England) (0.15 and 0.3 mg/kg ip). Number of animals dead in each group at the end of 1 and 24 hours after cocaine injection were noted. The statistical significance of the dose-effect curves and confidence limits of LD_{50} were analyzed by the method of Litchfield and Wilcoxon. Similarly, naloxone (10 mg/kg, 15 min before) (Sigma) and naltrexone (3 mg/kg, 15 min before) (Sigma) were also tried against LD_{50} dose of cocaine (100 mg/kg) and results were compared by chi square test.

Estimation of Lactate Dehydrogenase (LDH) activity: Saline or buprenorphine (0.3 mg/kg) was injected to different groups (n=10) of mice. Thirty minutes later sublethal dose of cocaine (80 mg/kg ip) was administered to all the treatment groups. Blood samples were collected by rupturing the retrobulbar venus plexus using heparinized micro hematocrit tubes at 0.5, 1, 2, 4, 8 and 24 hr after administration of cocaine hydrochloride from a saline and a buprenorphine treated groups at each time point. The plasma was separated and LDH activity was measured by spectrophotometric method using a commercial kit (Sigma). In a separate group of untreated animals (n=20) blood samples were collected and LDH activity was estimated same way to get basal values for LDH. The results were compared by analysis of variance (ANOVA) and separate variance at each time point. A $p < 0.05$ was considered as significant.

Results. Effect of buprenorphine on cocaine-induced lethality: Buprenorphine in a dose related way increased the LD_{50} values and decreased the potency of cocaine-induced lethality LD_{50} values (mg/kg ip) with 95% confidence limits at one and 24 hrs as compared to control (0) (Table 2).

Table 1. List of drugs which modulate the cocaine toxicity.

Category	Subcategory	Drug	Effect
Calcium Channel Antagonists	Dihydropyridines	Nifedipine	↑[15]
		Nitrindipine	↓[50,51,66,68]
		Nimodepine	↓[67,69]
		Nicardipine	↓[67]
	Verapamil Type	Verapamil	↓[4], ↑[15], −[67]
		Diltiazem	↓[67]
	Diphenylalkylamines	Flunarizine	↓[67]
Adrenergic Drugs	α₁ antagonists	Prazosine	↓[12], −[67]
	α₂ antagonists	Yohimbine	↓[37], ↑[74], −[12]
		Idazoxan	−[35]
		RX811059A	−[35]
	α₁,₂ antagonist	Phentolamine	↓[37,67], −[12,61]
		Ergotamine	−[26]
		Dibenamine	−[26]
	α₂ agonist	Clonidine	↓[12]
	β antagonist	Propranolol	↓[12,17,57-59,61], ↓[33,40,56], −[7,8,67]
		Esmolol	↓[53]
	α & β antagonist	Labetalol	↓[12,24,30], −[62,67]
	uptake blockers	Amitriptyline	↓[1]
		Desipramine	↓[35]
	storage depleter	Reserpine	↑[12,26]
Cholinergic Drugs	agonists	Physostigmine	↓[77], ↑[77]
		Neostigmine	↑[77], −[77]
		Oxotremorine	↑[77], −[77]
		Nicotine	↑[77], −[77]
	antagonist	Atropine	↓[23], ↑[77], −[77]
Dopaminergic Drugs	D₁ antagonist	SCH 23390	↓[19,76]
	D₂ antagonist	Haloperidol	↓[17,18]
		Pimozide	−[8]
	non-selective	Chlorpromazine	↓[7,8,33], −[26]
Anticonvulsant Drugs	hydantoins	Diphenylhydantoin	↓[26], ↓[13]
	barbiturates	Phenobarbital	↓[13,26,34,39], −[75]
		Barbital	↓[22,39,64,65], −
	iminostilbenes	Carbamazepine	↓[72], −[13]
	succinimides	Ethosuximide	−[13], −
	GABA mimetics	Valproic acid	↓[13]
		SKF 100330A	↓[13]
	benzodiazepines	Diazepam	↓[8,13,14,17,25,62,75], −[33,67]
		Chlordiazepoxide	↓[25]
	aminobenzamide	LY 201116	↓[13]
	miscellaneous	Acetazolamide	−[26,49]
Miscellaneous Drugs		Hydralazine	↓[12]
		Progesterone	↑[54]
		Hydroxylamine	↓[26]

	Pyridoxine	-[26]
	Ethanol	-[26]
	Flumazenil	↓[13]
	Methadone	↑[36]
	Paraldehyde	↓[39,65]
	Chloralhydrate	↓[39]
	Urethane	-[39]
	Ether	-[39]
angiotensin modulators	Enalaprilat	↓[50,67]
	[Sar-1-ile-8]ANGII	↓[67]
	[Sar-1-thr-8]ANGII	↓[67]
NMDA antagonist	MK 801	↓[13,75]
	Phencyclidine	↓[75]
	Dextromethorphan	-[75]
	CPP	↓[75]
	NPC 12626	↓[75]
glycine antagonist	7CKA	↓[75]
	ACPC	↓[75]
non-opioid antitussive anticonvulsant	Dextromethorphan	-[75]
	Caramiphen	-[75]
	Carbetapentane	-[75]
local anesthetic (antiarrhythmic)	Lidocaine	↑[16]

↑=increase, ↓=decrease, -=no effect, suprascripts=reference number

Table 2. LD_{50} values (mg/kg ip) with 95% confidence intervals of cocaine in control (0) and buprenorphine treated mice.

Buprenorphine (mg/kg ip)	LD_{50} (95% Confidence limit) of cocaine mg/kg	
	1 hr after	24 hrs after
0	100.61 (93.55-108.21)	97.73 (89.54-106.66)
0.15 Potency ratio	113.57 (103.86-124.19) 0.89 (0.79-0.99)**	106.83 (97.03-117.62) 0.91 (0.80-1.04)
0.30 Potency ratio	118.16 (111.17-125.58) 0.85 (0.77-0.94)**	110.56 (102.06-119.76) 0.88 (0.78-0.99)**

**$p < 0.05$

However neither naloxone (10 mg/kg, 15 min before) nor naltrexone (3 mg/kg, 15 min before) showed any significant effect.

Effect of buprenorphine on cocaine-induced increase in LDH activity: In the drug naive control animals the basal plasma LDH level was 297=45 (U/I, mean±SE). Buprenorphine (0.3 mg/kg) pretreatment significantly ($p < 0.05$) attenuated cocaine-induced increase in plasma LDH activity at 0.5, 1, 2, 4 hours after administration of cocaine as compared to its respective saline-treated group (Table 3).

Table 3. Effect of buprenorphine (0.3 mg/kg) on cocaine-induced (80 mg/kg) increase in lactate dehydrogenase (LDH) activity.

Hours after cocaine	LDH (U/l, mean$\pm$SE)	
(80 mg/kg, ip)	Saline	Buprenorphine
0.5	564$\pm$50	405$\pm$43[*]
1	618$\pm$67	364$\pm$36[*]
2	602$\pm$51	432$\pm$40[*]
4	2429$\pm$746	369$\pm$50[*]
8	6378$\pm$1741	6153$\pm$1799
24	15109$\pm$3125	8862$\pm$1947

[*]$p < 0.05$

Discussion: Buprenorphine an opioid agonist/antagonist suppresses cocaine self administration by Rhesus monkey[46,47]. Our study showed that buprenorphine treatment in a dose related manner increased the LD_{50} values and decreased the potency of cocaine-induced lethality.Our results also demonstrated that there was increase in plasma lactate dehydrogenase activity with toxic dose of cocaine.Toxic doses of cocaine produce massive damage to neurological, cardiovascular, gastrointestinal and pulmonary systems[31]. The release of lactate dehydrogenase from dying or metabolically deranged cells is generally considered a likely source of abnormal lactate dehydrogenase in the body fluids[28]. So the protective effect of buprenorphine was further strengthened by our observation that, pretreatment with buprenorphine significantly reversed the cocaine-induced increase in lactate dehydrogenase activity.

Mechanism by which buprenorphine gave protection against cocaine induced toxicity is not clear. Buprenorphine neither binds with high affinity to cocaine receptors sites, nor it enhances the in vitro binding of cocaine receptor ligand[38]. Other opioid agonist-antagonist like methadone increases the toxicity of cocaine[36]. On the other hand, it is speculated that classical opioid drug like morphine increases the toxicity of cocaine by increasing the respiratory depression[27]. Conversely, cocaine also increases the convulsant and acute lethal toxicity of morphine[5]. Our results showed that even opioid antagonists naltrexone and naloxone did not show any protective effect against cocaine-induced toxicity.

Cocaine toxicity is produced through numerous complex mechanisms including hyperstimulation of dopaminergic, noradrenergic pathways, interference with serotonergic, interference at selective sites with neuronal cell membranes as well as other peripheral effects[19]. Drugs which modulate one of these neurotransmitter systems, alter the cocaine-induced toxicity (Table 1). Neurophysiological, neuroendocrine, behavioral studies suggest that opiates modulate the dopaminergic system and converse[46,47]. Buprenorphine has high affinity for mu and kappa opiate receptors[42]. Mu agonist increases whereas kappa agonist decreases the release of dopamine[20]. In in vivo microdialysis study, low doses of buprenorphine or cocaine produced increase in extracellular dopamine in nucleus accumbens and this effect of cocaine was significantly potentiated by co-administering buprenorphine[6]. But in this study peak effect of buprenorphine reached in five hours, whereas for cocaine it took thirty minutes. The dopamine uptake complex is responsible for uptake of dopamine from the synaptic cleft following its release[10,11]. Results from cocaine binding studies have suggested the presence of multiple binding sites on this complex which may be distinct from the binding site of other drugs on the complex[45]. There is complex interaction of cocaine with dopamine uptake carrier complex[3]. There are two or three binding sites for cocaine on this complex and their role is not clear[60]. Desipramine inhibits the uptake of catecholamines, binds at the dopamine uptake complex[60] and also shows protection against cocaine-induced toxicity[35]. The protective effect of buprenorphine in our study may be related to some interaction at dopamine uptake complex, which needs further investigation.

The other possibility in mechanism of protective effect of buprenorphine is the involvement of calcium mediated event. Calcium channel blocker like nimodipine inhibits cocaine-induced dopamine release and motor stimulation[52] and also protects against cocaine-induced toxicity[67,69]. Buprenorphine increases the mitochondrial protein bound calcium and decreases the free intracellular calcium in the different areas of brain[78]. Moreover electrophysiological and biochemical studies have shown that kappa agonists have calcium channel blocking activity[2,44].

It is unlikely that the protective effect of buprenorphine in our study is due to some pharmacokinetic interaction with cocaine. Cocaine is metabolized by liver and plasma cholinestrases[71], whereas buprenorphine is largely inactivated by conjugation with glucuronic acid[55].

To conclude, our results indicate: a) buprenorphine effectively antagonizes cocaine-induced lethality and could be of potential advantage over naloxone in the management of "speed ball toxicity"; b) the mechanism of protective effect of buprenorphine is neither Mu opioid nor a cocaine receptor mediated event; c) in studies on the pharmacotherapy of cocaine-induced toxicity, LDH levels may be used as a biochemical marker to access the protective effects of drugs.

References:

1. Antelman SM, Kocan D, Rowland N, Giovanni LD, Chiodo LA (1981) Amitriptyline provides long-lasting immunization against sudden cardiac death from cocaine. Eur J Pharmacol 69:119-120

2. Attali B, Saya D, Nah S-Y, Vogel Z (1989) k Opiate agonist inhibit Ca^{2+} Influx in rat cord-dorsal root ganglion cocultures. J Biol Chem 264:347-353

3. Berger P, Elsworth JD, Reith MEA, Tanen D, Roth RH (1990) Complex interaction of cocaine with the dopamine uptake carrier. Eur J Pharmacol 176:251-252

4. Billman GE, Hoskins RS (1988) Cocaine-induced ventricular fibrillation: protection afforded by the calcium antagonist verapamil. FASEB J 2:2990-2995

5. Blumberg H, Ikeda C (1978) Naltrexone, morphine and cocaine interactions in mice and rats. J Pharmacol Exp Ther 206:303-310

6. Brown EE, Finlay JM, Wong JTF, Damsma G, Fibiger HC (1991) Behavioral and neurochemical interactions between cocaine and buprenorphine: implications for the pharmacotherapy of cocaine abuse. J Pharmacol Exp Ther 256:119-126

7. Catravas JD, Waters IW, Walz MA, Davis WM (1977) Anidotes for cocaine poisoning [Letter]. N Engl J Med 297:1238

8. Catravas JD, Waters IW (1981) Acute cocaine intoxication in conscious dog: studies on the mechanism of lethality. J Pharmacol Exp Ther 247:350-356

9. Catravas JD, Waters IW, Walz MA, Davis WM (1978) Acute cocaine intoxication in conscious dog: pathophysiologic profile of acute lethality. Arch Int Pharmacodyn 235:328-340

10. Coyle JT, Snyder SH (1969a) Regional differences in ^{3}H-norepinephrine and ^{3}H-dopamine uptake into rat brain homogenates. J Pharmacol Exp Ther 165:78-85

11. Coyle JT, Snyder SH (1969b) Catecholamine uptake by synaptosomes in homogenates of rat brain: stereospecificity of different areas. J Pharmacol Exp Ther 170:221-231

12. Derlet RW, Albertson TE (1990a) Acute cocaine toxicity: antagonism by agents interacting with adrenoceptor. Pharmacol Biochem Behav 36:225-231

13. Derlet RW, Albertson TE (1990b) Anticonvulsant modification of cocaine-induced toxicity in the rat. Neuropharmacology 29:255-259

14. Derlet RW, Albertson TE (1989b) Diazepam in the prevention of seizures and death in cocaine-intoxicated rats. Ann Emerg Med 18:542-546

15. Derlet RW, Albertson TE (1989a) Potentiation of cocaine toxicity with calcium channel blockers. Am J Emerg Med 7:464-468

16. Derlet RW, Albertson TE (1990c) Potentiation of cocaine toxicity with lidocaine (abstract 65). Ann Emerg Med 19:180

17. Derlet RW, Albertson TE, Rice P (1990a) Antagonism of cocaine, amphetamine and methamphetamine toxicity. Pharmacol Biochem Behav 36:745-749

18. Derlet RW, Albertson TE, Rice P (1989) The effect of haloperidol in cocaine and amphetamine intoxication. J Emerg Med 7:633-637

19. Derlet RW, Albertson TE, Rice P (1990b) The effect of SCH 23390 against toxic doses of cocaine, d-amphetamine and methamphetamine. Life Sci 47:821-827

20. DiChiara G, Imperato A (1988) Opposite effects of *Mu* and *Kappa* opiate agonists on dopamine release in the nucleus accumbens and in the dorsal caudate of freely moving rats. J Pharmacol Exp Ther 244:1067-1080

21. Doris C, Asgar K, Brown R (1988) Preface. In: Doris C, Asgar K, Brown R (eds) Mechanisms of cocaine abuse and toxicity NIDA Res. Monograph 88 (United States Department of Health and Human Services, Rockville) pp IX-X

22. Downs AW, Eddy NB (1932) The influence of barbital upon cocaine poisoning in the rat. J Pharmacol Exp Ther 45:383-387

23. Dragstedt CA, Lang VF (1928) Respiratory stimulants in acute cocaine poisoning in rabbits. J Pharmacol Exp Ther 32:215-222

24. Dusenberry SJ, Hicks MJ, Mariani PJ (1987) Labetalol treatment of cocaine toxicity (letter). Ann Emerg Med 16:235

25. Eidelberg E, Neer HM, Miller MK (1963) Anticonvulsant properties of some benzodiazepine derivatives. Neurology 15:223-230

26. Eidelberg E, Lesse H, Gault FP (1965) An experimental model of temporal lobe epilepsy: studies of convulsant properties of cocaine. In: Glaser GH (ed). EEG and Behavior. Basic Book Inc Publishers, New York London, pp 272-283

27. Ellinwood EH Jr, Eibergen RD, Kilbey MM (1976) Stimulants: interaction with clinically relevant drugs. Ann NY Acad Sci 281:393-408

28. Erickson RJ, Morales DR (1961) Clinical use of lactic dehydrogenase. N Engl J Med 265:531-534

29. Fleming JA, Byck R, Barash (1990) Pharmacology and therapeutic applications of cocaine. Anesthesiology 73:518-531

30. Gay GR, Loper KA (1988) The use of labetalol in the management of cocaine crisis. Ann Emerg Med 17:282-283

31. Goldfrank LR, Hoffman RS (1991) The cardio vascular effects of cocaine. Ann Emerg Med 20:165-175

32. Griesemer EC, Liu Y, Budd RD, Raftogianis L, Noguchi TT (1983) The determination of cocaine and its major metabolite, benzoylecgonine, in postmortem fluids and tissues by computerized gas chromatography/massspectrometry. J Forensic Sci 28:894-900

33. Guinn MM, Bedford JA, Wilson MC (1980) Antagonism of intravenous cocaine lethality in nonhuman primates. Clin Toxicol 16:499-508

34. Guttman MR (1928) Acute cocaine intoxication: prophylaxis and treatment with phenobarbital. JAMA 90:753-755

35. Jackson HC, Ball DM, Nutt DJ (1990) Noradrenergic mechanisms appear not to be involved in cocaine-induced seizures and lethality. Life Sci 47:353-359

36. Jaffe JH, Witkin JM, Goldberg SR, Katz JL (1989) Potential toxic interactions of cocaine and mazindol. Lancet 2:111

37. James RC, Schiefer MA, Roberts SM, Harbinson RD (1987) Antagonism of cocaine-induced hepatotoxicity by the alpha adrenergic antagonists phentolamine and yohimbine. J Pharmacol Exp Ther 242:726-732

38. Kamien JB, Bergman J, Madras BK, Spealman RD (1990) Buprenorphine potentiates behavioral effects of cocaine in squirrel monkeys. FASEB J 4:A593

39. Knoefel PK, Herwick RP, Loevenhart AS (1928) The prevention of acute intoxication from local anesthetics. J Pharmacol Exp Ther 33:397-411

40. Lang RA, Cigarroa RG, Flores ED, McBride W, et al (1990) Potentiation of cocaine-induced coronary vasoconstriction by beta-adrenergic blockade. Ann Intern Med 112:897-903

338

41. Lewin NA, Goldfrank LR, Weissman RS (1986) Cocaine. In: Goldfrank LR, et al (eds) Goldfrank's Toxicológic Emergencies. Appleton-Century-Crofts, Norwalk pp 477

42. Lewis JW (1985) Buprenorphine. Drug Alcohol Depend 14:362-372

43. Lie JT (1990) Medical complications of cocaine and other illicit drug abuse stimulating rheumatic disease. J Rheumatol 17:736-737

44. MacDonald RL, Werz MA (1986) Dynorphine decreases voltage-dependent calcium conductance of mouse dorsal root ganglion neurones. J Physiol (Lond) 377:237-249

45. Madras BK, Fahey MA, Bergman J, Canfield DR, Spealman RD (1989) Effects of cocaine and related drugs in non-human primates. I. ^{3}H-cocaine binding sites in caudate-putamen. J Pharmacol Exp Ther 251:131-141

46. Mello NK, Mendelson JH, Bree MP, Lukas SE (1989) Buprenorphine supresses cocaine self-administration by rhesus monkeys. Science 245:859-862

47. Mello NK, Mendelson JH, Bree MP, Lukas SE (1990) Buprenorphine and naltrexone effects on cocaine self-administration by rhesus monkey. J Pharmacol Exp Ther 254:926-939

48. Mendelson JH, Mello NK, Cristofaro P, Skupny A, Ellingboe J (1986) Use of naltrexone as a provocative test for hypothalamic-pituitary harmone function. Pharmacol Biochem Behav 24:309-313

49. Mennear JH, Rudzik AD (1966) Potentiation of the anticonvulsant action of acetazolamide. J Pharm Pharmac 18:833-834

50. Nahas GG, Trouve R, Manger WM (1990) Cocaine catecholamines and cardiac toxicity. Acta Anaesthesiol Scand 34(Suppl 94):77-81

51. Nahas GG, Trouve R, Demus JF, Von Sitbon M (1985) A calcium-channel blocker as antidote to the cardiac effects of cocaine intoxication (letter). N Engl J Med 313:519-520

52. Pani L, Carboni S, Kusmin A, Gessa GL, Rossetti ZL (1990) Nimodipine inhibits cocaine-induced dopamine release and motor stimulation. Eur J Pharmacol 176:245-246

53. Pollan S, Tadjziechy M (1989) Esmolol in the management of epinephrine- and cocaine-induced cardiovascular toxicity. Anesth Analg 69:663-664

54. Plessinger MA, Woods JR (1990) Progesterone increases cardiovascular toxicity to cocaine in nonpregnant ewes. Am J Obstet Gynecol 163:1659-1664

55. Rance MJ, Shillingford JS (1976) The role of gut in the metabolism of strong analgesics. Biochem Pharmacol 25:735-741

56. Ramoska E, Sacchetti AD (1985) Propranolol-induced hypertention in treatment of cocaine intoxication. Ann Emerg Med 14:1112-1113

57. Rappolt RT, Gay G, Inaba DS, Rappolt NR (1976a) Propranolol in cocaine toxicity (letter). Lancet 2:640-641

58. Rappolt RT, Gay G, Inaba DS (1976b) Propranolol in the treatment of cardiopressor effects of cocaine. N Engl J Med 295:448

59. Rappolt RT, Gay GR, Soman M, Kobernick M (1979) Treatment plan for acute and chronic adrenergic poisoning crisis utilizing sympatholytic effects of the B^1-B^2 receptor site blocker propranolol (Inderal) in concert with diazepam and urine acidification. Clin Toxicol 14:55-69

60. Richfield EK (1991) Quantitative autoradigraphy of the dopamine uptake complex in the rat brain using [^{3}H]GBR 12935: binding characteristics. Brain Research 540:1-13

61. Robin ED, Wong RJ, Ptashne KA (1989) Increased lung water and ascites after massive cocaine over-dosage in mice and improved survival related to beta-adrenergic blockage. Ann Intern Med 110:202-207

62. Spivey WH, Schofftall JM, Kirkpatrick R, Fuhs L (1990) Comparison of labetalol, diazepam and haloperidol for the treatment of cocaine toxicity in swine model. Ann Emerg Med 19:467-468

63. Stewart DJ, Inaba T, Tang BK, Kalow W (1977) Hydrolysis of cocaine in human plasma by cholinestrase. Life Sci 20:1557-1564

64. Tatum AL, Collins KH (1926) Acute cocaine poisoning and its treatment in the monkey (Macacus Rhesus). Arch Int Med 38:405-409

65. Tatum AL, Atkinson AJ, Collins KH (1925) Acute cocaine poisoning, its prophylaxis and treatment in labotatory animals. J Pharmacol Exp Ther 26:325-335

66. Trouve R, Nahas GG (1986) Nitrendipine: an antidot of cardiac and lethal toxicity of cocaine. Proc Soc Exp Biol Med 183:392-397

67. Trouve R, Nahas GG (1990) Antidot to lethal cocaine toxicity in the rat. Arch Int Pharmacodyn 305:197-207

68. Trouve R, Nahas GG, Maillet M (1987) Nitrendipine as an antagonist to the cardiac toxicity of cocaine. J Cardiovasc Pharmacol 9[Suppl 4]:549-553

69. Trouve R, Nahas GG, Manger WM, Vinyard C, Goldberg S (1990) Interaction of nimodipine and cocaine on endogenous catecholamines in the squirrel monkey. Proc Soc Exp Biol Med 193:171-175

70. Trouve R, Nahas GG, Manger WM (1991) Catecholamines, cocaine toxicity and their antidotes in the rat. Proc Soc Exp Biol Med 196:184-187

71. Vitti TG, Boni RL (1985) Metabolism of cocaine. In: Barnett G and Chiang CN (ed) Pharmacokinetics and pharmacodynamics of psychoactive drugs: a research monograph. Biomedical Publication, Foster City, CA, pp 427-440

72. Weiss SRB, Post RM, Szele F, Woodward R, Nierenberg J (1989) Chronic carbamazepine inhibits the development of local anesthetic seizures kindled by cocaine and lidocaine. Brain Research 497:72-79

73. Werz MA, MacDonald RL (1985) Dynorphine and neoendorphine pepides decrease dorsal root ganglion neuron calcium-dependent action potential duration. J Pharmacol Exp Ther 234:49-56

74. Wilkerson RD (1989) Cardiovascular effects of cocaine: enhancement by yohimbine and atropine. J Pharmacol Exp Ther 248:57-61

75. Witkin JM, Tortella FC (1991) Modulators of n-methyl-d-aspartate protect against diazepam- or phenobarbital-resistant cocaine convulsions 48:PL-51-PL-56

76. Witkin JM, Goldberg SR, Katz JL (1989a) Lethal effects of cocaine are reduced by the dopamine-1 receptor antagonist SCH 23390 but not by haloperidol. Life Sci 44:1285-1291

77. Witkin JM, Goldberg SR, Katz JL, Kuhar MJ (1989b) Modulation of the lethal effects of cocaine by cholinomimetics. Life Sci 45:2295-2301

78. Zhao XN, Liao H, Shi SL, Wang JJ, Xing J, Chen J, Zhang ZX, Chen RS (1990) Effects of buprenorphine on mitochondrial protein bound Ca^{2+} in the some brain regions. In: Collery Ph, et al (ed) Metal ions in biology and medicine. John Libbey Eurotext, Paris, pp 135-137

Criminal Law and AIDS

W. Bottke

Lehrstuhl für Strafrecht, Strafprozeßrecht und Kriminologie, Universität Augsburg,
Universitätsstraße 2, D-W-8900 Augsburg, Federal Republic of Germany

I. Introduction

Few social problems present the lawyer with difficulties such
as those in the question of 'AIDS prevention'.

1. All social issues allot to the lawyer the task of applying
his specific domestic law to a 'case' which he has formulated
on the basis of a 'real life situation' according to his
domestic 'legal rules'. Such a process, for instance, implies
interpretation of statutory law provisions, definition of the
ratio decidendi of legal precedents, limitation of the
infinite details of the 'real life situation' to the
'relevant facts', careful distinction of the 'case at hand'
from previously decided cases, and submission of the case at
hand to the established legal rules. A lawyer accustomed to
statutory law generally applies the legal rules without
questioning whether their application makes 'the best sense'
or whether other legislatorial decisions could resolve the
social problem in a better way. He abides by legal rules
which are enacted by a democratically legitimatized
legislator. He has only to ask whether those rules are
compatible with the constitution, but he has not to
scrutinize or reject the policy of a legal rule which
fulfills the constitutional requirements. Criminal law
provisions must also be applied in this way.

2. In a real life situation where the HIV might be transmitted, an *'apolitical' application of criminal law provisions* raises doubts. If the transmissivity of the HIV is caused by a sexual action, based on eternal or momentary love between monogamous, polygamous or promiscuitive, heterosexual or homosexual partners[1] who agree to the sexual act[2], application of a criminal law provision would appear to be an intrusion into the private life of people who are entitled to enjoy their sexuality[3]. There is little reason to believe that criminal law will prevent people from searching for sexual fulfillment in a non-aggressive way[4]. Instead of applying criminal law as a repressive measure of AIDS prevention, it seems preferable to strengthen the self-responsibility of all persons who are interested in having sexual contact, by offering them information about, and stimulating them, in a non-repressive way to 'safer sex'[5]. If transmission of the HIV is caused by two intravenous fixers

---

1 Application of a valid criminal law provision is more acceptable in cases where the AIDS-virus transmissive behaviour is based on an act of physical aggression.

2 The mutual agreement to the sexual act does not necessarily mean that both are aware of the risks involved.

3 Constitutions which guarantee an all-encompassing right to human freedom (e.g. Article 2 I German Constitution), acknowledge also a human right to sexuality, whether homo- or heterosexual, promiscuitive, polygamous or monogamous.

4 The criminalization of rape or other ways of aggressive sexuality is not a counter argument. A rapist does not primarily want 'to make love'. He wants to master and to command his victim, by using physical force. Compare to the criminology of rape CLARK/LEWIS, Rape: The Price of Coercive Sexuality, Toronto 1977; EISENBERG, Kriminologie, 3. Aufl. 1990, § 45 Rz 34 ff.

5 Compare RÜHMAN, Aids und Recht: Zur Geschichte des Gesetzes zur Bekämpfung der Geschlechtskrankheiten, in: PRITTWITZ (Hrsg.), Aids, Recht und Gesundheitspolitik, 1990, S. 31 ff.; SCHMACKE, Aids und Seuchengesetze: Anmerkungen zu historischen Erfahrungen bei der "Bekämpfung" von Infektionskrankheiten, in: PRITTWITZ (Hrsg.), Aids, Recht und Gesundheitspolitik, 1990, S. 17 ff.; SCHÜNEMANN, Die Rechtsprobleme der Aids-Eindämmung, in: SCHÜNEMANN/PFEIFFER (Hrsg.), Die Rechtsprobleme von AIDS, 1988, S. 373 ff..

using a contaminated syringe[6], application of a criminal law provision could resemble a helpless attempt to change the attitude of people who have shown an often immalleable disposition to self-endangering behaviour and have no fear of the 'poena naturalis' which threatens their fate. Finally, in all cases where an AIDS infected person is convicted for having put the life or health of his partner at an intolerable risk, penalization of his deed is harsh. Although the AIDS infected person is a human being who is suffering from a terrible disease and deserves care and help, his conviction and sentencing in court define him as a malefactor.

3. In order to speak in realistic terms about the behaviour of AIDS infected persons which puts other individuals at a risk of infection, it is advisable to discuss not only the question of which criminal law provisions are applicable but also the applicability of criminal law itself. I will therefore first discuss the *criminalpolitical sense of applying criminal law* and then focus on the *principles valid for 'intralegal' discussion*.

II. Legitimatization of the application of criminal law

1. Criminal law cannot be legitimatized by its *'positive special preventive impact'* on the future behaviour of the prosecuted and convicted person. There is no empirical proof that criminal law enforcement helps to educate, socialize or rehabilitate the defendant. On the contrary, incrimination damages his social reputation, conviction stigmatizes him, and imprisonment has often no positive therapeutic effect upon the inmate[7].

---

6 Compare e.g., KREUZER, Strafrecht als Hinderniss sinnvoller Aids-Prophylaxe?, in: NStZ 1987, S. 268 ff..

7 On the efforts to improve social rehabilitation work in prisons compare GLASER, The Effectivness of a Prison and

Although it is true that the AIDS infected person is not helped by being prosecuted, convicted and sentenced for criminal behaviour according to the rules of law, this is no argument against the application of criminal law, provided it can be legitimatized for other criminalpolitical reasons.

2. Under the theory of *integrative prevention*, or of *positive general prevention*[8], prosecution of crimes is reasonable because it strengthens people's readiness to respect the legally protected interests and furthers common reluctance to break criminal law prohibitions.

a) The severity of possible penal sanctions generally has no proven influence upon crime commission. However, social behaviour, whether legal or illegal, is learned through observation and positive association, imitation and internalization. The more potential delinquents truly calculate or even overestimate the risk of their future prosecution, the less willing they are to commit crime. Although criminal prosecution does not prevent the 'secret' commission of crime, it reduces 'open' crime commission and thereby the possibility of a potential delinquent's association with other criminals and criminal behaviour. Since criminal proceedings reduce the number of blatant bad examples, they are an effective means of social instruction and a working means of *social learning*.

b) The chances of integrative prevention are of course diminished when virus-transmissive behaviour is committed in private. Definition and prosecution of criminal behaviour still reinform, however, the public and other potential delinquents of the interests which are protected by the applied criminal law provisions. The *communication* of legal values endangered by criminal behaviour might be called

---

Parole System, 1964; HAWKINS, The Prison, 1976; SYKES, The Society of Captives, 1958.

8 Compare MÜLLER-DIETZ, Integrationsprävention im Strafrecht. Zum positiven Aspekt der Generalprävention. Ergebnisse und Chancen der Forschung, 1989.

344

ritualistic or symbolistic. But it is also a realistic and
necessary contribution to common legal behaviour in a
secularized society where religious beliefs have lost guiding
force.

3. Even though the hypothesis about the communicative
function of criminal prosecution in virus-transmissive cases
is questionable, *justice* demands equal treatment of equal
cases. If the legislator classified certain submissions of
another person under an intolerable risk as a criminal deed,
it would be ('lying silence' and) a *breach of law* if (his
spoken words were not repeated[9] and) his legal provision
were not applied in a case where all elements of the
statutory law provision are fulfilled. The AIDS phenomenon
has no legislative power. It does not derogate the general
will expressed in criminal law provisions.

III. Principles of Criminal Law Application on AIDS-Virus Transmissive Behaviour

The *'intralegal' questions* presented by the various domestic
legal systems cannot be discussed here in detail[10]. I will
therefore attempt to reveal the *common principles of the
evaluation of AIDS-Virus transmissive behaviour* which are

---

9 Statutory criminal law provisions might be called commands
   which have to be reinforced by verbal repetition and real
   application. They can be interpreted as 'legislatorial
   speech', hereby falling under the obligation of any
   communicative action to speak consistently and to speak the
   truth.

10 Compare e.g. BOTTKE, Transmission of Infective Ejaculate
   in Unprotected Sexual Intercourse by HIV-infected Persons
   to Minors, in: AIFO 1988, S. 628 ff.; BOTTKE, Transmission
   of the AIDS Virus as a Criminal Law Problem, in: AIFO 1989,
   S. 152 ff.; BOTTKE, Rechtsfragen beim ungeschützten
   Geschlechtsverkehr eines HIV-Infizierten, in: AIFO 1989, S.
   468 ff.; EBERBACH, Rechtsproblem der HTLV-III-Infektion
   (AIDS), 1986; PRITTWITZ (Hrsg.), Aids, Recht und
   Gesundheitspolitik, 1990; SCHÜNEMANN/PFEIFFER (Hrsg.), Die
   Rechtsprobleme von AIDS, 1988. Further information in:
   DREHER/TRÖNDLE, StGB, 45 editn., 1991, § 223 Rz 6a.

valid in all western democracies with a statutory criminal law system.

1. Punishment of a *completed criminal offence* which is characterized by the actually caused *damage* of an individual's legally protected interest such as life or health, presupposes that the *causality* of the act can be proven in court beyond all reasonable doubt.

a) This is barely possible in instances of hetero- or homosexual contact between promiscuous persons or of joint use of a syringe by intravenous fixers. The possibility that a member of such a risk group has been infected by another contact either before or after the alleged criminal act, can practically never be excluded. Moreover, the AIDS virus cannot be diagnosed immediately after presumed transmission. The seropositive result of a blood test only discovers the development of antibodies, but does not connect this finding with a particular person or act. Finally, an AIDS infected person, alledgedly responsible for the 'criminal' infection of another, can only be prosecuted if his personal state of health does not hinder him from defending himself in court.

b) The aforementioned dogmatic and forensic monita do not only exclude the conviction of an AIDS infected person who is aware of the risks involved or is even evil minded, for having committed an intented violation of an individual's interest (e.g. of health by causing bodily harm[11]). The necessity to demonstrate in court the link of causality between the virus transmissive act committed by the AIDS infected 'first victim', and the infection of his partner as the 'second victim', also makes practically impossible the conviction for having committed a reckless or neglient

---

11 Even though a person infected with the AIDS virus may not feel unwell and will perhaps have had a long period of incubation, from the moment of his own infection he is infectious to others. The infection alone causes actual injury and suffices for the assumption of 'bodily harm', see e.g. BGHSt. 36, S. 1 ff.; Further information in: DREHER/TRÖNDLE, StGB, 45 editn. 1991, § 223 Rz 6b.

346

violation of an individual's interest. Dogmatic attempts to substitute the requirement of causality between transmissive act and infection with the transmissivity of the act in cases of reckless or negligent behaviour[12], have to be rejected. They would lead to the establishment of an illegitimate 'special law'. They would be a violation of the 'nullum crimen sine lege'-principle[13] which makes any affirmation that a crime has been committed, dependent on the fulfillment of all elements of the criminal law provision. As to crimes of the aforementioned kind, the legal rules defining e.g. 'real injury' or 'reckless killing', demand more than 'risk aggravation' or 'risk submission'. They claim for the proof of 'risk realization', i.e. of causality.

2. Punishment of a *completed criminal offence*, however, is possible as far as the domestic law criminalizes the mere *endangerment* of a legally protected interest which may belong to an individual or to the society.

a) For instance, the domestic law could define AIDS as a contagious and/or venereal disease and penalize the exposition of another person to the risk of being infected by sexual intercourse[14]. A risk exponent whose virus transmissive behaviour[15] fulfills all elements of the

---

12 Attempts to substitute the requirement of causality with the lesser requirement of proven risk aggravation have been unsuccessful; compare on the one hand OTTO, Risikoerhöhungsprinzip statt Kausalitätsgrundsatz als Zurechnungskriterium bei Erfolgsdelikten, in: NJW 1980, S. 417 ff., on the other hand LACKNER, StGB, 18. Aufl., 1989, vor § 13, Anm. III 1 c dd.

13 Compare KREY, Keine Strafe ohne Gesetz, 1983; SCHÜNEMANN, Nulla poena sine lege?, 1978.

14 In the Federal Republic of Germany AIDS was not included in the 'numerus clausus' of such contagious and/or venereal diseases, compare § 1 BSeuchG.

15 Which forms of sexual behaviour are relevantly 'virus transmissive', is an empirical question. One might ascribe a relevantly riskful behaviour to all forms of penetration with the real or possible intromission of contagious bodily secretions, especially of male ejaculate but also of pre-ejaculative fluids, compare e.g. BGHSt. 36, S. 1 ff..

statutory law provision, may be convicted and sentenced according to the domestic legal rule[16] which protects the 'health of the public' from endangerment. A legal system which provides such a *legis specialis*, facilitates the juristic evaluation of behaviour which submits a sexual partner of the HIV carrier to a relevant risk; it bars the discussion whether or not acts of risk exposition by sexual intercourse must be regarded as criminal attempts (see III 3).

b) Law provisions which penalize any contribution to the traffic and/or consumption of illegal drugs, should not be enforced in cases where a 'disposable' or 'one-way' syringe is sold or otherwise offered to an AIDS-infected drug addict[17]. A free democratic society which does not patronize its members but respects their rights to self-determination and self-endangerment, does not criminalize drug dealing in order to prevent people from consuming drugs. It criminalizes in order to control the production and the trade of drugs[18]. A free democratic society need not penalize a pharmacist who sells 'one-way' syringes to a drug addict. Such rigid law enforcement would be counter-productive to a reasonable AIDS prevention policy. 'Needle sharing', however, by common use of a syringe is submissive to those rules of criminal law which penalize any offering of technical means of drug abuse.

3. Law systems without a 'legis specialis' criminalizing all AIDS transmissive behaviour leave it up to further consideration whether all potentially infectious contacts can

---

16 The Austrian Penal Code offers with §§ 178, 179, ÖStGB, § 2 I AIDS-Gesetz (ÖBGBl. 1986, S. 293) a legal provision to which the exposition to the risk of HIV infection committed by sexual intercourse is submissive, compare BITTMANN, Strafrechtliche Probleme im Zusammenhang mit AIDS, in: ÖJZ 1987, S. 486 ff..

17 KREUZER, Besonderheiten von AIDS und Drogenabhängigkeit, in: PRITTWITZ (Hrsg.), Aids, Recht und Gesundheitspolitik, 1990, S. 171 ff., S. 175 ff..

18 BOTTKE, Strafrechtliche Probleme von AIDS und der AIDS-Bekämpfung, in: SCHÜNEMANN/PFEIFFER (Hrsg.), Die REchtsprobleme von AIDS, 1988, S. 171 ff., S. 221.

348

be regarded as a *criminal attempt* to cause bodily harm[19] or even to commit manslaughter (presupposing that such attempts are criminalized by domestic statutory law).

a) Any criminal attempt requires that the infectious person has the 'wrongful intent' to transmit the HIV to his partner. It is questionable when 'wrongful intent' might be affirmed.

aa) There is no wrongful intent as long as the infected person is ignorant of his own infection and also has no reasonable cause to assume that he is infectious. There is wrongful intent as soon as the infected person is evil minded and aware of his one infectiousness, of his virus transmissive behaviour and of the fact that he endangers a person who is ignorant of the risks involved.

bb) It is, however, disputable whether there is wrongful intent if the 'first victim' of the AIDS epidemic is not 'evil minded' but *only conscious* of his own contamination and of his transmissive behaviour.
On the one hand, such a person hopes or even believes that 'everything will turn out well'; he does not 'want' to do bodily harm to his partner. On the other hand, a person who is aware that he is infected with AIDS, but nevertheless comes into virus transmissive contact with another by needlesharing or by sexual intercourse, presupposedly puts the health, and in the long run, the life of his partner at risk. If the infectious person is the only one who is conscious of the risks involved, he should remember the commandment "Thou shalt not (harm or) kill" and abide by it as a command of law. He should also follow the Golden Rule[20] stating that one should do to others as he would have others

---

19 The Courts in the Federal Republic of Germany affirm that the possible intromission of infectious bodily fluids into a partner by sexual intercourse must be regarded as a 'qualified criminal attempt to cause bodily harm', §§ 22, 223 a StGB , compare e.g. BGHSt. 36, S. 1 ff.. Further information in: DREHER/TRÖNDLE StGB, 45 editn. 1991, § 223a Rz 5a.

20 Compare Mathew 7:12

do to him (In other words: to avoid the dangerous act, to attenuate the risk, e.g. by using 'safer sex', or to inform his partner of the risks involved and to give him the chance to choose between dangerous, less dangerous or riskless contacts).

cc) Nota bene: There is *no wrongful intent* if a person knows that he exposes another to an intolerable risk but is insouciant or perhaps even disapproves, the fulfillment of the known risk. This is also valid in cases of HIV transmissive behaviour.

aaa) The criminal law of a specific country *may* use 'wrongful intent' as a synonym for 'on purpose', especially in cases of a completed criminal act which caused real harm. On the contrary, the *combination of cognizance* (of mere possibility, for instance, of 'virus transmissivity') *and disapproval* (of result realization, e.g.: of 'virus transmission') is considered to be reckless.

bbb) The criminal law of a specific country *may*, however, also evaluate the *awareness of the subjection of another to an intolerable risk*, as 'criminal intent'. Firstly, in cases where only the infectious person is conscious of the risks involved, he is the 'master of the situation' who can atually choose between 'dangerous contact', 'avoidance of contact', 'delegation of choice' by information or opting for means which 'reduce the extent of the risk from intolerable to tolerable' (e.g.: by using a condom). Secondly, the difference in the extent of criminalization and in the severity of the penalty for 'intended', 'reckless' and 'negligent' criminal acts, should not be legitimatized by the degree of 'consent' to the realization of the known risk or by other 'volitive' attitudes. The difference may be legitimatized by the existence or non-existence of 'cognition', i.e., the awareness that a person would be exposed to an intolerable predicament if he is the only incogniszant of his subjection to the danger. The affirmation of 'wrongful intent' secures the right of a person to veto a risk which he did not procure unlafully and for which he is not otherwise responsible.

dd) In summation, *if* the domestic law defines 'criminal intent' without refering to 'volitive' moments, a risk exponent who consciously subjects another to an intolerable risk by virus transmissive behaviour, may be punished for attempted violation of an individual's legally protected interest. Such punishment presupposes that the domestic legal rules criminalize a specific attempted violation (e.g.: penalize attempted bodily harm either generally or under certain circumstances, such as the use of one's body as a 'deadly weapon').

b) No criminal *'exposure'* of another to an intolerable risk must be affirmed if the infectious person shares his knowledge of the riks involved with his partner. A free democratic society guarantees the right to self determination[21] and principally entitles its members even to self endangerment[22]. Any criminal law provision of such a society is only legitimately applicable as far as its enforcement finally serves an individual's freedom and rights or the functioning of the society as a whole. If the AIDS infected person deliberately refrains from informing his partner of the risks involved, he violates his partner's right of self determination, that is to say, the right to decide freely whether there is a risk and, if so, whether he is prepared to accept the risk and the danger to which he is being exposed. The duty to inform, the right to be informed and the criminalization of omitted information assure that both the infectious person and his partner are equally aware of the risks involved in the virus transmissive behaviour.

---

21 BOTTKE, Strafrechtliche Probleme von AIDS und der AIDS-Bekämpfung, in: SCHÜNEMANN/PFEIFFER (Hreg.), Die Rechtsprobleme von AIDS, 1988, S. 171 ff., S. 186 f..

22 BOTTKE, Strafrechtliche Probleme von AIDS und der AIDS-Bekämpfung, in: SCHÜNEMANN/PFEIFFER (Hrsg.), Die Rechtsprobleme von AIDS, 1988, S. 171 ff., S. 186 f..

The rules of law do not demand that homosexual or heterosexual persons be in love with the partner with whom they are sexually intimate. The legal order of a free democratic society does, however, insist on 'cognitive honesty', which constitutes a 'symmetric' awareness of the relevant risks involved and secures the partner's right to self determination, i.e. to either accept the risk of virus transmission, or to refuse any contact with virus transmissive behaviour, or to reduce the risk. If the infectious person fails to share his available information about his infectiousness with his partner, his behaviour is unlawful and might fulfill all necessary elements of a criminal attempt to do bodily harm.

c) The primary purpose of the verdict of any trial is to 'speak the truth' and to define accurately which rule of law prescribing social behaviour, was broken by the convicted, and which damage or endangerment was caused by the criminal deed. Verdicts must be 'in full truth with all relevant facts'. Convictions must 'truly and truthfully' communicate those legally protected values which were endangered by the wrongful behaviour, and reinform other potential delinquents as to how they should behave in similar situations.

aa) At first sight, a judge who considers the 'communicative' function of verdicts, might even speak in terms of criminal law about the lethal risk, consciously caused by virus transmissive behaviour. Contingent intent can not only be based on the awareness of the primary risk to cause bodily harm, but also on the cognition of the final risk to cause death. This risk is already exposed to the partner at the moment of secure intromission of infectious fluids. The risk cannot be prevented from realization by medical treatment as long as no cure for AIDS exists. If, horribile dictu, the 'intromitter' knowingly subjects his incognizant partner to the lethal risk, he has begun and tried 'to kill'.

bb) At second sight, however, it is objectionable whether conscious virus-transmissive behaviour fulfills all elements of statutory law provisions which penalize 'attempted

352

manslaughter[23]. 'Manslaughter' may demand more than just the
unlawful killing of another human being without expressed or
implied malice. According to its second word, 'man-slaughter'
is the 'slaughtering' of another. It conveys the connotation
of killing "in a bloody or barbarous manner"[24] and may
require some action which soon causes the death of the
victim. An AIDS infected person who consciously exposes his
incognizant parner to the finally lethal risk, hardly
'slaughters' or 'slays' if the virus transmissive behaviour
lacks physical force or another form of violence. The lethal
risk is typically not realized in the near future. Generally,
the risk exponent does not 'attempt to slaughter' and has not
to be convicted for having committed 'attempted
manslaughter'[25].

23 Compare HERZBERG, Die Strafandrohung als Waffe im Kampf
   gegen AIDS? in: NJW 1987, S. 1461 ff.; GEPPERT, Strafbares
   Verhalten durch mögliche AIDS-Übertragung, in: JURA 1987,
   S. 668 ff.; KREUZER, Aids und Strafrecht, in: ZStW 100
   (1988), S. 786 ff.; MEIER, Strafrechtliche Aspekte der
   Aids-Übertragung, in: GA 1989, S. 207 ff.. The German
   Supreme Court did not exclude 'attempted murder' according
   to §§ 22, 212 StGB, BGHSt. 36, S. 1 ff., S. 16. Further
   information in: DREHER/TRÖNDLE, StGB, 45 editn., 1991, §
   223 Rz 6b.

24 Compare Websters Third New International Dictionary Of The
   English Language , Unabridged, and Britannica World
   Language Dictionary, Volume III, 1971, "slaughter".

25 It might be that there is a difference between the 'rules
   of social behaviour' which prevent the AIDS infected person
   from killing his partner (i.e., not to expose the
   incognizant partner to a lethal risk) and the criminal law
   provision penalizing only such cases of 'lethal risk
   exposure' which show some kind of violence or force. Open
   to further discussion is whether these objections are only
   of 'linguistic value'. Compare BOTTKE, Rechtsfragen beim
   ungeschützten Geschlechtsverkehr eines HIV-Infizierten, in:
   AIFO 1989, S. 468 ff, S. 468 f..

IV. Summary

Criminal law is a repressive means and the last option of AIDS prevention. Its application has to comply with the rules of domestic law. Possible conviction for criminal attempt in cases of conscious risk exposure by virus transmissive behaviour assures the right of self-determination. Such judgement strengthens the duty to inform the endangered partner of the risks involved. If 'attempted manslaughter' is denied and no special criminal law provision exists, the legislator should enact such a legal rule crminalizing conscious virus transmissive behaviour.

Criminal law enforcement does not 'solve' the problem of AIDS. Such law enforcement is only acceptable if all members of society are active in administrating care and help to all people suffering from AIDS.
Legislatorial measures should foster common readiness to support AIDS infected persons. For instance, people who help AIDS infected persons in recognized social services should have a legalized right to refuse to give evidence[26].
A law against unreasonable employment discrimination is recommendable. The legal order should also provide a form of 'protective cloak' for AIDS infected persons!

---

26 KREUZER, Konflikte zwischen Strafjustiz und Drogen - sowie Aids-Beratungsdiensten, in: PRITTWITZ (Hrsg.), Aids, Recht und Gesundheitspolitik, 1990, S. 181 ff..

Reference List

BITTMANN Strafrechtliche Probleme im Zusammenhang mit AIDS
in: ÖJZ 1987 S. 486 ff

BOTTKE Transmission of Infective Ejaculate in Unprotected
Sexual Intercourse by HIV-infected Persons to Minors in:
AIFO 1988 S. 628 ff

BOTTKE Transmission of the AIDS Virus as a Criminal Law
Problem in: AIFO 1989 S. 152 ff

BOTTKE Rechtsfragen beim ungeschützten Geschlechtsverkehr
eines HIV-Infizierten in: AIFO 1989 S. 468 ff

EBERBACH Rechtsproblem der HTLV-III-Infektion (AIDS) 1986

GEPPERT Strafbares Verhalten durch mögliche AIDS-Übertragung
in: JURA 1987 S. 668 ff

HERZBERG Die Strafandrohung als Waffe im Kampf gegen AIDS?
in: NJW 1987 S. 1461 ff

KREUZER Strafrecht als Hinderniss sinnvoller Aids-Prophylaxe?
in: NStZ 1987 S. 268 ff

KREUZER Aids und Strafrecht in: ZStW 100 (1988) S. 786 ff

MEIER Strafrechtliche Aspekte der Aids-Übertragung in: GA
1989 S. 207 ff

PRITTWITZ (Hrsg.) Aids, Recht und Gesundheitspolitik 1990

SCHÜNEMANN/PFEIFFER (Hrsg.) Die Rechtsprobleme von AIDS 1988

The Crisis and Opportunity of AIDS and Drug Misuse

J. STRANG

Consultant Psychiatrist in Drug Dependence, Drug Dependence, Drug Dependence
Clinical Research and Treatment Unit, National Addiction Centre, The Bethlem Royal
and Maudsley Hospital, London SE 5, United Kingdom

INTRODUCTION

Let us start at the point where we recognise crisis: what conclusions do we reach?
The Chinese ideogram for crisis comprises two parts - one denoting danger and the
other denoting opportunity. The rhetoric in both informed and ill-informed public
and scientific debate has been dominated by consideration of danger, with attempts
to define both the quality and quantity of this danger. However AIDS is also forcing
a fundamental reappraisal of the attitudes of treatment services to the wider drug
using population; and with this re-examination by service-planners and providers, a
similar re-appraisal must necessarily be undertaken by the broader society within
which both the drug users and the carers exist.

To what extent will opportunity be seized in this new re-appraisal, or will the
paint on the canvas relate mainly to depictions of the danger? As yet the picture is
still being constructed and the paint is certainly not yet dry: thus we have
opportunities to influence both the content and the portayal of the picture. We
would be well advised to remember that in years to come, our successors will judge
us harshly according to the extent to which we succcessfully harness the creative
energy of crisis.

PUSHING AT THE FRONTIERS

Major advances are taking place in diverse areas at a pace hitherto unseen - and HIV
has been the catalyst to this process. True to the function of a catalyst, the areas or
reactions themselves are not new, but the speed with which the changes are taking
place are truly of a new order.

Basic and applied scientific work is already helping us to understand the
nature of the virus and the interactions between virus, host and community which

have a bearing on its individual transmission and penetration within communities. With the development and application of new tests and imaging techniques it is now possible to undertake more specific study of the virus itself and its mutations - such as enabled by the development of the polymerase chain reaction (PCR) test. Ongoing work is charting the areas around disease progression so as to identify not only markers of the disease status but also factors which may hasten or retard the process of HIV disease progression itself. With the arrival of effective anti-viral treatments, the need for more efficient and widely applied immunological monitoring of individuals becomes self evident - but remains currently all too rare. In particular on-going work is contributing to our understanding of the inter-relationship between drug misuse and HIV disease. It has long been known that drugs such as the opiates and cannabis cause moderate reductions in immunological responses - even in the absence of any secondary infections, but it is not yet clear whether this reduced immune response will have a major influence on the unfolding epidemic of HIV amongst injecting drug users.

The practice of medicine itself - especially medical care to drug users - is being altered fundmentally. And here we have an example of where the new order, the new balance, the new holistic practice is one in which traditional physical care comes back centre stage after many years on the margins of the play. And with this move into the limelight, it then becomes evident that the relative absence of this physical care has led to insufficient attention being paid to other physical complications - notably the much-overlooked endemic hepatitis B. The drug worker of tomorrow can no longer legitimately shrug off responsibilities for attention to physical complications and monitoring of health care. It is not that the old sets of skills are redundant - rather that they must now exist within a wider range of tools in the armamentarium of the drug worker of tomorrow. Many drug workers will not have received formal medical training, but there remains considerable scope for such drug workers to enhance the competence of the monitoring by themselves and their clients of the health status of their clientele (for wider description see Brettle, Farrell and Strang, 1990).

THE PECULIAR CASE OF CASENESS

Central to much of the current confusion and debate is the uncertainty about the criteria which define a suitable case for treatment. From the heterogeneous population of individuals who may have used one or more drugs, towards which of these individuals might treatments (medical, social, public health, etc) be legitimately directed? In the U.K., drug workers and users will often refer to different levels of relationship with drug use as being either as experimental, recreational or compulsive/dependent.

Experimental drug users are led to drug use by curiosity about the nature of the drug effect is therefore time limited - lasting until the knowledge has been obtained. It is mainly a peer group activity and is unlikely to be associated with any pharmacological drive to seek the particular drug effect.

Recreational drug users are those who having experimented with drugs continue to take drugs in order to obtain a known effect (typically perceived as positive at this stage).

Compulsive/dependent drug users are those recreational users who develop dependence and/or other problems; for example the dominant position of pursuit and use of the drug may be accompanied by a tolerance of damage to personal or family well-being and as the use of the drug becomes a more exclusive pursuit and activity it may no longer be associated primarily with the pursuit of positive effects but may be taken mainly for the abolition of negative physical or psychological effects (Yates, 1984).

Two terms have been widely used which are, or relate to, the condition under consideration. Other sociological terms have become widely used in consideration of the problem drinker (see Kessel Report (Advisory Committee on Alcoholism) 1978) and problem drug taker (Advisory Council on the Misuse of Drugs, 1982) in which the problem drug taker is defined as "*any person who experiences social, psychological, physical or legal problems related to intoxication and/or regular excessive consumption and/or dependence as a consequence of his/her own use of drugs and other chemical substances ..... *". Much work has also been done to define more precisely the dependence itself; Edwards and his colleagues have explored this concept widely in the alcohol field (Edwards and Gross, 1976; Stockwell et al, 1979) and more recently, but less extensively, in the opiate field (Sutherland et al, 1986; Phillips et al, 1986). Often it is mistakenly thought that these two terms and linked areas of understanding merely reflect a medical or sociological term for the same phenomenon. However, when studied more closely it becomes clear that there may be value in considering them as largely independent dimensions (insofar as each of them might legitimately be considered as a single dimension). Consideration of two individual drug users, therefore, might find one scoring highly on problems but low on dependence, whilst for the second the loading was reversed.

The many perspectives and levels of understanding of drug use are seen in the diversity of terms. In different centres and with different professions the terms will often be interchanged, as though they merely reflect current fashion and one group's penchant for a particular term. Often, however, this approach fails to provide clarification for the different component parts of the drug taking behaviour which are the subject of treatment or study. In an effort to identify a limited set of terms and concepts around which consensus might form, the World Health Organisation prepared a memorandum on terminology. In this Edwards et al (1981) put forward proposals for more specific terms for the various phenomena under study. Terms such as "abuse" and "misuse" seemed prejorative and hence unsatisfactory in a scientific context. They suggested that the underlying meaning could be more effectively conveyed by using the following four terms :

(i) Unsanctioned use: Use of a drug that is not approved by a society, or a group within that society. When the term is used, it should be made clear who is responsible for the disapproval. The term implies that we accept disapproval as a fact in its own right without having to determine or justify the basis of that disapproval.

(ii) Hazardous use: Use of a drug that will probably lead to harmful consequences for the user - either dysfunction or to harm. This concept is similar to the idea of risky behaviour. For instance, smoking 20 cigarettes each day may not be accompanied by any present or actual harm but we know it to be hazardous.

(iii) Dysfunctional use: Use of a drug that is leading to impaired psychological or social functioning (e.g. loss of job or marital problems).

(iv) Harmful use: Use of a drug that is known to have caused tissue damage or mental illness in the particular person.

Edwards et al take up the increasing dissatisfaction with the apparent division between physical dependence and psychological/psychic dependence. They suggested the use of the term "neuroadaptation" which covers the changes associated with physical and psychological withdrawal phenomena and also with the

Therapie des alkoholbedingten Entzugsyndroms

Sedieren allein ist zuwenig…

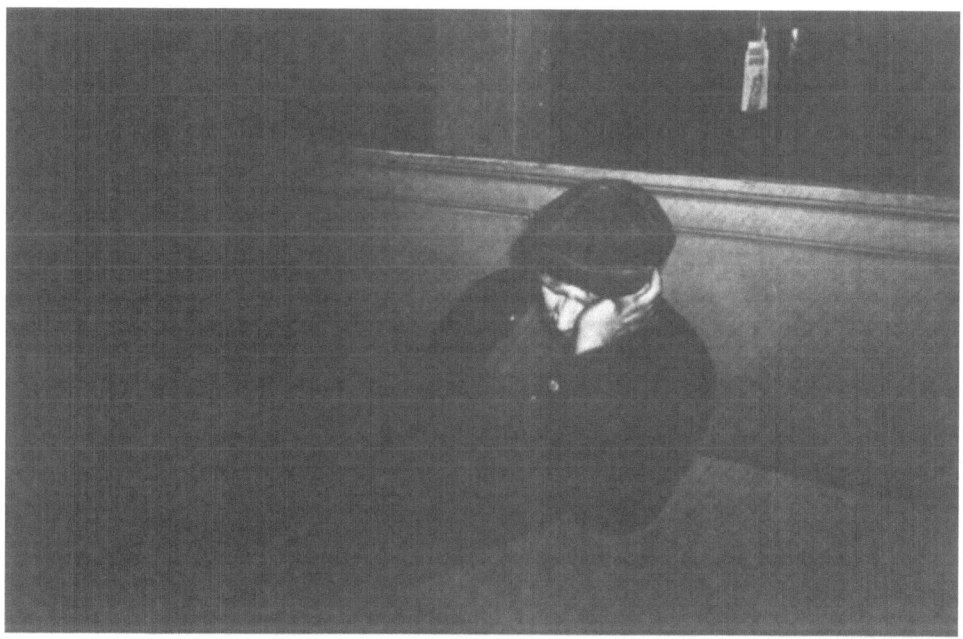

…nur ein klarer Kopf erkennt die Hilfe.

Nootropil®

● Aufhellung des Bewußtseins – statt übermäßiger Sedierung

● Vermeidung einer Suchtverlagerung – von einer Abhängigkeit auf andere

Wirkstoff: Piracetam. **Indikationen:** akute und chronische Hirnfunktionsstörungen. **Dosierung:** oral: 3x 1 Filmtablette 800 mg/die, parenteral: im allgemeinen 6 g–12 g/die. In der Therapie des alkoholischen Prädelirs werden des öfteren jedoch auch höhere parenterale Dosierungen, nämlich 12 g–24 g Piracetam, empfohlen. (Z. B. Mentzel H. [1], Moghaddan H. [2] bzw. Ulbricht B. [3].) **Nebenwirkungen:** selten auftretende Nebenwirkungen sind psychomotorische Agitation und Aggressivität, die eine Verringerung der Dosis erforderlich machen könnten. **Kontraindikationen, Wechselwirkungen:** sind bisher keine bekannt. **Darreichungsformen bzw. Packungsgrößen:** 1 Infusionsflasche zu 12 g/60 ml Z. Nr. 1-1811 · 30 Ampullen zu 3 g/15 ml, Reg. Nr. 17.051 · 12 Ampullen zu 1 g/5 ml, Reg. Nr. 15.622 · 60 Filmtabletten zu 800 mg, Reg. Nr. 17.031 · 60 Kapseln zu 400 mg, Reg. Nr. 15.621 · **Literatur:** 1. Mentzel H., Medical Tribune 7, 37 (1982) · 2. Moghaddan H., Therapiewoche 32, 2605 (1982) · 3. Ulbricht B., Med. Welt 27, 1912 (1976). UCB Pharma Gesellschaft m.b.H., Wien, A-1121 Wien, Altmannsdorfer Str. 104.

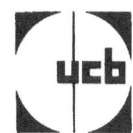

development of tolerance. Thus neuroadaptation covers the cellular, metabolic and behaviour adaptations to use and to continued use of the drug. It may also be extended to the concept of reciprocal neuroadaptation to discover the phenomenon previously described as cross-tolerance.

Thus the issue of caseness would not seem to be a simple binary phenomenon - either on or off, either present or absent. There may be public health or education interventions for one drug user (e.g. public information about the risks of needle sharing for the occasional hedonistic injector) which may need to be considered across a different population from more orthodox treatment populations (e.g. the regular heroin user who has become physically dependent). Here again, it is not that one type of case has disappeared as another has been defined: rather what is required is a careful scrutiny of the potential target population whilst considering the potential benefits (and harms) which may result from proposed and existing interventions.

THE NECESSARY RE-EXAMINATION OF CLINICAL PRACTICE

The most fundamental shift of opinion in contemporary analyses of the drugs/HIV problem is the extent to which it has become acceptable to consider second-best options - options which may bring about significant beneficial change in the nature of on-going drug use whilst falling short of going for abstinence. It is remarkable the extent to which this has been acceptable within the U.K. so that government departments and politicians now carefully explain to their colleagues how benefits may be accrued which fall short of the optimum goal. Somehow, going for gold is no longer all-important: going for silver or bronze has now become the popular - presumably on the grounds that a successful outcome may be more likely. The way forward was forged in large part by the official U.K. report on AIDS and Drug Misuse (Advisory Council on the Misuse of Drugs, 1988) which introduced the concept of intermediate goals. A contemporary commentary described in the following terms the need to concentrate on key changes in drug taking behaviour during the longer journey of treatment: "*There is an urgent need for injecting drug users to travel hastily down the section of the road from injecting to not injecting: as a second best, they may make the journey from at-risk injecting to safer injecting (insofar as the latter place may exist)*" (Strang, 1988). Later descriptions outlined how the overall course of treatment might be seen as a cascade of processes of change, with each process of change leading to an intermediate goal (e.g. from sharing to non-sharing of needle and syringe; from injecting to non-injecting; from high dose intoxication to low-dose background maintenance; etc) (Strang, 1990). Suddenly it had become acceptable once again to concentrate on benefits other than abstinence. This focus was not entirely new as it had previously been one of the areas of attention around the time of the creation of the drug clinics in the U.K., at which time policy documents from the Ministry of Health clearly lay out the brief for the new clinics efforts to reduce the harm resulting from the drug use, alongside efforts to promote abstinence. However the speed with which change has taken place should not be under-estimated. During the first half of the 1980s, there were major criticisms of a document from the Institute for the Study of Drug Dependence entitled "Teaching about a volatile situation" which gave advice to teachers on how to educate persistent glue sniffers so as to reduce the likelihood of harmful consequences if they continued with the behaviour (ISDD, 1982); and a similar document from the Lifeline Project in Manchester entitled "Sniffing for Pleasure" likewise attracted marked criticism (Lifeline, 1982). And yet other documents were tolerated or even encouraged: at around the same time the Lifeline Project developed an overdose aid leaflet giving advice to drug users and their friends of ways of managing inadvertent overdose; and in 1984/85 the North Western Regional Health Authority convened a group to prepare a booklet of specific advice to drug users on reducing the risks of their continued drug use ("Risk Reduction for Drug Users", North Western Regional Health Authority, 1986). However the more rapid change in attitudes and practice occurred alongside changing public and professional opinion on the availability of needles and syringes. Key influential practitioners such as Dr Roy Robertson in Edinburgh began to provide clean needles and syringes on an exchange basis to his drug injecting patients (see "Treating Drug Misusers" video, Roussel Medical Television, 1986), whilst at the same time the Pharmaceutical Society of Great Britain issued a position statement altering the balance of its advice to community pharmacists and thus creating a more sympathetic climate to the commercial sale (at low cost) of needles and syringes to presume drug injectors (Pharmaceutical Society of Great Britain, 1986). At around the same time the first U.K. needle and syringe exchange schemes were established in Liverpool and Kingston near London, modelled on the Amsterdam exchange schemes of recent years, and the opening of these exchange clinics undoubtedly sharpened and accelerated the pace of debate about needle and syringe provision in particular and harm minimisation in general. The

Department of Health in England then moved promptly to establish a grant-aided experiment in which 15 pilot needle and syringe exchange schemes were set up in England and Scotland, and were simultaneously the subject of audit and study (Stimson et al, 1988; 1989a, 1989b, 1990; Lart and Stimson, 1990; Donaghue et al, 1991).

There would appear to be areas in which clinical practice has not yet adapted sufficiently. Lip service is now routinely paid to the need for HIV education and promotion of behaviour change, and yet all too often the drug user and client enter into a collusive agreement to put off addressing these issues until a time when the drug taker feels better prepared to deal with them: one can only hope that the virus is similarly sympathetic to the niceties of a convenient frame of mind. Other areas of health care continue to be overlooked including the routine monitoring for the presence of hepatitis B, including the detection and treatment of chronic hepatitis B carriers who may have ongoing silent liver disease. It is also surprising that the provision of hepatitis B vaccination to injecting drug users and their partners remains so rarely available and provided (Farrell, Battersby and Strang, 1990). Until drug workers mature and translate the rhetoric of harm minimisation into the practice of actually reducing these harms, the full benefits from these new areas of work may not be accrued.

THE ROLES OF PRESCRIBING

The possible benefits and hazards of prescribing drugs to drug users has recently become a reinvigorated area of review (see for example Druglink, 1987; Advisory Council on the Misuse of Drugs, 1988; Strang, 1990a). In their second report on AIDS and Drug Misuse (1989), the Advisory Council on the Misuse of Drugs endorsed the principle prescribing should never be undertaken without an identified goal, and go on to identify four criteria which have a bearing on the decision whether or not to prescribe to an individual drug taker: "*(a) to attract seropositive drug misusers into regular contact with services; (b) to promote behaviour change away from practices which carry a risk of transmitting HIV infection; (c) to promote behaviour change in such a way as to maximise personal health and stablity; and (d) to encourage compliance with medical treatment, including regular check ups, and the regular self-administration of antiviral drugs, such as Zidovudine (AZT). The first of these goals is not an end in itself, but rather the platform on which the others are founded*" (ACMD, 1989). The ACMD has already emphasised elsewhere that services to drug users should be the same irrespective of HIV status. A widespread misinterpretation of these four factors relates to the first one - increasing contact with drug users. As is clear from the quotation this is regarded as a sufficient criterion for prescribing only insofar as it provides the opportunity for the other three criteria to be effected. Drawing drug users into contact with services is surely of little benefit if the nature of their drug taking behaviour is not altered in significant identifiable ways: if the transmission of hepatitis B, HIV or bacterial infections occurs by the sharing of State supplied pharmaceutical drugs through a State supplied sharp needle and syringe, then it must surely be questionable whether any of the criteria have been met apart from the platform criterion (a).

The prescribing of injectable drugs has been recently reconsidered within a new harm-minimisation perspective. There would appear to be two distinct forms of the argument. One form of argument proposes that by the State rationed supply of injectable drugs it should be possible to preserve the health of the injecting drug user until such time as they mature out of their drug addiction (arguments along these lines have been put forward by Marks, 1987; Dally, 1988, 1990; and these arguments are further considered by Brewer in this volume). The alternative approach for prescribing injectable drugs is one in which it occurs in an explicitly time limited context during which time there is active coaxing, cajoling and sometimes coercion to promote movement away from injecting so as to establish the drug taker stably on oral-only substitute drugs (for an account of this approach see Advisory Council on the Misuse of Drugs, 1989; Strang, 1990b). However a word of caution is necessary at this stage. Despite the enthusiasm of some practitioners and the reassurance given by their patients who are in receipt of injectable drugs, objective examination cases serious doubts on the validity of these claims and indicates that many of these patients may make little changes in their drug taking behaviour and may continue to use frequent additional supplies of other blackmarket drugs (see for example Strang, Johns and Gossop, 1990; Battersby et al (submitted for publication)).

MISSED OPPORTUNITIES FOR PHYSICAL CARE

If care is to be balanced and appropriate, then the care providers of tomorrow will find that they need to adopt an approach with much higher levels of vigilance for physical complications as well as involvement in monitoring of physical well-being, which may be achieved through routine rapid health checks (see for example Brettle,

Farrell and Strang, 1990); regular laboratory monitoring of HIV status and progression (see Moss, 1988; Webber, 1990) surveillance and intervention for hepatitis B (see Strang and Farrell, 1991) or alternatively through the establishment of separate well users clinics or health clinics for drug users (Strang, Farrell and Orgel, 1989; Datt and Feinmann, 1990). Unfortunately, at the present time, it is clear that the opportunities for provision of physical health care are currently being overlooked or ignored. If this continues, then services will find them ill prepared for the necessary introduction of new elements of health care with the arrival of more widespread of availability of anti viral treatments - just as they have been ill prepared and deficient in their response (or at least slow on the uptake) of the new developments in prevention and treatment of hepatitis B.

CONCLUSION

There can be no doubt that we are in the middle of a revolution in our understanding of AIDS and drug misuse. But revolutions come and revolutions go: what are we going to do about it that's what we need to know. Although the greater international traffic of modern times may have contributed to the rapid spread of the HIV epidemic, it is the same modern times which have brought us the scientific advances that permit more detailed study of the virus and its transmission, the framework for study of the social behaviour and context within which at risk behaviours occur and self-help strategies emerge, the technological ability to communicate internationally as never before so that discoveries here this morning can be with colleagues elsewhere this afternoon. Thus we are privileged to find ourselves at a point in the epidemic when our own actions and inactions are likely to have a real impact on the unfolding course of the continued HIV epidemic amongst drug users. Let us hope that in this crisis we may not only examine the danger, but also exploit the opportunity.

REFERENCES

Advisory Council on Alcoholism (Kessel Report) (1978) The pattern and range of services for problem drinkers. London: Her Majesty's Stationery Office.

Advisory Council on the Misuse of Drugs (1982) Treatment and Rehabilitation Report. London: Her Majesty's Stationery office.

Advisory Council on the Misuse of Drugs (1988) Report on AIDS and Drug Misuse, Part 1. London: Her Majesty's Stationery Office.

Advisory Council on the Misuse of Drugs (1989) Report on AIDS and Drug Misuse, Part 2. London; Her Majesty's Stationery Office.

Battersby, M., Farrell, M., Gossop, M., Robson, P. and Strang, J. "Horse Trading": prescribing injectable opiates to opiate addicts - a descriptive study (submitted for publication).

Brettle, R., Farrell, M. and Strang, J. (1990) Clinical Features of HIV Infection and AIDS in Drug Takers. In: Strang, J. and Stimson, G. (eds) AIDS and Drug Misuse: the challenge for policy and practice in the 1990s. London: Routledge.

Dally, A. (1988)

Dally, A. (1990) A Doctor's Story. London: Macmillan.

Datt, N. and Feinmann, C. (1990) Providing health care for drug users? British Journal of Addiction, 85: 1571-1575.

Donaghue, M. (1991) Syringe exchange: has it worked? Druglink, January/February: 8-11.

Druglink (1987) Series of articles by Strang, Rathod, Chang, Dally and Marks about the Prescribing Debate. Druglink.

Edwards, G. and Gross, M.M. (1976) Alcohol dependence: provisional description of a clinical syndrome. British Medical Journal, 1: 1058-1061.

Edwards, G., Arif, A. and Hodgson, R. (1981) Nomenclature and classification of drug and alcohol related problems: a shortened version of a WHO memorandum. British Journal of Addiction, 77: 287-306.

Farrell, M., Battersby, M. and Strang, J. (1990) Screening for hepatitis B and vaccination of injecting drug users in NHS drug treatment services. British Journal of Addiction, 85(12): 1657-1659.

Lart, R. and Stimson, G. (1990) National survey of syringe exchange schemes in England. British Journal of Addiction, 85: 1433-1444.

Marks, J. (1985) Opium, the religion of the people. The Lancet, June 22: 1439-1440.

Moss, A. (1988) Predicting who will progress to AIDS. British Medical Journal, 297: 1067-1068.

Phillips, G.T., Gossop, M., Edwards, G., Sutherland, G., Taylor, C. and Strang, J. (1987) The application of SODQ to the measurement of the severity of opiate dependence in a British sample. British Journal of Addiction, 82: 691-699.

Stimson, G., Dolan, K., Donoghoe, M. and Alldritt, L. (1988) Syringe Exchange 1. Druglink, May/June.

Stimson, G., Alldritt, L., Dolan, K. and Donoghoe, M. (1988) Syringe exchange schemes for drug users in England and Scotland. British Medical Journal, 296: 1717-1719.

Stimson, G., Dolan, K., Donoghoe, M., Alldritt, L. and Lart, R. (1989b) Syringe Exchange 3: can injectors change? Druglink, January/February: 10-11.

Stimson, G., Donoghoe, M., Lart, R. and Dolan, K. (1990) Distributing Sterile Needles and Syringes to people who inject drugs: the syringe-exchange experiment. In: Strang, J. and Stimson, G. (eds) AIDS and Drug Misuse: the challenge for policy and practice in the 1990s. London: Routledge.

Stockwell, T., Hodgson, R., Edwards, G., Taylor, C. and Rankin, H. (1979) The development of a questionnaire to measure severity of alcohol dependence. British Journal of Addiction, 74: 79-87.

Strang, J. (1988) Changing Injecting Practices: blunting the needle habit. British Journal of Addiction, 83: 237-239.

Strang, J., Orgel, M. and Farrell, M. (1989) Well users clinic for illicit drug users. British Medical Journal, 298: 1310.

Strang, J. (1990a) The roles of prescribing. In: Strang, J. and Stimson, G. (eds) AIDS and Drug Misuse: the challenge for policy and practice in the 1990s. London: Routledge.

Strang, J. (1990b) Intermediate goals and the process of change. In: Strang, J. and Stimson, G. (eds) AIDS and Drug Misuse: the challenge for policy and practice in the 1990s. London: Routledge.

Strang, J., Johns, A. and Gossop, M. (1990) Social and drug taking behaviour of 'maintained' opiate addicts. British Journal of Addiction, 85: 193-196.

Strang, J. and Farrell, M. (1991) Hepatitis B amongst drug users - the overlooked epidemic. Druglink (in press)

Sutherland, G., Edwards, G., Taylor, C., Phillips, G., Gossop, M. and Brady, R. (1986) The measurement of opiate dependence. British Journal of Addiction, 81: 485-494.

Weber, J. (1990) HIV: the virus and laboratory tests. In: Strang, J. and Stimson, G. (eds) AIDS and Drug Misuse: the challenge for policy and practice in the 1990s. London: Routledge.

Yates (1984)

Observed Patterns of HIV Related Risk Behaviour Amongst Intravenous Drug Users Attending a Dublin Needle Exchange in Its First Year

M. Scully, L. Pomeroy, Z. Johnson, H. Johnson, and A. Barry

AIDS Resource Centre, 19 Haddington Road, Dublin 4, Ireland

Introduction

The problem of serious drug use in Dublin started in the mid 1960s
with abuse of drugs such as amphetamines, barbiturates and tranqullisers.
The situation changed in the late 1970s with the onset of an opiate
epidemic, somewhat later than in other European cities, which reached a
peak in 1983. (Dean et al 1985) The areas most affected were the inner
city areas where there were also high levels of unemployment and poor
social conditions. With the finding that the majority of drug users were
injecting rather than sniffing or smoking, (Dean et al 1987), the potential
risks for spread of H.I.V. and Hepatitis B were obvious.

The need for an innovative approach to targeting this vulnerable group
was acknowledged by the Eastern Health Board which launched it's "Outreach
Project" in March 1988. The needle exchange was opened in June 1989 as
part of this project. The objectives are

1. to reach as many I.V.D.U.s in the Community as possible, particularily
   the young who have not yet contacted the existing services;
2. to educate and encourage I.V.D.U.s in risk reduction both with regard
   to needle use and sexual behaviour; and
3. to facilitate this by encouraging attendance at the AIDS Resource
   Centre, where needles, syringes and condoms are provided after
   appropriate counselling.

Methods

The needle exchange sessions are held at the AIDS Resource Centre,
located in a city centre community hospital complex. The centre was
developed to be as "user friendly" as possible, with comfortable waiting

area with easy chairs, coffee and tea facilities, individual counselling rooms and minimal data collection which is on a confidential first name basis. Attenders are not asked for their addresses, but give a postal number location. The data is kept on cards and each attender has access to his/her card.

Data is collected on age, sex and duration of intravenous drug use at the first visit, and, at this and subsequent visits, information is collected on needle sharing and condom requirements. A record of needles and syringes given out and returned is also kept.

Results

During the first year a total of 433 I.V.D.U.s attended; of these 85% were male and 15% female. The median age was 25 years, with 66% aged between 20 and 30 years. (Fig 1)

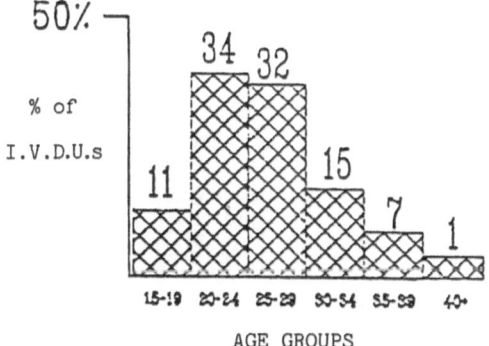

Figure 1   AGE DISTRIBUTION OF ATTENDERS

Approximately 55% of this 433 had been using drugs intravenously for 5 years or more, and of these 45% had been injecting for 10 years or more. It is encouraging, however, from the point of view of the "Outreach" activities that almost 12% had been injecting for less than 1 year with a further 12% injecting for approximately 1 year. (Fig 2)

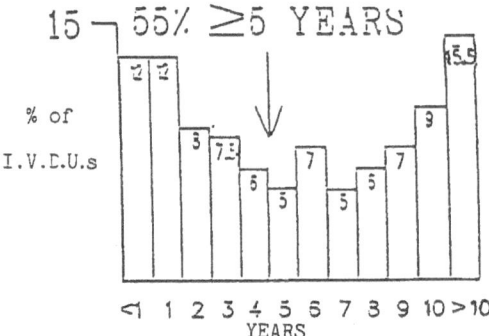

Figure 2   NUMBER OF YEARS INJECTING DRUGS

Data on the 217 I.V.D.U.s who had attended the centre on two or more occasions during the year was then reviewed. At their first visit 32% admitted to current or recent needle/syringe sharing and 50% accepted condoms following counselling. In order to assess changes in behaviour, data from the last visit, that is the most recent visit to 31st May 1990, was reviewed and it was found that while the proportion admitting to needle sharing had decreased to 12%, there was also a decrease in the proportion who accepted condoms, from 50% to 45%. (Fig. 3)

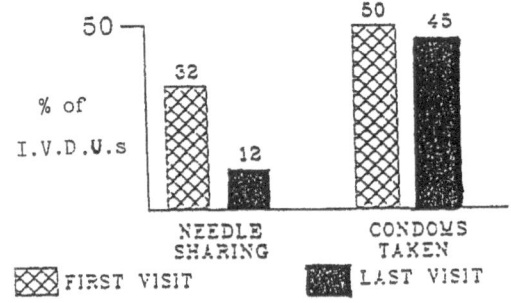

Figure 3   RISK BEHAVIOUR:FIRST AND LAST VISIT

As condoms are offered to attenders on each visit, the pattern of accepting them over the year was used as a guide to changes in sexual risk behaviour. Those I.V.D.U.s who accepted condoms on more than half of their visits were defined as "regular" takers; 27% of the 217 were in this group; 24% never accepted condoms and the remaining 49% accepted them "sometimes", that is at a frequency between the first two groups. (Fig. 4)

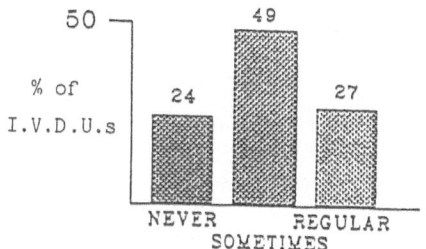

Figure 4   ACCEPTANCE OF CONDOMS : PATTERN OVER 12 MONTHS

Conclusions

    The service at the AIDS Resource Centre is new and it was therefore
necessary to balance the service needs of I.V.D.U.s against the need to
collect data for research and evaluation. Because of this, these results
are only a guide to the trends in risk behaviour in the group attending.
However, the perception of staff at the centre was that there was greater
willingness to change risk behaviour with regard to needle use than sexual
behaviour. The results support this view. As a result greater emphasis
is now placed on the risks of sexual transmission, and data collection
has been amended to permit monitoring of actual risk behaviour. Future
analysis will reflect more accurately the trend in risk behaviour and the
impact of the service on this

References

1. Dean G, O'Hare A, O'Connor A, Kelly M, Kelly G, (1985), The "Opiate
    Epidemic" in Dublin 1979-1983, I.M.J. 78 (4) 197-110
2. Dean G, O'Hare A, O'Connor A, Kelly M, Kelly G (1987). The "Opiate
    Epidemic" in Dublin: Are we over the Worst?
    I.M.J. 80 (5) 139-142

Outreach Work as a Strategy for Risk Reduction in Hard-to-Reach Populations. For Example: Injecting Drug Users

W. Heckmann, G. Krauss, B. Gusy, G. Schott-Ben Redjeb, and Y. Seyrer

Sozialpädagogisches Institut, Berlin, Federal Republic of Germany

The AIDS crisis has created a worldwide situation necessitating immediate and effective action. This is just as true in the area of research as it is in initiating counselling services for the people affected, watching the epidemic development and avoiding further infection.

The problem has spread worldwide, even if all continents are not affected to the same extent. The Federal Republic of Germany was one of the first European countries hit by the first epidemic wave and has reflected the typical epidemiological situation from the very start. The groups most severely affected were the homosexual and bisexual men and drug addicts. Heterosexuals have still not been affected to the same extent, though there is an upward tendency. The number of incidents resulting in hemophiliacs and in recipients of transfusions are declining since the blood donations and blood products are being screened for HIV.

Basically three conceivable strategic concepts have been put to discussion in the Federal Republic of Germany ever since the people affected, the politically responsible and the experts have had to cope with the problem of AIDS. These three concepts are:

- Medical strategy

- the strategy related to compulsory measures and public order

- psychosocial strategy.

To obtain only a vague idea of the complex political dynamics behind these strategic concepts concerning health care, the sciences and training in the professions, anyone wanting to become involved in fighting AIDS should be required to read:

George Orwell's "1984," in which the attempt is made to solve individual problems and social conflicts by exaggerating controls and regimentation – a strategy that is being officially practiced with fighting AIDS in only a few countries, but which scrutinizes ever ything and – as Big Brother's watchful eye – can be put into action without warning;

Aldous Huxley's "Brave New World," in which all human needs and all social and health problems could be miraculously cured and solved by a drug – a strategic concept that still cannot be used against AIDS despite scientific advances, but which is being tried in drug addiction – only that "Soma" is being marketed under the names of Methadone or Polamidone and is being promised to the other inflicted;

Albert Camus' "La Peste," in which methods of formal controls, such as quarantining, proved to be useless and the people were subjected to an absurd existence reflecting the forces of nature and society. The character, Dr. Rieux, sets out working against these forces with all his energy, fantasy, humanity, fortitude, and sensitivity. The only strategic concept that can be presently regarded as realistic gaining global importance as psychosocial strategy against AIDS.

For many of his readers, since the time that Camus wrote it opposing nazi terror as a member of the French resistance, "La Peste" has become synonymous for fascism, suppression, cold war, nuclear threat or environmental destruction. Within this context, the reference of any threat to human and social existence by HIV is Sisyphean.

The Ministers of Health from most countries of the world accepted an invitation to attend an AIDS conference in London at the beginning of 1988. They met to confer on their mutual concern and to establish congruous strategic concepts. There was great consensus expressed in the reports of this conference in giving priority to prevention through medical and pedagogic measures as opposed to mandatory ones.

Prevention Strategy in the Federal Republic of Germany

In the Federal Republic of Germany as well, there is the so-called psychosocial strategic concept that has been agreed upon by the Federal Government (under the auspices of the Federal Ministry of Health) and the Länder with respect to dealing with the illness and the inflicted. This strategic concept promotes the priority being given to preventive measures instead of rigid controls and compulsory measures. Because, at least for the time being, we cannot anticipate a cure for AIDS or a vaccine against HIV, most of the German experts believe that considerable efforts will be required in avoiding new infections by convincing not only those groups at risk but all of the sexually active populus to change their sexual behavior in favor of drastically reducing the risk of infection.

A general prevention optimism prevails in those countries, in which the psychosocial strategy has been put most consequently into practice. The Northern European countries are leading in this respect. Besides, the epidemiological development in the Scandinavian countries, Great Britain, the Netherlands and the Federal Republic of Germany confirms this optimism. The early intervention in mass media and education, the influence of the peer groups and the measurable change in behavior in the groups mainly at risk have led to a unique epidemiological development throughout the world. Although the therapeutic expectations for those, who have become infected still are to be regarded as somewhat pessimistic, standards and practical success have been implemented in the area of primary prevention, i.e., avoiding infection, so that there is reason for hope.

The prerequisite for any amount of success in prevention, i.e., the "changing behavior that becomes stable over a period of time" (Rosenbrock), particularly in connection with sexual behavior, but also in other areas of risk, such as drug consumption, are the joint decisions made in a free society.

Since most risky situations are part of the extremely private aspects of life, and because of the partial tabus still existing when topics concerning sexuality and addiction crop up (particularly homosexuality and promiscuity) making public discussion difficult, it becomes very important to influence individuals – besides educating the public. The function of social work in the AIDS crisis and its influence on social change as a result of AIDS can still not be evaluated conclusively. They also will be dependent upon how the protagonists take sides in this field.

It is certain that the positive results that have been obtained in most parts of the world with respect to knowledge concerning HIV and AIDS, means of transmittal and avoiding infection are by themselves no reason for optimism in the fight against this epidemic. In the case of this particular infection, which is transmitted as a social disease, there are significantly larger gaps to be bridged by active influence, education, good example, identification, fortitude, motivation and cooperation than are found elsewhere separating knowledge and opinion and between opinions / convictions and behavior.

Public services and professional organizations have continually learned from the inflicted when trying to cope with the AIDS crisis. The inflicted are mainly homosexual men in this country; then come the drug addicts and, when seen on a worldwide scale, predominantly poor people from all parts of the globe, especially from the Third World. Homosexual men in North America and Northern Europe have established their own particular methods of coping with the problem. They have developed many specific forms of peer counseling and peer care and have put these into practice with a great deal of success. We were able to learn about many important aspects for use in professional AIDS counselling and health care.

The situation is similar in primary prevention. The studies on behavior and changes of behavior in both of the groups mainly at risk in this country, homosexuals and drug addicts, fortunately reflect a strong tendency toward modifying behavior in favor of safer sex and safer use. On the other hand, they prove to us that the strongest influence comes from the groups' own peers. In his repeated studies on homosexual men, Bochow (1990) comes to the conclusion that acceptance and practice of safer sex is proportionate to the amount of involvement the persons questioned in the gay community had in politically interested groups, AIDS counselling centers and other groups dedicated to helping the inflicted. Kleiber et al. (1990) were able to demarcate lasting changes in behavior even among drug addicts, if their social ties were moderately stable.

The significance of these observations is that not only explicit periods and favorable conditions are necessary for the process of transition from knowledge to application, but above all suited mediators are required to present and to develop the process. This means, within the process of planning measures of primary prevention that the peers have to have a greater influence, that self-help groups organized by the inflicted more support and that training by peers will have to be adapted as a method of professional assistance.

Pilot Projects in the Federal Republic of Germany

Taking the predominant situations of risk into consideration, there is theoretically no problem in obtaining effective protection. You take precaution not to let the blood of others get into your own system and you always use a prophylactic when sexual behavior could be risky. This becomes more difficult when trying to put this into practice and only one partner wants to protect himself and the other construes this as having been betrayed. This develops into a difficult situation when a man, who is willing to use a condom, encounters disgust or resistance from his partner. It is also difficult for some to see their manhood packed in latex after decades of freedom. It is particularly difficult for anyone lacking experience, e.g., youths, in reaching for mechanical protection as a matter of course at the decisive moment without loosing face or potency. Following the revolution of "the pill," hardly anyone was concerned with explaining "the facts of life," not to mention making an effort at sensually integrating the prophylactic into their sex life.

At the moment, a more suited alternative to using condoms does not exist. Whoever protects himself against the main risks (e.g., in the area of sex) is just about one-hundred-percent protected against infection. Whoever neglects this protection is running an ever increasing risk of becoming infected.

With the onset of AIDS, it became necessary for all who have sexual intercourse frequently with new partners or who are inclined to come into contact with blood to change their behavioral patterns objectively and notably. The nature of the potential risk situation (sexuality and illicit drug consumption) makes it futile to try to influence behavior exoterically, that is by taking mandatory or control measures. Self-motivated learning is the only help public campaigns can provide particularly in the area of prevention offered as social work at various levels.

If you look at the primary prevention measures that have been taken since the start of the AIDS crisis, i.e., those aimed at avoiding new infections, then we see much activity that has been churned out as more of the same. We have information leaflets for every household in the country, posters and TV spots. But, there is hesitation about getting group-specific measures going, such as using the media unique to the gay community or by linking with the needs of drug addicts.

Involved in a good deal of excitement and especially innovative in their methodological aspects are the projects that learn from the self-help groups, that are oriented to mediator concepts and finally cash in on the principles of individualized prevention (Heckmann 1981). These programs are essentially involved in outreach work or in streetwork. This is a method of using a communicator to convey a message on prevention directed at a particular group, found in their customary environment.

Outreach work, streetwork and street-corner work are methods, which resulted from social work with problematic minorities, such as street gangs, drug addicts, soccer fans. These are the groups aimed at that the streetworkers are usually confronted with. Further, it is normally the goal of this kind of work to calm these groups down, to make them more peaceful and to reintegrate them more or less into productive society. As far as we can tell, this is the first attempt in the Federal Republic of Germany to use methods of outreach work for intensive health education and counseling. Health promotion has attained an entirely new dimension with some different pilot programs. One of the projects is to be described in the following.

Streetwork (funded by the Federal Ministry of Health)

It is intuitive that forms of work are applied that seek out the clients when dealing with AIDS and the risk of AIDS, and that these forms of work help either to eliminate or lessen the hurdles involved in obtaining medical assistance, going to a health-care center or to any other kind of help center. The street-work method means looking for those at risk at the places, where they gather and are exposed to their particular type of risk. This applies to both of the major groups at risk – the homosexuals and opiate addicts – because they do exactly that. They socialize in their circles, and one of the main reasons for doing this is either to have sexual intercourse or to use i.v. drugs at that place and time or within the immediate vicinity or shortly thereafter. Although there are large qualitative and quantitative differences between both groups, the willingness to take risks is characteristic of many homosexuals and the majority of opiate addicts. When seen from this point of view, streetwork is equally as necessary and difficult and certainly not very successful in very many cases, at least not when success is measured only in rudimentary behavioral changes.

The experiences we have had with streetwork as a method in the area of drug addiction cannot be uncritically adapted to streetwork in the area of those at risk of contracting AIDS. Although in the drug scene, it is usually necessary to establish a contact that either immediately or eventually culminates in the individuals' entering the rehabilitation system – counseling, detox, psychologically breaking the habit and reentering the gainfully employed population – the situation of the streetworker in the gay community is entirely different. We cannot conjecture that there are any large differences between those giving and those receiving advice. Normally in the gay community, there is no evidence of deficiencies, which might be in need of any compensation. Outreach work must be conducted in an atmosphere of mutual respect, lending an open ear to problems, even for the most trivial ones. The worker can establish his proficiency by having a larger and better knowledge of AIDS risks and safer sex, but also by lending a helping hand in practic ing safer sex, by counseling on preventive medicine and possibly by establishing the necessary contact to official agencies. This helps us develop a link based on the purely human aspects of counselling.

Many pilot projects are being sponsored in the field of psychosocial strategic concepts in the prevention of AIDS. One of these projects is the "Streetworker Model," for which the Federal Ministry of Health correctly defined the objectives as "personal contacts, education and counseling individual members of the groups at risk, particularly from among the main groups at risk, the homosexuals . . . Establishing a stable network of communication among the people, who have regular profession al and personal contact to members of the groups at risk, and who are willing to inform and counsel them."

There are two points here worth mentioning.

– First, the intention of not using the streetworker as the customary helper of individuals but as a multiplier, they are meant to work in the scene as a type of procreator, who motivates others working in related services, e.g., at the health offices just as wel l as members of the group at risk itself, e.g., certain opinion makers from the scene, to work in educating others and becoming an intricate part of a communications system. The streetworkers only offer actual assistance and counseling in certain isolated cases.

– Secondly, it is our conviction that the streetworker's effectiveness in the field cannot be measured with a yardstick. This requi res a qualitative evaluation and can particularly be assessed in categories such as levels of information within the community, acceptance of the safer-sex campaigns or to what extent the streetworker is known.

However, as a result of practical application, the streetworker delves into his field of operation establishing contacts to individuals and groups, in order to become their direct partner for talks, contact and mediator for assistance programs and counselor. This basis then provides the multiplication effect, when individual cases are referred to consulting services or when yesterday's advice seeker has become today's co-consultant.

Other fields of endeavor, in which the methods of outreach work have been documented and discussed, have always been in groups that are strongly ambivalent in their attitudes and behavior. This means, for example in the case of opiate addicts that, several times each day, they give up their behavior patterns, which are endangering their health and want to detox, but at the same time they let themselves be enticed each day by dope and want nothing more adamantly. Streetwork can lock onto this very low level of ambivalence and get started.

However, streetwork among those at risk of contracting AIDS means that this kind of ambivalence cannot be expected at least in the group mainly at risk and that the streetworkers have to fulfill the demands for more and more qualified information and have to rec on with all kinds of reactions of fear. Therefore, there are a sequence of special aspects to be taken into consideration when reaching out to members of the gay community. The people in the scene are suspicious. Both of the groups at major risk are socially repressed minorities, which have become organized to varying degrees in the course of their existence, have gotten together assertive movements or have openly identified themselves with using subversive tactics for coping with life. In any case, they are suspicious of anyone not belonging to their groups and who shows up without being invited.

An everyday problem is posed by acceptance or by the prerequisites for acceptance within the group. At the beginning of the pilot project, we assumed that it would be easiest for homosexual men to accept streetworkers in the gay community. Yet, as time went on, other aspects, such as, to which organization the workers belonged and his or her personal qualifications began to become important for their acceptance.

–   Homosexual men naturally have a better approach to their "own" clients for safer sex. They behave less inhibited in homosexual bars, saunas etc. than do straights and have fewer troubles making contacts. On the other hand, as streetworkers, they come into a certain conflict of interest, because they are in fact on duty and not there privately looking for intimate contact, as the people they are talking to might expect. Conversely, heterosexuals have difficulties in establishing contact at all in strictly gay bars or meeting places and occasionally get into dubious situations that even put their professionalism into question.

–   The problem is similar in the drug scene. Streetworkers cannot approach addicts as a matter of course, because they are regarded as possible undercover narcotics agents or anybody else capable of harassing them. The less removed from the scene the professionals are, the easier the contact. This also means that the more they identified with the problems encountered by the addicts, the more they have had to cope with their own ambivalence with respect to addiction. On the other hand, there is always the danger of blending in, of over identification and the burn out shortly thereafter.

–   The question of being affiliated to institutions has proven to be very important in the initial phases of the pilot project. Those from the "AIDS-Hilfe" (self-help counseling service) or any other non-government organization found it easier to become introduced into the scene than anyone working for the Health Offices, the later being put immediately under suspicion (this mainly stems from direct previous experience). Many streetworkers are able to compensate for this, because they may be regarded as useful resulting from their working for a governmental agency or due to their personality.

–   This is a major aspect. The most important factor for becoming accepted by the target groups is the personality of the streetworker – his or her ability to convey their capability, credibility, understanding and their facility of listening, just to mention a few. We also would like to point out here that the safer-sex message can be conveyed best by people, who relay a certain love of life, and who can speak from their own experience that sex with latex is not necessarily the end of all sensuality.

During the pilot project, we collected many examples of how streetwork was more effective in putting the safer-sex campaign into practice, than were the one-sided messages presented by posters or TV spots. The streetwork activities included distributing prophylactics in Easter eggs, as tree ornaments at Christmas time, in lockets on key chains etc. The streetworkers took part in the festivities and demonstrations of the gay community, established round-table discussions, "positive nights" or safer-sex parties to name a few. The catalog of activities makes it very impressively clear that you cannot even consider having this amount of influence on the target groups without actively reaching out, that is not while sitting at a desk at the Health Office.

Summary

Whoever is concerned with the effectiveness of the HIV/AIDS prevention programs cannot escape the fact that

- the psychological problem of transferring knowledge via attitudes and convictions into taking action is also valid for this field,

- checking for any actual changes in behavior is much more difficult than testing knowledge you can ask questions about or verbally expressed behavioral attitudes. This is mainly due to the privacy and tabus surrounding incidents touching upon sex and addiction,

- traditional unidirectional communication such as brochures, posters, TV spots at their best only increases the attention paid to the topic but hardly ever have a direct influence on behavior relevant to health,

- the influence of peer groups is much larger in relatively closed subcultural groups, such as homosexual men or drug consumers, than it is in other areas of society and is innately effective when used in HIV/AIDS prevention programs.

Based on the information – aside from campaigns for the general public – gained in a series of pilot projects, we are headed in a di rection in the Federal Republic of Germany that permits any individual to protect himself from becoming infected with HIV. By reaching out, we were able to work with specific target groups, i.e., homosexual men, male and female prostitutes, drug consumers and adolescents. This made it possible to develop and evaluate a truly innovative method of conducting HIV/AIDS prevention programs, health education and health care.

382

The experience gained in these projects show that

-   the programs for individual protection can directly influence behavioral changes and stabilize these changes over a longer period,

-   groups that are considered to be difficult to reach, are willing to communicate when the talks are based on their life style and are oriented toward their environment,

-   health-oriented demeanor can become inured into specific environments and life styles,

-   health-oriented behavior also can be trained and practicing with dry runs that can improve the transfer into everyday life,

-   a psychosocial moratorium can be achieved, in which preventive behavior can be worked into many groups simultaneously without causing any disturbing effects,

-   placing maximized demands on the development of preventive behavior is almost always detrimental, but that a hierarchy of minimal to optimal behavior has to be offered for safer sex and safer use, from which the individuals select their own patterns fitting to their situation.

References

Bochow M (1990) Zeitstabilität von Änderungen im Sexualverhalten und Zielgruppenspezifik der Aids-Präventionsarbeit. In: Rosenbrock/Salmen (Hg.) (1990): Aids-Prävention. Sigma. Berlin

Böhm/Heckmann/Michel/Seyrer (1989) Lernen am Kondom. Zur Entwicklung von Wissen, Einstellungen und Verhalten Jugendlicher angesichts der Gefährdung durch AIDS. Sozialpädagogisches Institut. Berlin

Camus A (1975) Die Pest (German translation of "La Peste"). Rowohlt. Düsseldorf

Heckmann W (1981) Suchtprävention als Gemeinschaftsaufgabe. In: Suchtgefahren 3/1981

Heckmann W.(1987) AIDS als Herausforderung der Sozialarbeit. In: BewHi 2/1987

Heckmann W (1987) AIDS und Schule. In: Jugendwohl 6/1987

Heckmann W (1989) Streetwork-Modell in der AIDS-Prävention. In: Steffan W (Hrsg.) Straßensozialarbeit. Eine Methode für heiße Arbeitsfelder. Beltz. Weinheim Basel

Heckmann W (1989) AIDS-Prävention als Aufgabe sozialer Arbeit. Sozialpädagogisches Institut. Berlin

Heckmann W (Red.) (1990) Zielgruppe: Jugend. Eine Recherche über jugendspezifische AIDS-Prävention in Bund und Ländern. Sozialpädagogisches Institut. Berlin

Huxley A (1953) Schöne Neue Welt (German translation of "A Brave New World"). Suhrkamp. Frankfurt/Main

Kahlki R, Heckmann W (Hrsg.) (1989) Sozialpädagogische Modelle der AIDS-Prävention in Schule und Jugendarbeit. Sozialpädagogisches Institut. Berlin

Kleiber D (1990a) Erfordernisse der AIDS-Prävention bei i.v. Drogenabhängigen. Prävention 13/1990

Kleiber D (1990b) HIV-Prävalenz bei Drogenabhängigen in der Bundesrepublik Deutschland. BewHi 2/1990

Orians W (1987) Die Brückenbauer. In: Sozialmagazin 10/1987

Orwell G (1962) 1984. Rowohlt. Reinbek

Rosenbrock R (1986) AIDS kann schneller besiegt werden. Gesundheitspolitik am Beispiel einer Infektionskrankheit. VSA. Hamburg

Schneider W (1987) Die Kondomisierung der Gesellschaft. Streetwork mit AIDS-Risikogruppen. In: sozial extra 4/1987

AIDS Risk Behavior Among Intravenous Drug Users Hospitalized in a Public Psychiatric Hospital

G. BONDOLFI and P. BOVET

Clinique Psychiatrique Universitaire de Cery, CH-1008 Prilly-Lausanne, Switzerland

Introduction

Among the numerous papers devoted to the epidemiology of AIDS risk behavior, those focusing on psychiatric inpatients seem to be very few - in fact, our attempts to find such literature remained sterile. This represents an important lacuna, as psychiatric inpatients might have different patterns of behavior from non-psychiatric populations, at least for some diagnostic categories, thus requiring specific preventive measures. We tried to conduct a pilot study on such a population, and we shall present here a part of it, concerning intravenous drug abusers.

Aims and methods

Our aim was to get epidemiological data from a population hospitalized in the Psychiatric University Hospital of Lausanne, which is the only general psychiatric inpatient facility for a population of ca. 250'000 inhabitants. Thus, it does not select any particular psychopathology (but it selects in the age range of 18 to 65 y.). The following items were investigated: HIV-screening test, intravenous drug use, sexual behavior, and change in the risk behavior (increased use of condoms and/or reduction of the number of sexual partners; reduction of syringe and needle sharing) linked to the prevention campaign (which, in Switzerland, started in 1986).

During a period of 6 months (1.8.1990 - 31.1.1991), every new admission was proposed a structured questionnaire through his/her resident physician, under the guarantee of anonymity. Out of the 450 patients admitted during that period, 408 fulfilled the questionnaire, and among those, 31 acknowledged to be intravenous drug users (IVDUs). We shall present our findings in breaking up this group of 31 patients following diagnostic categories. Diagnosis, in our clinic, is attributed to each patient by an experienced senior psychiatrist, following ICD-9 categories, and using clinical criteria stemming from the Swiss and German tradition in psychopathology more than from DSM-III criteria. Due to the small number of patients, we formed three diagnostic categories : Psychotics (N = 5, of which one schizophrenic), Borderline and Prepsychotic Personality Disorders (B&P PD, N = 19), and Other Personality Disorders (OPD, N = 7).

Findings

1. Age and sex distributions

The subgroup of IVDUs were born between 1950 and 1970 (median 1962, mean 1961,7, mode 1960). It comprises 21 males (2/3) and 10 females. This is to be compared to the age and sex distributions in the whole population of 408 patients (range of birth year from 1918 to 1972, median 1952; 209 males and 199 females).
To allow for the important difference in age distribution, some of the findings will be compared to those of the 236 patients, in the entire admitted population, who were born 1950 and over (comprising 54 % of males).

2. HIV-screening test

In the subgroup of IVDUs, all patients *except the schizophrenic one* had performed at least one HIV screening test in the previous months. Of these 30 tested patients, 7 were seropositive (2 Psychotics, 4 B&P PD, 1 OPD).
Comparison: 37,4 % of the 236 patients of the comparison group had performed a screening test.

Thus, IVDUs seem prone to perform a screening test.

3. Sexual behavior

None of the 31 IVDUs were pure homosexuals. 6 were bisexuals (1 psychotic, 5 B&P PD), the remaining 25 had only heterosexual activity.
Only 3 of the 31 patients had one stable sexual partner (none of whom were Psychotics); the remaining 28 had multiple, casual or prostitute partners (5 Psychotics, 18 B&P PD, 5 OPD). Thus, 28 (90 %) of the IVDUs have a risk sexual behavior.

Comparison: 32,2 % of the 204 patients of the comparison group, and having bi- or heterosexual activity, keep to one stable partner.

4. Changes in the risk behavior

a. In the sexual behavior

Of the 28 patients who have a risk sexual behavior, 13 did not change anything to their sexual behavior (2 Psychotics, 10 B&P PD, 1 OPD). 4 patients reduced the number of partners, 5 increased their use of condoms, and 6 performed both. Thus, precautions in the sexual domain are taken only by half of the IVDUs who have a risk behavior.

But it is worth mentioning that, among the 7 IVDUs who were seropositive, 5 had a risk sexual behavior, and all of the latter but one changed it by reducing the number of partners and/or increasing their use of condoms.

b. In the syringe and needle sharing

Due to a methodological shortcoming, a clear-cut answer could not be given for 14 patients. Of the remaining 17, 13 had reduced their sharing, and 4 did not (all of them B&P PD, none of them seropositive).

c. Overall change

Out of the 16 patients with sexual risk behavior and for whom we know whether they reduced or not their needle and syringe sharing, 1 did not change anything (neither "a", nor "b"), 8 made a partial change (either "a" or "b"), and 7 changed both.

Discussion

Syringe and needle sharing on the one hand, sexual behavior on the other hand, represent the main risk factors among IVDUs (Robertson et al., 1988). Nevertheless, most HIV transmission studies among IVDUs have focused on drug-use related behavior, and little is known about sexual risk factors in that population (Harris et al., 1990; Nemoto et al., 1990). Our findings confirm that the risk linked to sexual behavior should not be underestimated. As our sample is drawn from an inpatient psychiatric population, we could assess a diagnosis to each IVDU, and we think that the risk due to sexual behavior is particularly striking in the *psychotic* drug users, even though our figures are small.

IVDUs seem to be concerned by the risk of HIV-infection, as is shown by the almost general performance of a screening test, but only one out of four changed adequately his/her behavior (both in the sexual and in the needle and syringe sharing). We cannot point to any difference in the change of behavior linked to psychiatric diagnosis but, as has been shown by Robertson et al. (1988), seropositive IVDUs seem more prone to change their behavior, both in the drug-related and in the sexual domains.

Conclusion

Our study, which should be replicated on a larger sample, points to the fact that a more thorough attention should be paid to the risk linked to sexual behavior among IVDUs. In our small sample, we found that *psychotic* IVDUs were at a particularly high risk linked to their sexual behavior. Thus, a psychiatric evaluation could help to identify among IVDUs a subgroup of very high-risk individuals, for whom specific educational and preventive measures should be taken, notably in the sexual domain.

References

Harris RE, Langrod J, Hebert JR, Lowinson J, Zang E, Wynder EL (1990) Changes in AIDS risk behavior among intravenous drug abusers in New York City. NY State J Med 90: 123-126

Nemoto T, Brown LS, Foster K, Chu A (1990) Behavioral risk factors of human immunodeficiency virus infection among intravenous drug users and implications for preventive interventions. AIDS Education and Prevention 2: 116-126

Robertson JR, Skidmore CA, Roberts JJK (1988) HIV infection in intravenous drug users: a follow-up study indicating changes in risk-taking behaviour. Br J Addict 83:387-391

Campaigns of Fear and Behaviour Change in UK Drug Users

L. Sherr

Principal Clinical Psychologist, St Mary's Hospital, Pread Street, London W2 1NY,
United Kingdom

INTRODUCTION

In the UK drug users (DU) form a sizeable proportion of those
infected with HIV and those with AIDS.   Furthermore if one
examines the statistics in depth the picture that emerges is
of grave concern.   In the gay community the percentage of new
infections is reducing, yet the drug using community shows a
dramatic increase.   The situation is further exacerbated by
the fact that, in Europe generally, drug users contribute
direct and indirectly to both the heterosexual spread of HIV
and to paediatric infection.

This urgent challenge has been known from the start yet many
of the efforts to combat spread in this group have fallen
short of their target.   There are many reasons for this.
Firstly, unlike the gay community, the DUs are not necessarily a community as such, with little or no cohesion, scant
resources and limited access to organisational and health
care outlets.   DUs on the whole, have many life crises and
HIV infection can often represent yet another crisis without
being the major focus.   They are already indulging in a self

injurious behaviour and many of the messages may not have salience to their value systems. Furthermore, their links with health care agencies are often limited or haphazard. Problems and prejudices from society may also present hurdles. For example the availability of clean needles has been contentious in many countries and much ground had to be laid before some workers could accommodate the notions of harm reduction and minimisation. At least a third of HIV +ve DUs are women and the majority of these are in their childbearing years. The infection rates in women closely parallel those in children and can be used as a predictor of subsequent paediatric infection. This can also be compounded with the impact of drugs on pregnancy and a potentially compromised infant may have to struggle against HIV, drug withdrawal as well as social and economic challenges.

This urgent agenda has seen a catalogue of reactions from health education sources. It is of note that the worldwide reaction to HIV has seen the production of enormous quantities of literature and health education attempts, often with high profile, yet with little examination of efficacy and impact. Also of note is the appearance of visions of gloom and doom, grim reapers and skeletons, coffins and blood. This paper sets out to examine, both theoretically and empirically, the role of fear arousal in this applied area and the extent to which it facilitates or hinders the quest for behaviour change as a partial containment of HIV.

It is invariably meaningless to ask whether health education works or not - despite the fact that this is an oft posed question. Rather it is the academic task to understand the nature of effects which can be anticipated via various media sources in particular situations on different groups. Mass media provides, by its very nature an immediate and massive audience, yet devoid of interpersonal communication and limited in terms of its immediate feedback. The form of input of the mass media differs considerably in terms of its cost, its methodology, the audience it reaches, salience and impact. In addition despite planned goals mass media may have addtional unanticipated effects (Cantril 1958).

Health education has drawn heavily on commercial marketing notions. However, the very nature of the difference in the products and aims of the promoters may need in depth application of the theory rather than simple adoption of techniques which may have been useful in the promotion of soap powders. Workers such as Solomon (1981) point out the need for campaigns to meet consumers' needs, the importance of making the "product" real, attractive and accessible (Tones 1990), the hierarchy of communication effects, the need to understand and target different segments of the market appropriately, a requirement to understand the needs and responses of the market, to provide and react upon feedback all within the constraints of resources, competing elements and the expectations of the target population in the first place.

Based on these notions health education literature suggestscaution and understanding that the mass media is limited when called upon to convey complex messages, teach motor tasks or provide support to facilitate or encourage change.In the United Kingdom a series of campaigns were launched as a Government response to HIV. These were often hurriedly compiled and although they were of high profile, there was little recorded behaviour change in the short term (Sherr 1987, Sherr 1990). After the initial round there was a decided need to target such campaigns. In response the UK Government set up a series of campaigns, ostensibly targetted at the drug using groups, using, in the main, fear arousal.

Fear arousal has often been used despite weak theoretical underpinning. Janis (1977) and Leventhal (1970) found that some levels of fear could facilitate attention, but excess fear may encourage denial. As far back as 1974 Sternthal and Craig concluded that fear arousal was ineffective in behaviour change. It is unclear whether this is because fearful subjects simply do not respond or if ostensibly frightening messages did not scare the subject. The former explanation would suggest the abandonment of fear arousing techniques, yet the latter would encourage higher levels of fear provocation. No studies utilising fear messages have yet measured if their target subjects are indeed frightened.

In this series of campaigns targetting was not carried out by clear thought out placement of material or attempts to reach this population. Rather there was a need for those to whom the message was aimed to self select. The campaign utilised bill board posters (visual) and television advertisements (audio visual). The initial set of posters (with some slight variations) presented a scene of bloody gauze, used syringe and needle, bent metal teaspoon with a warning caption (fear vision plus fear message). A later set of posters showed a giant syringe puncturing five arms with a caption "Sharing your mate's works means sharing with everyone he's ever shared with" and pictures of three needles in an outstretched hand. The two television advertisements also used fear arousal techniques. One portrayed a couple and vividly showed a scene of needle sharing and injecting. The second showed a worried young man attending hospital, surrounded by ill wheelchair bound patients, being told he was HIV positive. The adverts culminated in a visual portrayal of needles piercing a doll to emphasize the message.

In the light of these considerations, two studies were set up to examine the impact of this material on the drug using population and students.

METHODOLOGY

Study 1:- 111 subjects (59 students - mean age 21.7; 49% male - and 52 drug dependency unit (DDU) attenders - mean age 30.9; 60% male) were contacted at the initiation of the government public campaign. Clinical anxiety measures (Spielberger 1974) were taken and subjects were subsequently exposed to either the first visual or audiovisual campaigns (randomly chosen). Post exposure anxiety was measured so that change scores could indicate the impact of the material, together with details of drug using behaviour, sexual behaviour, perceptions of risk and appraisal of the problem.

Study 11. This study involved only drug users (n=53) with a mean age of 29.2 years. These subjects were randomly divided into four groups. A baseline group (n=14) completed clinical anxiety questionnaire. Group 2 saw the early bill board posters (n=14) group 3 saw the later posters (n=11) and group

4 saw the TV commercials (n=11). Similarly to study 1 post exposure anxiety, sexual and drug using behaviour, perceptions of risk and attitudes were completed by all.

RESULTS Study 1

ANXIETY :- Prior to exposure students were significantly less anxious than DU (t=6.1 p<.0001). Exposure to the material increased anxiety significantly for students (t=3.8 p<.0001) but had no effect on DU. Anxiety scores for all groups were not affected by medium of exposure -visual or audiovisual. DU appraised the adverts significantly less likely to be shocking (t=1.5 p <.01) or frightening (t=2.4 p<.01 table 1).

VARIABLE	MEAN		SIG
	DDU	STUDENTS	
Age	30.9	21.7	**
Anxiety (pre v and av)	51.3	38.1	**
Anxiety (post v and av)	49.9	41.7	**
7 pt ratings:-			
Realistic Ads	3.7	5.0	**
Ads change thoughts	2.8	3.4	NS
Ads shock you	2.3	3.9	**
Ads made you anxious	2.8	3.2	ns
Ads frighten you	2.4	3.2	*
Ads change your sex behaviour	2.7	2.2	ns
Ads apply to you	3.2	1.9	**
Perceived personal risk HIV	2.7	2.4	ns
How worried about AIDS	4.1	3.5	ns

TABLE 1. COMPARISONS BETWEEN STUDENTS AND DRUG USERS.

GROUPS:- The DDU were significantly older than the students. Students were more shocked by the adverts, yet behaviour change did not differ between the groups and was reported as low. Targetting was ineffective in that not one single subject in either group thought the advertisements were aimed at them personally. Opinions varied, some thought them aimed at current users, some at non users and some at adolescents.

394

Surprisingly 42% of the drug users thought they were not
personally at risk for HIV as did 24% of the students despite
the fact that many students reported some drug use in the
past 6 months (72.4% cannabis, 25.5% narcotics and 2.3%
injecting). Most subjects (84.6% DDU and 83% students)
reported no change in their drug using behaviour. Those who
had changed reported both decreases and increases.

MEDIUM:- Both groups were equally likely to report noticing
visual material (43 and 47%) but DUs were less likely to
notice television (41.5% versus 25%) due, in all probability
to their socioeconomic situation which may limit their access
to television sets. Planners should clearly take this into
account. DUs rated the material significantly lower when
appraising how realistic they were (t=3.8 p<.001).

RISKS:- Perceived personal risk was low. The emphasis on
needle sharing may overlook risks from sexual exposure as 35%
DDU and 32% students reported more than 2 partners in the
preceding 6 months. Over half said the campaign had not
changed their sexual behaviour at all despite personal knowledge of someone with AIDS (65% DDU 37% students).

RESULTS STUDY II

ANXIETY:- No significant differences were found between the
baseline DU group and those exposed to all three conditions.
Average anxiety levels for the sample was 48.02 which is
considerably higher than other groups (Spielberger 1970: eg
undergraduates 36.35, prison inmates 45.96) which may have
implications for use of fear arousal with an anxiety vulnerable   group   (see   table   2)

VARIABLE	BASE	2(POSTER 1)	3 (POSTER 2)	4 (AV)
Anxiety	49.3	49.5	46.1	46.2
Worried re AIDS		4.6	3.3	4.0
Personal risk		2.4	2.4	2.9
Change behaviour		2.6	2.8	2.6
Apply to you		2.9	2.6	3.2

TABLE 2. SCORES ACCORDING TO GROUP.

BEHAVIOURAL MEASURES:- One way analysis of variance revealed no significant differences between groups in response to any behavioural questions. 48.2% stated the advertisements had little effect on their thoughts about drug use and AIDS/HIV infection. 63% thought the adverts did not apply to them at all. 75.9% stated the adverts would have little effect on their behaviour and a further 50% thought it would not effect the behaviour of others. 68.5% thought they were not personally at risk for AIDS. Less than half (39%) report any worry about AIDS at all. Over half the sample (55.6%) reported sex with more than one partner in the preceding six months.

DISCUSSION

This study shows that fear messages do frighten some (the students) but had no significant effect on the DUs. The anxiety norms of drug users were significantly higher than the students and that of other normative populations.

Behaviour change, for both students and DUs, was low in terms of drug use and sexual behaviour - both risk factors for HIV transmission. Fear arousal was limited. No long term follow up data was available but may be of interest. Public resources should be utilised with great care. Television advertisements (which are usually much more costly) had no greater impact in this instance and were not a source utilised by DUs who often had limited access to television or motivation to watch. It is also debatable whether attempting to increase the anxiety levels of a group who are already highly anxious is justifiable. The targetting of the campaign seemed ambiguous. Most subjects questioned, irrespective of group, felt that the campaign was not targetted at them which may partially explain the absence of anxiety. The problem may be a similar one to that identified by Woffinden (1988) - the advertisements are uncomprimisingly bleak and squalid. Whilst this may fit popular prejudices about drugs and thereby discourage their use in the population generally, it may have limited impact on drug users themselves who find the images at variance with their experience or too negative, and subsequently reject them. Indeed, some subjects reported, anecdotally, that the visual image of the needle in the advertisements triggered desires to inject.

Knowledge of someone with AIDS (unlike the San Francisco findings) was not predictive of behaviour change or perceived personal risk. This is consistent with Weinstein's (1980) notions that people tend to believe that negative events are less likely to happen to them whilst endorsing the notion that positive events are more likely to happen. This optimistic bias may result in a reluctance to take on board precautions or behaviour change.

From Health Education theory these campaigns were problematic. Goals and aims were unclear as was targetting. No pretesting was reported. These results suggest a need for alternative strategies to reach this population in the first instance and to engender sustained behaviour change in the second. Some effects have been clearly demonstrated by needle exchange units (Hart 1990), outreach projects (Stimson 1989) and reports of changed sharing behaviour from needle exchange attenders (Mulleady 1990). Fear arousing mass media campaigns have yet to prove their efficacy.

REFERENCES.

Cantril H (1958) The invasion from Mars in Readings in Social Psychology eds EE Maccoby TM Newcomb and EL Hartley Henry Holt New York pp 291-300

Hart G Woodward N & Carvell A (1989) Needle Exchange in Central London Operating philosophy and communication strategies AIDS Care Vol 1 no 2 pp 125-134

Janis IL Mann I (1977)Decision making a psychological analysis of conflict choice and commitment New York Free Press

Leventhal H (1970) Findings and theory in the studies of fear communictions in Adv in Exp and Social Psych 5, Acad Press

Mulleady G (1990) Paper presented at the British Psychological Society London Conference Symposium AIDS and Sex.

Sherr L (1987) Evaluation of the UK Health education capaign on AIDS Psychology Health 1, 61-72

Sherr L (1990) Fear arousal and AIDS Do shock tactics work? AIDS Vol4 no 4 pp 361-364

Solomon DS (1981) A social marketing perspective on campaigns in Public Communication Campaigns eds RE Rice and WJ Paisley Sage Beverly Hills.

Spielberger CD Gorsuch R Lusherne R (1974) The State Trait Anxient Inventory, Consulting Psychology Press, Palo Alto

Sternthal B Craig C (1981) Fear appeal revisited Journal of Consumer Research 3, 22-34

Stimson G (1989) Syringe exchange programmes for injecting drug users AIDS 3 pp 253-260

Tones K Tilford S & Robinson Y (1990) Health Education Effectiveness and Efficiency, Chapman Hall, London

Weinstein ND (1983) Reducing unrealistic optimism about future life events. Health Psychology 2, 11-20

Woffinden B (1988) Campaigns that die of ignorance The Listener March 3

Resocialization and AIDS-Prevention by Remedacen Substitution

R. Wille, H. Siegismund, and R. Pels Leusden

Klinikum der Christian-Albrechts-Universität zu Kiel, Arnold-Hellerstraße 12,
D-W-2300 Kiel, Federal Republic of Germany

We assume that all participants of this congress are well acquainted with the individual misery and the socio-political emotionality of both subjects concerned - AIDS and drugs. So doing without the usual theoretical or ethic preliminaries, we would therefore like to introduce to you here our empirical data about an uncommon substitution treatment of IVDA with Remedacen, a codein remedium.

As far as the method and the extent is concerned, this treatment program of the physician, Dr. Grimm deserves attention.

<u>Data and method:</u>

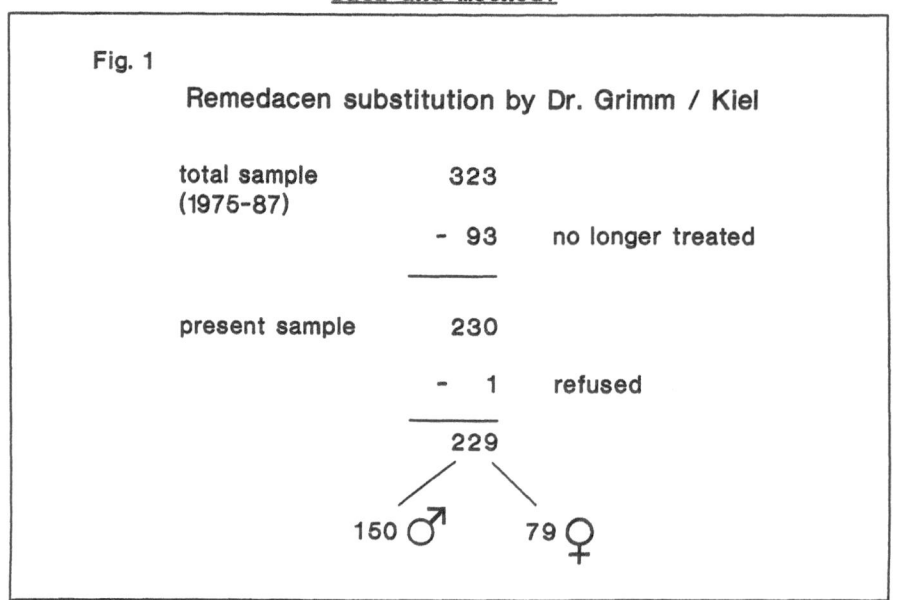

From 1975 to 1987 Dr. Grimm ambulatory prescribes Dihydrocodein, i.e. Remedacen, which is metabolized at a rate of approx. 10% into Dihydromorphine, but is not covered by the narcotics law, to drug addicts in his practice in Kiel. The efficacy profile is comparable to that of Methadon with longer effect duration without pronounced euphory and calling for more unpleasant feelings at the abstinence syndrome.

Dr. Grimm prescribes the capsules on demand and as a weekly ration, whereby 20 capsules daily stand for a low dosage, 50 capsules a medium and 100 capsules a maximum dosage. The actual taking is not medically or otherwise controlled. The same goes for the also prescribed Codein- phosphoric tablets.

Additonal psychotropic substances (benzodiacepines) on the other hand are only prescribed in limited amounts. We can confirm, that on joining the programm a drug anamnesis is ascertained and noted in the medical history data.

Principle requirements for treatment are:

-IVD (ab)use

-unsuccessful abstinence attempts or refusing of this.

-no psychotropic medication by other doctors.

-unexpected blood and urine controls.

-reliable accounts about illegal drug consumption.

Purpose of treatment:
decriminalization and social reintegration along with somatic, psychic and social healing.

```
Fig. 2
   total sample    323

                   - 93  no longer treated
                   ─────────────────────────

                     16  died
                       - 9  suicide/homicide
                       - 3  overdosage
                       - 1  AIDS
                       - 3  unclarified

                      9  imprisoned

                     19
                       - 5  abstinence therapy
                       - 4  maintenance therapy
                       - 9  quit prematurely
                       - 1  excluded by therapist

                     49  no longer abusing opiats
                          (not strictly controlled )
                       -44  since several years
                       - 5  since several months
                   ─────────────────────────
                     93
```

In this manner there were 323 patients treated between 1975 and 1987, 230 of those during the investigation period from december 1988 to summer 1989.

Fig. 3   Treatment Dr. Grimm

       Opiats: Remedacen = 30 mg Dehydrocodein
                 Codein compr.= 50 mg Codeinphosphate

       low dosage   20 capsules per day

       middle dosage   40-50 capsules per day

       maximum dosage   70-100 capsules per day

       Prescription weekly as demanded
       150-700 capsules
       Consume not controlled

       Additional prescription of benzodiazepines
       at limited dosage

The patients were informed by Dr. Grimm about the research project. 229 consented and turned out to be quite cooperative in all points of this survey. The statements made by the patients were not controlled by us, merely the working status was objectivated by documents.
Alongside the extensive interviews, we had all medical records in the practice at our unrestricted disposal.

This is therefore a retrospective, not controlled study based mainly on subjective information given by the patient with a rough orientation according to pragmatic aspects such as:

-demographic data (age and gender)

-illness revealed at the beginning of the treatment.

-medical anamnesis including HIV/AIDS.

-drug anamnesis, social anamnesis and sexual anamnesis.

-comparison prior to and following substitution.

-critical notes made by the patients.

Of all results first a survey covering the 93 patients already quit (see fig. 2). The statements about the 44 patients free of opiats are based on information by the practice Dr. Grimm; (so far) they have not been controlled by us.

```
Fig. 4                    HIV - positive IVDA

    total sample     323        35  HIV - positive ▪ 10,8%

                                 23  male

                                 12  female

    present sample  229         22  HIV - positive ▪ 9,6%

                                 14  male

                                  8  female
                                 ─────────────────────────
                                 11  with symptoms

                                 11  no symptoms
```

The HIV-test positiveness is revealed as follows:

35 of 323 = 11% taking the whole sample

22 of 229 = 9,6% taking the present sample

which is clearly u n d e r comparable surveys.

We suspect several causes:
In Schleswig-Holstein drug scene as well as AIDS are underrepresented in comparison to other states in the FRG. However, 30% of the patients are from Hamburg with a relatively high HIV-rate.

Considering that the substitution treatment averagely takes a period of 4 years, an HIV-prevention effect seems to us to be worth discussion.

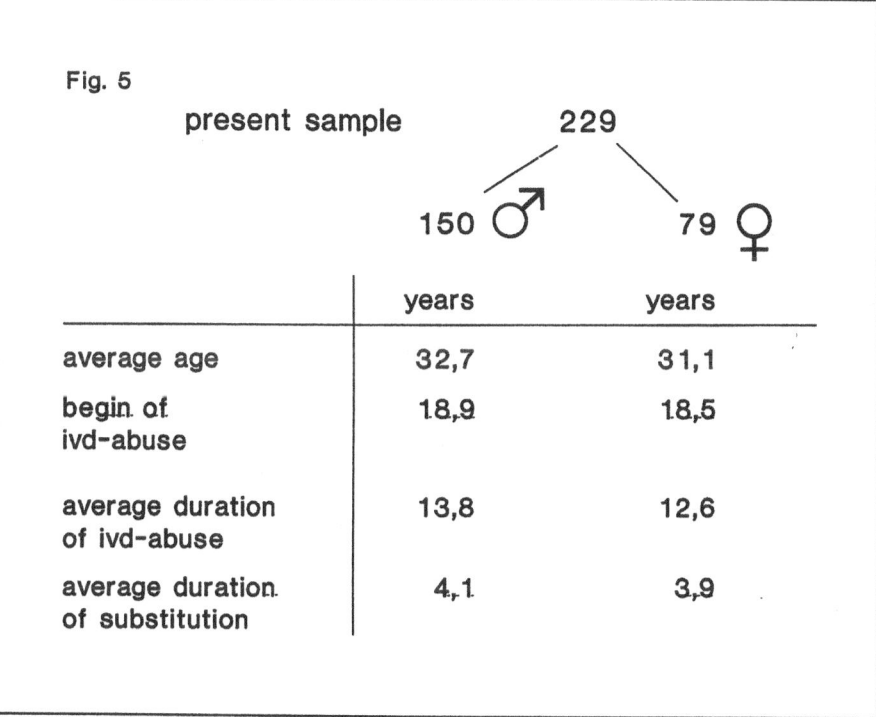

Fig. 5

present sample   229

150 ♂   79 ♀

	years	years
average age	32,7	31,1
begin of ivd-abuse	18,9	18,5
average duration of ivd-abuse	13,8	12,6
average duration of substitution	4,1	3,9

Age and gender relation are in accordance with the data of the drug-population.

The following tables show the results of comparison prior to and after beginning substitution and each relate to 229 patients, of these 150 male and 79 female with average ages of 32,7 (male) and 31,1(female).

The entrance into the drug-scene began for the males at the age of 18,9 and for the females at an age of 18,5 in average. The duration of substitution in the middle for the males was 48,7 month and for females 46,7. The times of substitution (4 years) are nearly a half of the 9 years drug career. In evaluation the data of substitution must be doubled.

Results

Fig. 6   Results

                        Frequency of IVD-abuse

                        pre   post

once per day   119   5

several times   59   7
per week

once per month   51   130
and less frequent

no iv-opiats   –   59

Needle sharing is regarded as a specific risk for ivd-users and
is the main pathway of transmission for the HIV-infection and
ranges far before sexual transfer.

Fig. 7   Results

                        Needle-sharing

                        pre   post

no   38   193

yes   188   36

no answer   3   –

More than 80% of the sample had experienced needle-sharing - of those 55% in less cases than 30% of the injections, 25% in more than 30%.

The pre and post treatment comparison shows a distinct decrease from 80% to 15%.

In the case of sexual transmission distinctions are made among sexual partnerships within as well as outside of the scene. Supply prostitution is regarded separately.

22 (= 9,6%) male and 17 (=22) female patients had had homosexual experiences, mostly in homes or prisons - usually by chance relationships with 2,1 and 1,6 partners in average.
The one male proband with homosexual identity referred to 95 partners, the one lesbian to 16 (female) partners.

Fig. 8   Results

                              Prostitution
                    pre   post
                   ♂ ♀   ♂ ♀

no prostitution   143 49   149 75

prostitution   6   28   -   3

answer refused   1   2   1   1

Very much lower than in comparable surveys (there 50% - 80%) was the number of 28 (= 35%) women and 6 (= 4%) men stating to have prostituted themselves in order to acquire the badly needed money for the drug supply averagely 19 months for men and 15 for women on the street. Monthly approx. 66 customers - therefore altogether 1500 for the females and 1000 for the males.

6 of the female supply prostitutes were HIV-positive , 3 reported experiences with anale , sado-masochistic and urine-fetishist practices.

One of the male prostitutes was HIV-positive.

After taking up the substitution, two women continued the prostitution, one of them being HIV-positive, the other having to "pay old debts" and therefore expecting a large customer frequency.

None of the male prostitutes continues this after the substitution.

Fig. 9	Results			
	Imprisonment			
	pre		**post**	
	male/female		male/female	
not imprisoned	53	39	132	76
imprisoned	97	40	18	3
average duration of imprisonment in weeks	124	49	33	13

Similarly impressing is the comparison prior to and after substitution in regard to decriminalization.

The most convincing stabilization is reported concerning the social situation. The chasing after the poison stops and along with that the distortion of the daily routine. The substituted ivd users can far more easily cope with the burdens of every-day-working life.

Fig. 10   Results

Occupation and training

	pre		post	
	male/female		male/female	
no occupation	79	41	64	36
jobbing	28	26	31	15
regular work	43	12	54	28
school, training	14	14	15	12

more than one answer possible

Our results do show some improvement, not a dramatic one, of the social and professional situation.

Although all patients felt stabilized in their psychic and social situation and felt obliged to Dr. Grimm's prescriptions - some even clearly showed emotional binding to him personally - approx. 75% criticize the shortcoming or even lacking of psycho-social attendance by their doctor.

It was always acknowledged that Dr. Grimm took time for his patients in crisis-situations but on the whole the lacking attendance was the main point of criticism.

408

Discussion

On the basis of patients' statements, distinct and positive effects of the Remedacen substitution are quite obvious: Some opponants' arguments become questionable. We are able to observe a decrease of convictions and prison sentences - even if only indirectly controlled. So substitution is liable to reduce criminality. Under the aspect of HIV prevention, a distinct reduction of needle-sharing and also of supply prostitution was to be observed.

If 10000 out of 20000 female IVD addicts prostitute themselves occasionally and approx. 1000 to 2000 are HIV positive and presuming 2 customers daily with 50% unsafe sexual contacts, you can estimate 1 to 2 infections each day. In order to reduce the number of approx. 300 to 500 infections annually, the substitution principally does seem a promising and sensible approach.

By this, the channels of the virus into the heterosexual population majority are narrowed. But even within the drug scene there are definitely less HIV and hepatitis infections to be expected thus also contributing to health, psychological and social stabilization.

Even if the subjective statements made by the patients themselves are judged to be incomplete and euphemic, the positive tendancy on the whole will only change in quantity.

As far as the mechanisms of influence are concerned, our retrospective approach does not allow for assertion about stabilization of the personality structure and also not about the psychic state of feelings on no more than the grounds of an indeed repeated but nevertheless only superficial impression dealing with a very inhomogenous group:

Many, perhaps even most of them continue their dealer habits during or after the substitution treatment: Not only the train fare to Kiel but also other requirements are paid by the sale of Remedacen capsules. It is no problem to have more than the personal supply prescribed by Dr. Grimm. We spoke to patients

who had hoarded several hundred (up to 1000) capsules which
they would put into use when needed as extra currency. ("I fly
to Mallorca for 500 capsules").

Reports from the drug scene outside of Kiel say that Remedacen
is also exchanged directly or indirectly into illegal drugs.

The emotionally stabilizing pharmacological effect enables a
more balanced daily routine without the hectic run for drug
supply; in individual periods of time it allows a "high by
injection" and can help to bring the abstinence syndrom under
control. Furthermore they mean financial aid for everyday-needs
but also for injection equipment and therefore reduce acute
crises which in the past would have lead to prostitution and
also supported needle-sharing.

Whether or not these effects outweigh the numerous serious
objections against substitution is not for us to say - each
individual should decide for himself. Considering the large
number of drug addicts (and also other) patients making an
individual attendance along with psychological and social
support as well as a sensitive perception or undesirable
developments nearly impossible thus causing the situation of
uncontrolled prescribing, does not help to reduce our
reservations regarding Dr. Grimm's method of treatment.

We are most sincerely grateful to our colleague, Dr. Grimm, for
his readiness to support this survey.

In our opinion, however, his mission-minded management with a
certain lack of self-criticism does not agree and come up to
our medical standards. This survey provokes the following idea:
If such a questionable substitution programm as this one shows
an HIV prevention effect, how much more convincing would this
be in the case of responsible, careful handling. This would, of
course, call for a financially extensive engagement of trained
therapeuts and a great deal of psychosocial ideas.

References

Angaro G, Pastore G, Monno L, Santantonio T, Luchena N, Schiraldi O (1985) Rapid spread of HTLV-III among drug addicts in Italy. Lancet II: 1302

Behrendt U (1979) Erkrankungen bei Drogenabhängigen vom Opiattyp. Inaugural-Dissertation, FU Berlin

Bornemann R, Bschor F, Kalinna V (1988) AIDS- und HIV-Progression 1982-1987 bei iv-Drogengebrauchern und -abhängigen in Europa. AIDS und Drogen, Deutsche AIDS-Hilfe e.V., Berlin

Grimm G (1985) Die Lösung des Drogenproblems. Verlag Wolf Pflesser

Harms G, Laukamm-Josten U, Bienzle U, Guggenmoos-Holzmann I (1987) Risk factors for HIV infection in German iv drug abusers. Kli Wochenschrift 65: 376-379

Harms G, Bienzle U, Schneider V, Bschor F (1987) HIV-Antikörperprävalenz bei Berliner iv-Drogenabhängigen. AIFO 7: 392-393

Hubbard RL, Allison M, Bray RM, Craddock SG, Rachal JV, Ginzburg HM (1983) An overview of client characteristics, treatment services and during-treatment outcome for outpatient methadone clinics in the treatment outcome prospective study (TOPS). National Institute on Drug Abuse (NIDA). Research on the treatment of Narcotic Addiction, State of the Art

Mielk A (1990) Weibliche Prostituierte und HIV-Ausbreitung: Diskussion der epidemiologischen Erkenntnisse. AIFO 4: 183-187

Oemichen M, Staak M (1988) Der Tod des Drogenkonsumenten: Geschehensablauf, Häufigkeit sowie Nachweisbarkeit und Prognose. Betäubungsmittelmißbrauch, Springer Verlag

Püschel K, Teicher M, Arnold W, Schmold A, Koops E, Beckmann E-R, Janssen W, Gessmann H, Dönnecke E, Plewka W (1984) Fornsisch-medizinische und kriminologische Aspekte der Hamburger Rauschgifttodesfälle bis Ende 1982. Suchtgefahren 3

Schoenbaum EE, Hartel D, Selwyn PA, Klein RS, Davenny K, Rogers M, Feiner C, Friedland G (1989) Risk factors for human immunodeficiency virus infection in intravenous drug users. N Engl J Med 321: 874-897

Uchtenhagen U (1987) Zehn Jahre Methadon-Programme in der Schweiz - zum Bericht der Schweizer Methadonkommission. Medikamentengestützte Rehabilitation bei Drogenabhängigen

Van den Hoek JAR, Coutinho RA, Van Haastrecht HJA, Van Zadelhof AW, Goudsmit J (1988) Prevalence and risk factors of HIV infections among drug users and drug-using prostitutes in Amsterdam. AIDS 2: 55-60

Velimirovic B (1987) AIDS und Drogenabhängigkeit aus der Sicht des Epidemiologen. AIFO 2: 323-332

A Treatment Model to Heroin Addicts in Italy

U. Avico[1], P. Castrogiovanni[2], A. Dell' Utri[1], I. Maremmani[2],
D. Meloni[3], P. E. Manconi[3], O. Zolesi[2], and A. Tagliamonte[3]

[1] Instituto Superiore di Sanità, Viale Regina Elena 299, I-00161 Roma
[2] Institute of Psychiatry, University of Pisa, Via Roma 67, I-53100 Pisa
[3] Institute of Pharmacology and Biochemical Pathology, University of Cagliari,
Via Porcell 4, I-09124 Cagliari, Italy

The heroin is the main hard drug of abuse among the illicit ones in Italy. The number of overdose episodes increase steadily year by year, indicating the danger of the phenomenon. The policy of several Authorities privileges drug-free treatment approaches and residential communities role while methadone programs still find a sort of ideological opposition.

On the ground of our experience a correct use of methadone, administered on a maintenace or long term base, produces complete heroin abstinence in 40% of the examined patients and it permits a controlled use of illicit narcotics in further 30% of them, resulting in a final 70% positive outcomes.

The issue of assistance to drug addicts in general and to heroin addicts in particular is still under debate in Italy. The available data from both Public Services (PS) and Residential Communities (RC), beginning from 1980, show a continous increase in the number of patients demanding treatment. A steady increase in the number of drug addicts treated from 1986 to 1989 in PS, RC and Prison (P) was recorded (tab. 1).

New patients increased in percentage, while the ratio (4:1) of males to females remained constant (tab. 2). The percentage of females treated in the PS was about half in respect of that treated in RC. Moreover, a marked increase in number of newly assessed RC from 1988 to 1989 and a tendency to decrease substitutive treatments emerged (fig. 1).

A better understanding of the apparent discrepancies observed in the previous data is possible. By the experience of sardinian facilities, we are aware that the figures may be the average of the data surveied at the end of the two semesters or of the four quarters each year. Then these figures represent the number of patients under treatment at the moment of the survey and do not reflect their month to month turnover. Similarly, the data from P reflect merely the number of drug addicts among inmates, some of which could be the same person arrested two or more times during the same year and submitted to treatment each time (tab. 3).

The tendency to use psycho-social, drug-free approaches is continuosly increasing, at expense of the multimodal ones in the PS (tab. 4). In 1990 only 15% of the heroin addicts demanding treatment at the PS received a methadone maintenance treatment.

Even if this criterion can signify the purpose of a global improvement of the intervention at a prolonged time, the fact remains that in Italy heroin is the leading drug of abuse among illicit compounds (tab. 5, 6) and the number of heroin abuse related deaths is steadily increasing year by year (tab. 7, 8).

Finally, it seems useful to envisage both the no. of the AIDS-cases drug abuse related (from 120-1986 to 1,615-1989) and their proportion to the no. of addicts anyhow mentioned (from 1,0%-1986 to 3.0%-1989) (tab. 9).

TABLE 1

DRUG ADDICTS TREATED BY PUBLIC SERVICES (PS),
RESIDENTIAL COMMUNITIES (RC) AND IN PRISON (P). (1986-1989)

YEAR	PS	RC	P	TOTAL
1986	20,137	5,927	6,015	32,079
1987	23,276	6,676	5,281	35,233
1988	27,906	8,017	7,500	43,423
1989	33,335	9,965	7,722	51,022

SOURCES: Drug Abuse Monitoring Department - Min. of the Interior
D.G. on Prisons - Min. Justice

Data processed by the Istituto Superiore di Sanità
Data presented to the CEWG meeting - Wash. D.C., Dec. 1990

TABLE 2

DRUG ADDICTS TREATED BY PS (1986 - 1989)

	1986	1987	1988	1989
TOTAL	36,000	45,000	51,000	60,000
NEW PATIENTS	31.0%	33.5%	35.0%	38.0%
MALES	78.2%	78.5%	81.0%	81.0%
FEMALES	21.8%	21.5%	19.0%	19.0%

SOURCE: D.G. on Social Medicine - Min. Health

Data presented to the CEWG meeting - Wash. D. C., Dec. 1990

FIGURE 1

PUBLIC SERVICES AND RESIDENTIAL COMMUNITIES , ADDICTS U. TREATMENT
AND DISTRIBUTION BY SEX . (1988 - 1989)

PUBLIC SERVICES

1988	1989	INC. %
Assessed centres = 479	Assessed centres = 488	+ 1.9
Total addicts = 27,000	Total addicts = 33,335	+ 18.4
% Females = 10.8	% Females = 10.8	-
% Substitutive treat. = 41.1	% Substitutive treat. = 39.4	- 2.0

RESIDENTIAL COMMUNITIES

1988	1989	INC .%
Assessed centres = 351	Assessed centres = 404	+ 15.0
Total addicts = 8,017	Total addicts = 9,965	+ 24.3
% Females = 18.8	% Females = 17.8	- 10.0

SOURCE: Drug Abuse Monitoring Department - Min. of the Interior

Data processed by the Istituto Superiore di Sanità
Data presented to the CEWG meeting - Wash. D.C., Dec. 1990

TABLE 3

DRUG ADDICTS TREATED BY PUBLIC SERVICES (PS), RESIDENTIAL COMMUNITIES (RC)
AND IN PRISON (P). (Regional distribution - 1989)

REGION	PS	RC	P	TOTAL
PIEMONTE	4,575	484	845	5,904
AOSTA	44	9	63	116
LIGURIA	1,969	293	187	2,449
LOMBARDIA	6,215	1,494	1,446	9,155
TRENTINO ALTO ADIGE	568	98	126	792
FRIULI V.G.	589	85	86	760
VENETO	1,997	570	319	2,886
EMILIA ROM.	2,810	2,143	596	5,549
TOSCANA	2,336	931	416	3,683
MARCHE	696	379	71	1,146
UMBRIA	721	624	108	1,453
LAZIO	2,425	595	822	3,842
ABRUZZO	300	158	204	662
SARDEGNA	1,120	202	415	1,743
CAMPANIA	1,594	231	918	2,743
PUGLIA	4,046	843	457	5,346
MOLISE	25	-	54	79
CALABRIA	452	160	93	705
BASILICATA	141	11	47	199
SICILIA	706	655	449	1,810
ITALY	33,335	9,965	7,722	51,022

SOURCES: Drug Abuse Monitoring Departement - Min. of the Interior
D.G. on Prison - Min. Justice

Data processed by the Istituto Superiore di Sanità.
Data presented to the CEWG meeting - Wash. D.C., Dec. 1990.

416

TABLE 4

TREATMENT TYPES IN PS. (1986 - 1989)

TREATMENT	1986	1987	1988	1989
METHADONE:				
Maintenance	-	-	17.0%	15.0%
Short term	-	-	59.7%	56.0%
OTHER OPIODS	-	-	2.1%	3.5%
CLONIDINE	-	-	3.2%	4.0%
OTHER PSYCHOACTIVE COMPOUNDS	-	-	18.0%	21.5%
DRUG-FREE PSYCHOTHER.	32.8%	31.9%	42.0%	45.0%
PHARMAC. DRUGS ONLY	42.6%	41.5%	40.0%	39.0%
PSYCHOTHER.+ DRUGS	24.4%	26.5%	18.0%	16.0%

SOURCE: D.G. on Social Medicine - Min. Health

Data presented to the CEWG meeting - Wash. D.C., Dec. 1990.

TABLE 5

PRIMARY SUBSTANCE OF ABUSE IN NEW PATIENTS. (1986-1988)

	1986	1987	1988
HEROIN	80.2%	89.7%	89.5%
CANNABIS	8.3%	5.2%	5.9%
BENZODIAZEPINES	4.7%	2.4%	1.6%
COCAINE	1.6%	0.6%	0.6%
OTHERS	5.2%	2.1%	2.4%
POLIDRUG ABUSERS	46.5%	56.6%	70.5%

SOURCE: D.G. on Social Medicine - Min. Health

Data presented to the CEWG meeting - Wash. D.C., Dec.1990

TABLE 6

SEIZURE TREND. (1989 - 1990 ; Jan 1st - Nov 30th)

SEIZED DRUGS (KG)	1990	1989
HEROIN	797.3	620.5
COCAINE	739.1	565.1
CANNABIS	7,777.4	23,125.0

SOURCE: Drug Enforcement Service-Min. of the Interior

Data presented to the CEWG meeting - Wash. D.C., Dec. 1990

TABLE 7

DRUG ABUSE RELATED DEATHS IN ITALY
DATA RELATED TO: RISK POPULATION (MALE + FEMALE, AGED 15-39)
AND DRUG ADDICTS (DA = PS+RC+P). (1986-1989)

PART OF	DEATHS/RISK POP. $(\times 10^5)$				DEATHS/DA $(\times 10^5)$ (mortality rate)			
ITALY	1986	1987	1988	1989	1986	1987	1988 (*)	1989
NORTH	1.8	3.7	5.1	6.1	9.2	19.2	-	19.7
CENTER	0.8	1.6	2.5	3.4	4.7	8.7	-	13.4
SOUTH +ISL.	0.7	1.3	1.8	2.2	6.7	12.1	-	17.5

(*) 1988 data were not available.

SOURCES: Drug Abuse Monitoring Department - Min. of the Interior
             D.G. on Prison - Min. Justice

Data processed by the Istituto Superiore di Sanità
Data presented to the CEWG meeting - Wash. D.C., Dec. 1990

TABLE 8

DRUG ABUSE RELATED DEATHS IN ITALY (*). (1986-1989)

REGION	1986	1987	1988	1989	1990
PIEMONTE	33	47	84	88	135
VAL D'AOSTA	-	4	2	-	3
LIGURIA	17	37	56	65	68
LOMBARDIA	81	115	213	292	263
TRENTINO					
ALTO ADIGE	4	12	12	17	14
FRIULI V.G.	3	9	5	5	13
VENETO	20	50	64	59	83
EMILIA ROM.	24	44	68	88	115
TOSCANA	9	16	46	43	65
MARCHE	2	7	10	14	20
UMBRIA	2	3	2	7	6
LAZIO	26	55	92	109	124
ABRUZZO	2	3	4	6	9
SARDEGNA	1	7	11	14	23
CAMPANIA	20	36	50	53	80
PUGLIA	15	29	38	58	59
MOLISE	-	-	-	3	-
BASILICATA	-	1	4	1	5
CALABRIA	2	6	7	12	20
SICILIA	15	24	18	27	44
ABROAD (**)	4	11	6	11	3
ITALY	276	516	792	972	1152

(*) Foreigners dead in Italy are included
(**) Italian dead abroad

SOURCE: Drug Enforcement Service - Min. of the Interior

Data processed by the Istituto Superiore di Sanità
Data presented to the CEWG meeting - Wash. D.C., Dec 1990

TABLE 9

NUMBER OF AIDS PATIENTS DRUG ABUSE RELATED; % INCREASE
AND RATIO TO THE CALCULATED NUMBER OF DRUG ADDICTS. (1985-1989)

	1985	1986	1987	1988	1989
AIDS (*)	120	309	706	1,272	1,615
% INCREASE		+158	+128	+80	+27
DRUG ADDICTS	27,301	32,079	35,233	43,423	51,022
RATIO AIDS/DA	0.4	1.,0	2.0	2.9	3.2

(*) Drug addicts + infants from DA mothers.

SOURCE: Istituto Superiore di Sanità

Data presented to the CEWG meeting - Wash. D.C., Dec. 1990.

The data from a PS in Cagliari, Sardinia active since October 1980 refer to more than 3,000 heroin addicts treated in the service. The "forced" approach proposed to such a large population of patients is that of a substitutive therapy with methadone. The patients are initially allowed to choose between a short term detoxification or a maintenance program. At the end of 1990 about 1,200 patients were under treatment and 1,000 of them were on methadone maintenance therapy.

On their request, the patients are assisted for HIV related problems in the same clinic where they receive treatment for heroin addiction.

The same staff has promoted and guarantees, in parallel with other institutions, a campaign of information on the danger and risks of heroin use and of potential infection with HIV. A decrease in the percentage (from an initial 75% to a scarce 35%) of drug addicts seropositive for anti-HIV antibodies at the first control was recorded in our clinic from 1985 to 1990 (Fig. 2).

On the other hand, the number of new patients entering the methadone program during the same period of time did not change as compared to the previous years. The percentage of patients under methadone who abuse other licit drugs reached 10% while another 13% of them had serious alcohol problems (Molari et al., 1987). Such figures, which do not include data on cannabinoids use, are in the average of other methadone programs (Liebson et al., 1973; Rounsaville et al., 1982). The therapeutic protocol proposed to these patients is based on gradual acquisition of privileges as a function of their agreement to the prescribed protocol. Patients are supposed to attend daily the clinic, to assume methadone in front to the nurse, and to report to a staff member any possible problem relevant to this situation.

Urine samples are taken weekly and analysed randomly for the presence of morphine. After a month of complete compliance and negative morphinuria, patients are allowed to take home methadone on sunday. A six monthly complete protocol agreement does allow the patients

FIGURE 2

PREVALENCE OF HIV INFECTION IN INTRAVENOUS DRUG ADDICTS. (1985-1990)

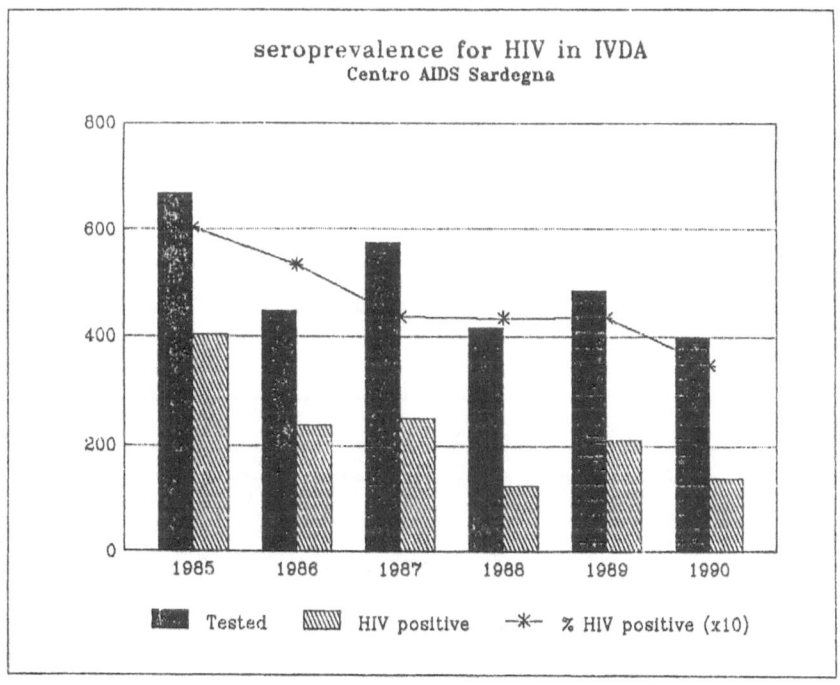

diagnosed as psychosis-free to be submitted once a week to due controls and staff interviews in the clinic, and to take methadone home for the remaining six days. Taking methadone home becomes a positive reinforcement which controls behaviour of a large number of patient and contributes to reduction and cessation of heroin use. Obviously, the privilege of taking methadone home remains linked to the absence of morphine in urine.

The patients population results divided into different categories on the basis of therapeutic compliance, subjects having to attend at the clinic daily and those who earned a relative self-sufficiency. About 20% of the patients presently under therapy, for a total of 186 subjects, started treatment 10 years ago. One hundred of them were randomly assigned to two groups, 40 weekly taking-home patients and 53 daily ones (7 were discarded because gave unreliable answers). The following parameters were controlled for each of them: sex, age, age of onset of heroin abuse, years while addicted, other abused drugs (alcohol, marijuana, central stimulants, benzodiazepines, hallucinogens), mean methadone dosage, protocol compliance, morphinuria, social adjustement and criminality rate at the first interview and during the last treatment year.

The 53 daily patients were further subdivised, on the base of therapeutic compliance, into two subgroups. The first one (28 subjects) includes addicts regularly attending daily at the clinic, and taking the prescribed dose of methadone; although 30% to 70% presented positive test for morphine they mantained a correct relationship with the staff. The second group (25 subjects) includes addicts absent from clinic more than twice a month and repeatedly trying to modify the methadone dosage; they had both a high rate of positive test for morphine, and a difficult relationship with the staff.

Thus three homogeneous groups of patients were defined, on the base of therapeutic compliance: 1. No-agreement to the program (25 patients); 2. Partial-agreement (28 patients); 3. Total- agreement (40 patients). Such classification appeared to be independent of patient's age, age of disease onset, duration of addiction (years), and other abused psychotropic drugs (tab. 10). Sex could not be taken in consideration, since only 4 subjects were female.

The mean methadone dosages were significantly different through groups. The 75% of group 1. used a dose from 30 to 60 mg a day. It is to notice that the over-60 mg dosages (16 subjects) concern merely the group 2. (9 subjects corresponding to 56%). On the whole, group 1.

TABLE 10

CHARACTERISTICS OF THE SAMPLE UNDER METHADONE TREATMENT

	GROUPS							
	1		2		3			
	No agreem. (n = 25)		Part. agreem. (n = 28)		Total agreem. (n = 40)			
	M	s	M	s	M	s	F	p
Age	34.0	3.5	33.1	3.4	33.0	4.3	0.67	0.51
Age of onset	19.0	3.0	19.3	3.1	18.1	4.3	1.10	0.33
Addiction years	15.0	2.9	13.8	1.8	14.9	3.2	1.81	0.16
Polidrug use	0.9	1.0	1.2	1.1	1.1	0.9	1.32	0.27
	%		%		%		CHI-SQ	p
Male	100.0		96.4		92.5		2.15	0.35

used the lowest mean dosage (tab. 11). Tab. 12 reports the Analysis of Variance (ANOVA) of two factor repeated measures applied to the social adjustment score of the three groups. Social

TABLE 11

MEAN METHADONE DOSAGES (mg) AND THERAPEUTIC COMPLIANCE.

	< 30	30-60	> 60	Total
No-agreem.	12.50%	75.00%	12.50%	100%
Part-agreem.	14.81%	55.56%	29.63%	100%
Total-agreem	40.00%	50.00%	10.00%	100%
Total	25.27%	58.24%	16.48%	100%

Chi Square = 11.89   p = .01

TABLE 12

SOCIAL ADJUSTEMENT SCORE IN PATIENTS CHRONICALLY TREATED WITH METHADONE
AS FUNCTION OF THERAPEUTIC COMPLIANCE

GROUPS			
1	2	3	
No agreem. (n=25)	Part. agreem. (n=28)	Total agreem. (n=40)	2 FACTOR repeated measures ANOVA
bas obs	bas obs	bas obs	GR(A): F = 12.6 $p < .001$ RM(B): F = 202.7 $p < .001$ AxB: F = 1.08 p = n.s.
1.04 2.12	1.25 2.64	1.45 2.83	

Baseline
1 Vs 3: Scheffe F-test = 3.87 p<.05
Observation
1 Vs 2: Scheffe F-test = 4.18 p<.05
1 Vs 3: Scheffe F-test = 8.86 p<.05

Paired T-test
1: T = -5.66 $p < .001$
2: T = -10 $p < .01$
3: T = -9.4 $p < .01$

adjustment was evaluated according to the 5th axis of the DSM-III-R, both before starting treatment (basal) and at observation time (obs).

The result of ANOVA in respect to the considered factors (group division and score changes as a function of time) showed significant differences within each factor. In fact, the basal social adjustment scored significantly higher in the group 3. as compared to group 1. Moreover, all groups had a significant improvement during the elapsed ten years.

However, the social improvement within each group as a function of time resulted independent of initial differences. Finally, the groups 2. and 3. presented a similar improvement in social adjustment, which resulted significantly higher in respect to the group 1.

The criminality score rate through groups, evaluated by the prevalence of crimes and arrests at the time of the first visit as compared to the last year of treatment does not show initial differences among the three groups. The evolution of criminality score paralleled that of social adjiustment. It was significant within each group, but it resulted markedly higher in groups 2. and 3. as compared to group 1. (tab. 13).

TABLE 13

CRIMINALITY SCORE IN PATIENTS CHRONICALLY TREATED WITH METHADONE
AS FUNCTION OF THERAPEUTIC COMPLIANCE

	GROUPS		
1	2	3	
No agreem. (n=25)	Part. agreem. (n=28)	Total agreem. (n=40)	2 FACTOR repeated measures ANOVA
bas obs	bas obs	bas obs	GR(A): F = 2.97 $p < .001$ RM(B): F = 66.28 $p < .001$ AxB: F = 1.04 p = n.s.
1.28 0.64	1.07 0.14	1.12 0.10	

Observation
1 Vs 2: Scheffe F-test = 3.99 $p < .05$
1 Vs 3: Scheffe F-test = 4.49 $p < .05$

Paired T-test
1: T = -5.66 $p < .001$
2: T = -10 $p < .01$
3: T = -9.4 $p < .01$

Moreover the available no-punitive service since 1985 did allow to contact 400-600 never previously studied intravenous drug addicts each year, and to provide useful informative-educational support against the HIV spreading. A progressive decrement of the prevalence of the HIV infection from 60% to 36% was observed, probably due to this campaign.

The present findings allow the following conclusions: a) informing and educational campaigns resulted useful for the prevention of HIV spreading infection, but seemed powerless against heroin use; b) patients showing an initial better social adjustment needed lower mean doses of methadone and were more likely to stop completely heroin use; c) from b) it may be inferred that the more precociously the treatment, is started the better outcomes can be expected; d) a satisfactory social adjustment and a low level of criminality may be reached under methadone maintenance independently of the complete cessation of heroin use. Which is to say that chronic use of methadone, in conditions of correct compliance, permits a diminished use of heroin.

REFERENCES

Liebson I, Bigelow G, and Flamer R (1973). Alcoholism among methadone patients: a specific treatment method. Am. J. Psychiatry, pp 483-498.

Molari A, Pani PP, Pili p, and Tagliamonte A (1987). Incidenza dell'abuso di alcool di una popolazione di eroinomani in terapia sostitutiva con metadone. Boll. Farmacod. e Alcolismo, pp 333-346.

Rounsaville BJ, Weissman MM, and Kleber HD (1982). The significance of alcoholism in treated opiate addicts. The Journal of Nervous and Mental disease, pp 479-488.

The Importance of IV Drug Users Personality Traits in AIDS Prevention

D. X. DA SILVEIRA and N. DA SILVA JR.

Departamento de Psiquiatria da Escola Paulista de Medicina,
Rua Botucatu 740, CEP 04023 Sao Paulo, Brazil

Intravenous drug users have been found to be the group who less effectively respond to profilatic measures concerning HIV infection. At first, this high-risk group concurred with a very few number of cases in the infected population. Its rates, however, are increasing and reaching significant numbers.

Whether prevention from HIV infection among this group is possible or not has been subject of considerable disagreement. One can observe that the same profilatic measures, which proved to be adequate to the other high-risk groups, are usually uneffective or even aggravating when drug-addicts are concerned. This contradictory behavior can be better understood if we take into account some of their personality traits.

Some experts considers that successful prevention is not possible since they regard drug abuse essencially as self destructive behaviour. On the other hand, several studies reported that basic information on AIDS spread both through the mass media as well as oral communication did result in effective behaviour changes. These changes, however, lead to a reducing risk of developing AIDS nevertheless, the reduction of risk has not been enough to decrease transmission in this ever progressing epidemic.

Intravenous drug-users play an increasingly important role in the growing of AIDS epidemic, since they are the second largest group of people who have been infected with HIV, as well as the most likely one to transmit the virus to heterosexual partners. Still, they constitute a major "reservoir" for perinatal transmission of the HIV from mothers to their children.

We can observe that in many instances the kind of information transmitted to IV drug users is not sufficiently effective since it does not take into account some personality traits of this very target population.

The same drug-addictive behaviour, which in young people may be considered as "healthy transgression", can be used pathologically as a defense mechanism of negation. This "pathological transgression" has a trait of omnipotence and bears the illusion that nothing can be lost. Now, if the individual's Ego is identified with omnipotent figure, the social rules tend to be deeply rejected. Thus, in a situation of pathological transgression, the authority figures that generally represent these rules cannot be accepted. As a consequence, the informations given by them will be neglected. It becomes, then, very easy to understand within this context, why authoritarian and moralistic Preventing interventions result in a complete failure among drug addicts.

It is important to remember that the urging need for efficient measures in Aids prevention does not allow innocent goals such as extinguishing the drug-addictive behaviour. The action should basically envolve the transmission aspects of the disease, leaving no place for moralistic speculations about drug use. This is specially true if we consider the paradoxical effect upon the drug addictive behaviour originated from moralistic and prejudicial attitudes. We can easily recognize the contradiction that lies behind these attitudes, when we realise that society stimulates the use of alcohol at the same time it condems the use of illegal drugs.

Another important aspect involves the employement of exclusively individual needles and syringes which, together with "safer sex", constitute important measures for the control of HIV transmission. Both preventing strategies, however, are hindered by two peculiar traits of the drug-addicts personality: lack of impulse control and identity disorder.

The employement of mass media represents useful instruments in the prevention of Aids. But, when drug-addicts are concerned, it is worthwhile to make some observations on how these informations should be given. For these individuals, drug-addiction is a means to change the perception of an unbearable reality. Drugs offer a way out of anxious and fearful situations. Thus, a campaign based on disseminating fear is inappropriate, for this fear could be appeased only by the drug itself. As a consequence, we know that while the advertisements and campaigns continue to spread fear and anxiety, there will be an induced increase in drug consumption by addicts.

The drug-addicts urge to consume immediately the newly aquired drug has already been emphasised in many studies (Des Jarlais, Friedman & Hopkins 1985). Claude Olievenstein (1987) describes the lack of impulse control in terms of "kinetic" and "intensity", which means a need for maximum pleasure, here and now, a pleasure that cannot be postponed and can be obtained only through the "rush". The drug will allow the drug addict to rescue his lost identity.

Similar to the already mentioned impulsive need to take the drug, we frequently detect the need to join a group as, again, a way to rescue identity. The need for identification, which impels the drug-addict to make use of drugs also as a way to share group communion, is realy experienced as a Holy Communion, once it repairs the individual's identify. Like in a symbolic ritual, the members of the group, when sharing the same syringe and mixing each-other's blood, feel like strengthening the bonds and compromises that tie them toghether.

Many countries have tried imaginative solutions for this problem. Operating with the drug-addicted's identification need, they show famous personalities admired by the psychodelic culture (rock stars, sportsmen, etc) talking about the benefits of safe drug self-administration, instead of repressively reinforcing the dangers involved in improper self-administration of drugs.

Going back to the strategies we have already discussed, if we aim at stopping the spread of the virus through shared drug injection equipment and through sexual activity of IV drug users, we need to go beyond than just providing information about AIDS and its ways of transmission.

We must mention the great difficulty anyone or anything playing the role of a third element will find to penetrate the bond established between the drug-addict and the drug. He considers this bond complete and perfect and will allow no interference with it, be it a psychotherapist or even self-protection measure. For instance, there is no possibility to begin whatever treatment before the onset of a crisis in this bond. By crisis we mean the moment when the drug stops to provide the same level of pleasure that established the dependence relatioship. The psychotherapist, until this this moment, has no means to compete with the seduction and the power to give the same immediate and intensive pleasure as that one rendered by the drug.

Nevertheless, drug users demonstrate they can change AIDS risk behaviour even if they cannot quit using drugs. As an example, many methadone maintenancy programs have succeeded in reducing HIV spread although they are known to be generally uneffective in terms of extinguishing addictive behaviour.

Risk reduction among IV drug users is expected to be successcul in an environment where a higher percentage of drug users are in contact with drug dependence treatment facilities. Risk reduction tends to occur easily in treatment services characterized by comprehensive approach of the subject, inclunding biological, sociological and psychodynamic knowledge on both AIDS and substance misuse. Some characteristics of treatment programs known to affect positively risky behaviour are:

1. Pharmacotherapeutic support, since it has been proved to reduce both dropping out and relapse.

2. Providing of face to face contacts to stimulate "safer-sex" practices.

3. Providing of legal sterile injection equipment.

4. Availability of a consistent psychological approach.

5. Substitution of repressive attitudes toward drug dependence for a more tolerant and complascent one when lower risk behaviours have been or are to be achieved, despite persistent addiction.

Drug misuse is a very complex phenomenon envoluving a large number of components. Any intervention must be based on deep knowledge on the subject. It is important to stress that addiction itself cannot simply be reduced to its biological aspects. In practice this can clearly be seen when, in some clinical situations, we can have a specific severe biological dependence when no addictive behaviour can be observed. Drug addiction phenomenon goes beyond the biological limits and in this sense we have always to consider the individual's personality traits. Drug addicts tend to establish different peculiar relations towards sexuality and death. Transgression, lack of limits and sexual ambivalence, all of them lead the drug addict to experiment with a wide range of different possibilities in the field of sexuality.

Omnipotence masks the drug addict's fragmented identity, what explains his peculiar attitudes towards death.

Considering these specific aspects, we begin to understand why drug addicts are a group with whom the regular AIDS prevention measures do not work as expected. Their psychological reactions before Aids will individually depend on their personality characteristics. For many drug addicts, AIDS is quite an abstract reality to trigger important reactions of anxiety. They remain indifferent and incredulous as a consequence of their denial before death. For others, there is an increase in the ammount of risky attitudes concerning AIDS, both through sharing injection equipment and intensification of sexual contacts. A third group of them, however, will react much differently toward AIDS. The possibility of contracting or having contracted AIDS will urge them to reflect about the underlying motivations of their addictive behaviour as well as their consequences. This explains why some individuals will quit addiction by the time they learn about their serum conversion. Searching and adherence to drug treatment units are also significantly higher among HIV infected drug users.

In summary, be it through information or be it through more drastic intervention, we know we can stem HIV epidemic among IV drug users more effectively as long as we consider the very characteristics of their personalities focused in their specific social and cultural environment. Our personal beliefs and prejudices toward drug addiction are to be overcome in such circunstances.

REFERENCES

Des Jarlais, D.C.; Friedman, S.R., Hopkins, W. (1985); Risk Reduction for the Acquired Immunodeliciency Syndrome Among Intravenous Drug Users, Annais of Internal Medicine; 103: 755-759.

Olievenstein, C. (1987); La Clinique du Toxicomane; Ed. Universitaires, Paris.